CONCEPTIONS & MISCONCEPTIONS

SECOND EDITION

CONCEPTIONS & MISCONCEPTIONS

SECOND EDITION

The Informed Consumer's Guide through the Maze of
In Vitro Fertilization *& other*
Assisted Reproduction Techniques

ARTHUR L. WISOT M.D., FACOG
DAVID R. MELDRUM M.D., FACOG

Hartley
&Marks
PUBLISHERS

Published by

HARTLEY & MARKS PUBLISHERS INC.

P. O. Box 147   3661 West Broadway
Point Roberts, WA   Vancouver, BC
98281   V6R 2B8

Text © 1988, 1997, 2004 by Arthur Wisot   Illustrations © 1997, 2004 by HARTLEY & MARKS, INC.

LIBRARY OF CONGRESS CATALOGING-IN-PUBLICATION DATA

Wisot, Arthur L.
    Conceptions & misconceptions : the informed consumer's guide through the maze of in vitro fertilization & other assisted reproduction techniques / Arthur L. Wisot, David R. Meldrum.—2nd ed.
        p.   cm.
    Includes index.
    ISBN 0-88179-203-9 pb
        1. Human reproductive technology.   2. Patient education.   I. Title: Conceptions and misconceptions.   II. Meldrum, David R.   III. Title.
    RG133.5.W55   2004
    616.6'9206—dc22   2003067758

Design and composition by The Typeworks
Cover design by Diane McIntosh
Set in SPECTRUM & TRAJAN

Printed in the U.S.A.

NOTICE TO THE READER

This book is meant to be a source of information for those who are interested in learning about modern and alternative fertility treatments, including their various components. Every person has different health problems and issues, based on age, sex, lifestyle, health status, genetics, diet, psychological state, and spiritual maturity. Our intent is to share our experience and offer guidelines to help you become more informed about your fertility choices and options. In cooperation with your physician and other healthcare providers, you can then take the necessary steps to maximize your fertility potential. This book is sold with the understanding that the publisher is not engaged in rendering medical or other professional services. If medical or expert assistance is required, the services of a competent professional should be sought. Neither the authors nor the publisher takes medical or legal responsibility for the reader who uses the contents of this book as a prescription.

This book is dedicated to the families—including our own—who make it all worthwhile: Phyllis, David, Andrew and Jeffrey Wisot, and Claudia, Erik, Tiffany, Nicole and Bret Meldrum.

And to parents—including our own—whose love and support made it all possible: Hilly and Helen Wisot, and Roy and Margaret Meldrum.

ACKNOWLEDGMENTS

Our deep appreciation goes to our editor, Susan Juby, and our publisher, Victor Marks, whose foresight was instrumental in the publication of this book; Dr. Gene Naftulin for his contributions in the field of male infertility; Claudia Meldrum for her support and sharing her own personal struggle with infertility; and Phyllis Wisot for her editing, which greatly improved the original manuscript and second edition revisions.

Our heartfelt thanks go to the members of the Reproductive Partners Medical Group, Inc. team, including Dr. Denise Cassidenti, Dr. Gabriel Garzo, Dr. Gregory Rosen and Dr. Bill Yee for their advice, support and contributions to the development of the protocols used in the book. We could not have written this book without the help of our office staff and others whose critical reading of portions of the original manuscript and ideas were vital: embryologist Minda Hamilton and administrator Willetta Allen. Michelle Weinbaum-Rosen provided valuable information on egg donation. Chapter 14, "Alternative Treatments in Infertility," was developed with the assistance of Daoshing Ni, L.Ac., D.O.M., Ph.D.; Tara Perry, L.Ac.; Richard Sternberg, M.D., Cheirel Gustavis-Person, R.N., RNP; Pat Vlahakis, R.N.; Jenny D'Alessandro, R.N., Sandra Topete, R.N.; and Dawn Erskine, R.N.

We especially appreciate the contribution of all our patients, many of whom offered suggestions and are anonymously represented in the book. However, certain individuals generously offered to share their stories publicly so that others may benefit from their experiences: Cheryl and Jeff Scruggs, Patty and Brad Woods, Jane and Terry Mohr, Nancy and Dick Woodka, Carol and Mike Wallensack, Penny and Roger Berry, Becky and Mike Ripley, and Beth Yates.

We would also like to thank Serono Laboratories, Inc. for permission to use their medical illustrations.

We could not have completed this project without the love and constant support of our families—Phyllis, David, Andrew and Jeff Wisot, Melanie Friedlander, M.D., Irving Bernstein, and Claudia, Erik, Tiffany, Nicole and Bret Meldrum.

CONTENTS

INTRODUCTION

"You do become desperate. You go through periods where you cry for no reason and you want someone to help you. If someone says they can help you, if they say stand on your head after sex you will try that. If your friends say, gee, I held a chicken foot up and it worked for me you will try that. If a man says, thousands and thousands of dollars, if you can afford it you will try it."

Actress JoBeth Williams, testifying before the U.S. Congressional subcommittee hearing on Consumer Protection Issues Involving In Vitro Fertilization Clinics, March 9, 1989

This statement, from a person who has struggled with an infertility problem, is not unusual. Also not unusual is the difficulty infertile couples have in obtaining valid information regarding the high-tech procedures that have become dispassionately known as assisted reproductive technology (ART). These couples are so desperate, the technology is so complex, and the means of gauging success are so confusing that, as Dr. Alan DeCherney, director of Reproductive Endocrinology at UCLA, testified at the hearing, "infertility patients are exceptionally vulnerable to exploitation." Subcommittee chairman Representative Ron Wyden (Democratic Party, Oregon) agreed, concluding that "infertile couples find it extremely difficult to obtain clear, understandable and unbiased information about the performance of in vitro fertilization (IVF) clinics. Many of these couples are desperate to have children. They have been on an emotional roller coaster for years, attempting to conceive through a variety of procedures. They are vulnerable to exploitation." Despite some changes as the result of legislation recommended by Rep. Wyden's subcommittee, his statement is still true today.

Precise, but unaudited, annual statistics do exist for clinics which do report as required, but statistics quoted by some centers in other formats may still be misleading or downright inaccurate. Some programs may quote national figures. Others may present their statistics in a favorable light. For example, they may cite a time interval when they did exceptionally well and quote a success rate that does not reflect their overall experience. But now, somewhat objective information is available if you know where to look for it. Statistics on individual U.S. centers are reported by the Society for Assisted Reproductive Technology (SART) of the American Society for Reproductive Medicine (ASRM) and the Centers for Disease Control and Prevention (SART/CDC). They are published in a medical journal as pooled statistics, as well as in individual reports available on the Internet at the Centers for Disease Control and Prevention (CDC) website (www.cdc.gov), giving the national rates as well as those for specific programs.

But statistics are not the only issue that infertility patients have to be concerned about. The last decade has revealed a number of ethical bombshells. These include a prominent fertility doctor convicted of using his own sperm for insemination, resulting in an estimated 75 pregnancies. Perhaps the most shocking allegation came when two of the nation's most heralded fertility specialists were alleged to have taken eggs from an estimated 80 patients without their consent and given them to others, as well as being accused of a variety of business fraud charges.

The scope of the problem is large since IVF clinics are a tremendous growth industry. The U.S. government's Office of Technology Assessment, in its latest report on the subject before it closed in 1997, estimated that more than a billion dollars was spent in 1987 on infertility treatment for an estimated 2.4 million couples in the United States. The report estimated that $30 to $40 million had been spent on IVF procedures alone at that time. Since then, the number of patients undergoing treatment has been increasing dramatically. According to a 1998 article in *Family Planning Perspectives*, the proportion of women in the U.S. who think they have a fertility problem increased from 5.7% in 1988 to 7.7% in 1996. Treatment cycles reported to the congressional survey increased from 8,167 in 1987 to 10,105 in 1988. By 1994 the SART IVF Registry recorded initiation of 39,390 cycles in that year alone. By 1995 the number of couples dealing with infertility increased to an estimated 5.3 million in the U.S., with the percentage of childless infertile couples trying to achieve pregnancy increasing from 14.4% in 1965 to 18.5% in 1995, according to the National Center for Health Statistics. In 2001 107,587 ART cycles were performed in the United States.

* * * *

These procedures are being performed in a variety of settings, from university centers to private centers, to single-doctor offices. There is a wide spectrum of qualifications—some of these practitioners have inadequate training or experience. In the U.S. at present there is no mandatory regulation of this industry. Any physician can hold himself or herself out as a fertility specialist. Embryo laboratories are only voluntarily subject to the accreditation process developed by the ASRM and the College of American Pathologists. Canadian centers can do voluntary accreditation as well.

* * * *

Yet, despite all these vital consumer and ethical issues, the technology can be successful. Some of the best programs are now legitimately reporting that well over 40% of their patients take home a baby for each patient under age 40 having an egg retrieval procedure. It is the prospective user of this technology who has the job of seeking information and finding those clinics that are achieving the best results. JoBeth Williams, who played the surrogate birthmother Mary Beth Whitehead in the TV movie *Baby M.*, concluded her testimony to the subcommittee: "We, the infertile couples, need to learn what questions to ask. We need to know where we can get the right answers."

In 1990 we published *New Options for Fertility* and in 1997, the first edition of *Conceptions & Misconceptions,* which tried to provide the "right answers" with a straightforward approach to the technology and the consumer issues of that day. Now, a few years into the new millennium, the technology is well developed with good success rates at the best centers. Still, the infertile couple faces not only dealing with the technology, but also a whole host of issues including deceptive advertising practices, centers still producing poor results, allegations of unethical practices, insurance coverage issues, payment methods, marketing schemes and other ethical concerns. Thus, what was *New Options* in 1990 became *Conceptions & Misconceptions* in the late 1990s. We are pleased to offer this second edition in the early 2000s, because with the proper information and knowledge regarding the pitfalls of technology, couples can successfully find their way through the labyrinth of assisted reproduction.

ABOUT THE AUTHORS

Co-author Dr. Arthur Wisot developed his interest in infertility as a resident physician in obstetrics and gynecology at the Long Island Jewish Medical Center in New Hyde Park, New York. As he worked in the various disciplines included in obstetrics and gynecology, he developed an affinity for the patients who were having trouble conceiving. Although infertility treatments were in their infancy at that time, he recognized the importance to the patients of overcoming their infertility problems.

His interest expanded during continuing education courses in all the new developments, including special training in microsurgery. He was instrumental, in conjunction with Dr. Meldrum, in the development of the In Vitro Fertilization Center at AMI-South Bay Hospital in Redondo Beach, California, which became the Center for Advanced Reproductive Care (CARC) and developed into Reproductive Partners Medical Group, Inc. (RPMG). In addition to helping Dr. Meldrum develop the center, Dr. Wisot learned all of the clinical monitoring protocols and procedures and has worked alongside Dr. Meldrum in one of the most successful IVF programs in the nation.

Along with his clinical interest in infertility and assisted reproduction, Dr. Wisot has long been involved in consumer issues relating to health care issues. He has worked to inform the public about these issues in many newspaper and magazine articles and as the consumer-health reporter for Channel 9, in Los Angeles. This media experience led to his serving as host and medical editor of "Physicians' Journal Update" and "Obstetrics and Gynecology Update" on Lifetime Medical Television, informing physicians on new medical and surgical developments. In addition, he is a clinical professor in the Department of Obstetrics and Gynecology at the UCLA School of Medicine.

Co-author Dr. David Meldrum's interest in infertility began with a personal circumstance. When he became engaged to his wife, Claudia, she informed him that she might not be able to have children and indicated that she would understand if he wanted to break off the engagement.

Childlessness would be devastating to her, so she felt that he should be aware of this possibility. But her fiancé realized that her problem (lack of ovulation) could probably be solved through drugs then available. Although the treatments could be difficult, he was relatively certain, as a young intern, that if they persevered they would be successful.

By this time (1973) David Meldrum had already decided to go into obstetrics and gynecology, but his and Claudia's own difficulty moved him in the direction of caring for patients with infertility. Claudia was initially given the drug clomiphene to try to stimulate ovulation. She showed signs of responding but apparently did not ovulate despite increasing doses. (A yet-to-be-discovered advance in the treatment of ovulatory problems—the combination of a simple injection of hCG with clomiphene—might have worked for her.)

After three failed cycles on clomiphene, Claudia and Dave made the decision to go on to treatment with hMG, a powerful hormone designed to stimulate the ovaries. A naturally occurring product, it is very expensive, requires daily injections and holds an increased risk of multiple births. We now have sophisticated ways of monitoring patients using this medication, such as observing estrogen levels and ultrasound examinations. But in those days, doctors monitored patients by following the changes in their cervical mucus, looking for indications that the patient's estrogen level was high.

Claudia went through six cycles of hMG before she finally became pregnant. During that successful cycle, Claudia was probably overstimulated—that is, she produced too many eggs, increasing the risk of multiple pregnancy. If she had been monitored with the methods we use today, this cycle would probably have been bypassed and pregnancy would not have occurred. In addition, this successful cycle happened after she resumed the hMG treatments following six relaxing months in Spain away from infertility treatments. Claudia feels that their trip minimized the importance of the problem and relieved much of the pressure by some time away from an anxious family.

An ultrasound in early pregnancy revealed the presence of twins. The Meldrums were delighted. By about 26 weeks, the ultrasound found a third baby. Triplets! The Meldrums were now getting nervous. The fourth baby was never discovered by the ultrasound. Bret, their fourth child, was a complete surprise to everyone. Claudia delivered prematurely at 34 weeks. All four babies were delivered normally and ranged in weight from 2.75 to 3.75 pounds. Their birth order was Erik, Tiffany, Nicole and Bret. Dave describes the experience as overwhelming. Claudia did not know that she had quads until she awakened from the emergency general anesthesia, given because of a prolapsed umbilical cord during the birth of Erik. She had not planned on an anesthetic and was hoping for a natural childbirth using the Lamaze technique. However, the Meldrum quads did very well and came home from the hospital one at a time, three to five weeks after birth.

The quads were born during Dave's first year on the UCLA faculty. At that point the focus of his practice was infertility, treated primarily with tubal microsurgery. He became interested in IVF as he realized that some patients clearly would be better treated with this new method. This was a natural outgrowth of his belief that the clinician had to find the best treatment for each individual patient. He felt that there should be no need for a patient to go through surgery if IVF could produce the same or better results with less risk.

Infertility was not as great a stress emotionally for Dave and Claudia as for some other couples because they always looked at it as a problem that could be solved. Although she was not as optimistic as Dave, Claudia feels his positive attitude was contagious. With the advances in infertility treatment and assisted reproduction since that time, he feels that almost every couple can approach the problem with the same confidence they did. He thinks that if couples maintain a sense of optimism, there can be less stress associated with infertility. He feels that this is a realistic approach, given today's technology. If a couple perseveres through four cycles of IVF or even egg donation, they will have an excellent chance to have their family. Perhaps this factor is best illustrated by a picture hanging in RPMG's office which was donated by one of our successful couples. It shows two gulls in flight with a quote from Virgil beneath: "They can because they think they can."

Dr. Meldrum learned IVF during a sabbatical in Australia in 1982 and set up both the clinical and laboratory aspects of the UCLA IVF program. After 12 years on the full-time faculty he moved the program to South Bay Hospital in 1986. The program became the Center for Advanced Reproductive Care and in 1995, along with Dr. Wisot, established an affiliation with Dr. Bill Yee and the University Infertility Associates in Long Beach. In 1998 both groups formally merged into Reproductive Partners Medical Group, Inc. and now have offices throughout Southern California.

Over the years, Dr. Meldrum has been a pioneer in many of the clinical and laboratory techniques involved with in vitro fertilization. He is a frequent lecturer and has published over 100 articles and chapters related to microsurgery, female hormone problems and assisted reproductive technology. In addition to his position as scientific director of RPMG, he maintains his affiliation with UCLA as a clinical professor in the Department of Obstetrics and Gynecology. He is also a past president of the Society for Assisted Reproduction Technology (SART) of the American Society for Reproductive Medicine (ASRM).

To provide a comprehensive picture of male fertility, Dr. Gene Naftulin assisted with the sections relating to male infertility. Dr. Naftulin is a urologist specializing in male infertility and is a clinical instructor in the Department of Urology at the UCLA School of Medicine and a past president of the Pacific Coast Reproductive Society.

We consulted two well-respected experts to help us navigate through the confusing and often contradictory subject of complementary and alternative treatments in infertility. We interviewed two of the leading practitioners of Traditional Chinese Medicine (TCM) in infertility in the Los Angeles Area—Daoshing Ni, L.Ac., D.O.M., Ph.D. of the Tao of Wellness and Tara Perry, L.Ac.—both of whom practice in Santa Monica.

WHY WE ARE WRITING THIS BOOK

We both believe that not enough information is available to the public regarding assisted reproduction. In addition, there is a great deal of confusion over ethical issues regarding this new technology, and especially about the validity of success rates and the place of these procedures in the treatment plan for infertility. We also strongly feel that most of the information the public receives is not presented in the proper perspective. We are writing this book to help infertile couples become better consumers by providing them with the right questions to ask and the means to interpret the answers.

In order to give you enough of an understanding to make the proper interpretations, we review basic reproductive science and describe all the alternatives for maximizing your chances of conception. You cannot understand this advanced technology without knowing the basics of reproduction. We discuss the conditions that cause infertility and how to test for them, and conventional fertility treatments because assisted reproduction should not even be considered until conventional treatments have been exhausted. All of the current assisted reproduction techniques are explored in detail and patients' experiences with these procedures are included. We provide criteria for selecting a program, including detailed information about how success rates are calculated and how they can be obtained and compared. We explore special considerations for the prenatal care of an IVF patient who is successful. And for those instances when the best medical science has to offer is not enough, we look at the use of donors for sperm and eggs as well as the use of surrogates. Finally, we look toward the future, considering both scientific and consumer issues, and at the current state of alternative treatments in infertility.

The book also contains appendices providing you with information on obtaining success rates of programs that report to the SART/CDC and the names and addresses of those programs, as well as Canadian fertility clinics, resources for further information and a glossary of terms and abbreviations. We've also provided 20 questions and answers for couples who want information at a glance.

HOW TO USE THIS BOOK

For the most detailed information, read the entire book. If you are already familiar with reproductive anatomy, read those chapters anyway because they will provide a good review. The sections on causes, diagnosis and conventional treatment will ensure that you have had all the proper tests and treatments before going on to assisted reproductive technology procedures.

Some may choose to use the book primarily as a reference. If that's your desire, the index will help you find the material you need. In this case, we recommend frequent use of the glossary to help you with abbreviations and terms that may not be totally familiar to you.

THE BOTTOM LINE

This book *can* help you get pregnant! As we will remind you throughout its pages, with persistence and proper choices you can maximize your chance to conceive. Of course, we can't guarantee that you'll succeed, but we can help you find the way to give it your best shot. We sincerely hope that each of you can fulfill your dream of having a baby.

CHAPTER 1

Conceptions

"IT'S A MIRACLE EVERY TIME"

"It's a miracle every time!" said Robert Young as the compassionate, caring Marcus Welby, M.D. just after he had delivered a baby in one of the weekly episodes of that popular television series.

That statement might sound like a cliché coming from the lips of Marcus Welby. But it's true. Once you understand all the complex processes that must occur to conceive and carry a baby to delivery, you will agree that it *is* a miracle every time a healthy baby is born.

The "little miracles" we talk about in this book are the healthy babies conceived through assisted reproductive technology (ART), such as Greta, the first baby born in the United States as the result of ultrasound-guided egg retrieval in an IVF procedure. The best-known ART procedures are in vitro fertilization (IVF) and gamete intrafallopian transfer (GIFT). When Greta was born, the use of ultrasound was a new technique to obtain the mother's eggs without surgery and was an important milestone in assisted reproductive technology.

ASSISTED REPRODUCTION

What exactly is "assisted reproduction"? The key word is *assisted*. Actually, any kind of help we give a couple in achieving a pregnancy could be called assisted reproduction, from simply maximizing a couple's chances of achieving a pregnancy by teaching them to properly time intercourse to using the most sophisticated techniques to help a single sperm fertilize an egg in the laboratory.

But the term usually refers to the more sophisticated types of infertility treatments, which can be identified by their acronyms—IVF, GIFT, ZIFT, ICSI, FET, PGD—abbreviations that may have no meaning to you yet.

If all of this doesn't sound sexy to you, it isn't! In fact, by the time you are involved in anything to do with assisted reproduction, you are probably living your life around your or your partner's menstrual cycle, taking daily injections, having almost daily ultrasound examinations and blood tests, producing semen on demand in a little room with appropriate reading material and perhaps even undergoing surgery. Any relationship between romance and reproduction went out the window a long time ago. But, if you want a miracle...

Little Miracles

Some would argue that the word miracle is overused in our field. But we find it frequently and justifiably applies to the type of work we do because many of the people who benefit from assisted reproduction thought they were hopelessly infertile before this technology was developed. When someone is desperate, with no expectation of remedy or cure, and succeeds, you can see how "miracle" readily applies.

We see this hopelessness every day. Patty was a young woman whose pelvic organs were left seriously damaged by infection from a Dalkon Shield IUD. She had suffered through tubal ectopic pregnancies, years of infertility and even multiple attempts at in vitro fertilization. Having her own baby appeared impossible. Finally, after her third transfer of frozen embryos, she achieved her dream with the birth of her son, Brian. Just moments after Brian was born, Patty's husband Brad sat at her bedside looking at his son and said with tears of joy in his eyes, "I can't believe it. It's a miracle."

But do we believe that we are really creating miracles? Of course not! The couples are creating the miracles through modern technology with the assistance of a team of professionals. That is why it is termed assisted reproductive technology. In fact, this is one of the few areas in medicine where clinical physicians and scientists, such as embryologists, bring together the art of the clinician and the science of medicine to benefit patients.

Patients often refer to ART conceptions as miracles.

OVER A QUARTER-CENTURY AND A MILLION BABIES LATER

Assisted reproductive technology in humans is relatively new. The term in vitro fertilization literally means "fertilized in glass" and was first demonstrated using rabbits in 1959 by Dr. M.C. Chang. In fact, much of the technology we now use was first used by scientists in animal husbandry many years before it was applied to humans. Physicians are relative latecomers to this technology.

The era of assisted reproduction in humans began in the 1970s with attempts at in vitro fertilization by teams in England and Australia. These efforts culminated in the first successful birth (of Louise Brown) in England on July 25, 1978. Drs. Patrick Steptoe and Robert Edwards achieved this milestone by obtaining an egg from the mother's ovary during a natural cycle, fertilizing it in the laboratory and then placing the resulting embryo back into the mother's uterus. That first success was followed fairly rapidly by assisted pregnancies in Australia (Royal Women's Hospital, Melbourne) in 1980 and in the United States (Eastern Virginia Medical School, Norfolk) in 1981. By Louise Brown's 25th birthday, reports estimated there had been one million assisted reproduction births worldwide and what once took years to achieve is now a routine medical treatment. In the United States, assisted reproduction has been responsible for over 200,000 births. In 2000, a total of 99,639 ART cycles resulted in 35,035 live babies born in the U.S. alone.

What took Steptoe and Edwards years to achieve is now an everyday occurrence.

In 1984, the first pregnancy as the result of gamete intrafallopian transfer (GIFT) was reported by Dr. Ricardo Asch in San Antonio, Texas. In this procedure the eggs are retrieved by laparoscopy, a procedure in which a telescopic device is inserted through the navel and the eggs are removed by means of a needle placed through the abdominal wall. These eggs are then placed with sperm directly into the fallopian tubes to allow fertilization to take place in the natural location. Also achieved in 1984 was the first human pregnancy resulting from an egg donated by another woman to treat premature ovarian failure. In 1986 Dr. Zev Rosenwaks of the Jones Institute, Eastern Virginia Medical School, demonstrated that IVF with donated eggs can be used to treat patients with a variety of causes of infertility. This showed that the chronological age of the uterus was not critical, breaking the age barrier for childbearing in females.

Originally, IVF was used to treat couples when a problem with the woman's fallopian tubes caused infertility, but in the early 1980s it evolved as a treatment option for couples with other fertility problems. In 1984 Dr. Jacques Cohen of the Reproductive Biology Associates in Atlanta, introduced IVF as a successful treatment for male factor infertility.

The first successful pregnancy from zygote intrafallopian transfer (ZIFT), which combines IVF (by retrieving the eggs and fertilizing them in the laboratory) with GIFT (by placing the resulting embryos in the fallopian tube), was reported in 1986. This procedure was designed to take advantage of the theoretical increased success rates of placing the more advanced embryos in their natural environment (the fallopian tube) at that stage of their development, rather than in the uterus.

Steptoe and Edwards' first pregnancy and those that followed shortly thereafter were achieved using the woman's natural cycle. The woman was allowed to ovulate normally, her cycle was monitored and one egg was retrieved before it would normally be released from the ovary. In order to make the process more efficient and successful, medication was used to produce multiple eggs based on the concept that you could improve success rates by implanting more than one embryo. Subsequently, much of the research in IVF has been devoted to finding efficient, yet safe, egg stimulation regimens. Another milestone was the discovery in Australia by Dr. Alan Trounson that since the eggs were being retrieved early, before they were ready for fertilization, a period of incubation of the eggs prior to adding sperm would dramatically increase fertilization and thus pregnancy rates.

The first successful IVF led to rapid developments such as GIFT and ZIFT.

While stimulation protocols and fertilization techniques were being refined, the method of obtaining the eggs was undergoing change. At the beginning, laparoscopy was used for all egg retrievals. This meant that patients had to go through outpatient surgery under general anesthesia. However, with the development of ultrasound techniques, most egg retrievals are now performed by an ultrasound-guided needle inserted into the ovary through the vagina. This can be done with sedation rather than under anesthesia and is not considered a surgical procedure. In addition, the ultrasound approach can generally be done in less time and has a low complication rate. The first ultrasound retrievals were performed in Sweden by Dr. Mats Wikland and in Denmark by Dr. Susan Lenz in 1981. The first ultrasound egg retrieval in the United States resulting in successful pregnancy was performed by Dr. Meldrum's IVF program, then at UCLA. The baby, Greta, was born in 1984.

Greta's parents, Nancy and Dick, are another example of the value of perseverance in achieving success. Their major infertility problem was endometriosis. Nancy was working as a consumer and health reporter with Dr. Wisot at KHJ-TV in Los Angeles at the time Dr. Meldrum was administering hormonal treatment for her endometriosis. Dick was working as a technical director at neighboring Fox Tape. Nancy not only had major surgery to remove substantial amounts of endometriosis, but also underwent hormonal treatments for the endometriosis and an additional operation to correct tubal problems. Still, she did not get pregnant.

She and Dick decided to try the new technique of IVF and went through an unsuccessful IVF cycle with the eggs retrieved by laparoscopy. At about that time, the first successful egg retrievals using abdominal ultrasound were being reported in Sweden and Denmark. Dr. Meldrum was preparing to use the new technique and Nancy and Dick decided to give it another try. Using ultrasound as a guide, the needle was placed through the bladder into the ovary. Two eggs were retrieved and fertilized and the resulting embryos were placed into her uterus, resulting in Greta's birth.

Nancy became pregnant again. But this time she and Dick did it on their own, without IVF. Nancy is one of a number of our patients with endometriosis who, after an IVF pregnancy, have conceived on their own. For decades doctors have believed that pregnancy can improve endometriosis and prevent its recurrence. Nancy and other similar patients are evidence of the correctness of that belief.

We are now over a quarter century and a million babies into the era of assisted reproduction. The development of this field has occurred rapidly, but we feel that the clinical methods we now use are unlikely to be dramatically different in the next decade. Rather, we are in a phase of fine-tuning laboratory techniques and evolving preferred methods that will result in consistently good results by many programs.

CHAPTER 2

Misconceptions

mis•con•cep•tion, n. an erroneous conception; mistaken notion.
[MIS_ + CONCEPTION]

Webster's Encyclopedic Unabridged Dictionary of the English Language

To this standard definition of misconception we would suggest adding, "misinformation on the part of an infertile couple which prevents their conceiving." In some cases the misinformation may be scientific. For example, a couple may not be aware of how to maximize their chances of conceiving and may actually be avoiding intercourse at the most fertile time of the cycle. These issues are explored in chapter 3 under Maximizing Your Chances.

But with infertility treatment rapidly becoming more technical and complex, the risk of misinformation is increased as people must now navigate through the maze of new technology, claims of success, marketing schemes and statistics. That's the reason we wrote this book—to guide you through the "infertility-industrial-complex." So without further ado, we present our countdown of the top 10 misconceptions regarding fertility treatment.

THE TOP TEN MISCONCEPTIONS

10. "Our goal is to become pregnant."

No. The goal is to have a baby. In fact, more exactly, the goal is to have a healthy, full-term baby who is discharged from the hospital with its mother. This may seem a trivial difference, but the difference between a pregnancy and a healthy baby is far from trivial. When you see all the things that can happen between the words "You're pregnant" and the birth of a healthy baby, you will understand why it is important to be mindful of your final goal as you make decisions throughout your treatment.

9. "Success isn't everything; it's the only thing."

We're sure the great Green Bay Packers' football coach, Vince Lombardi, would agree with this statement; he felt the same way about winning. We don't agree. When you are searching for a doctor or clinic to perform your assisted reproductive procedure, the success rate of that center is not the only factor to consider. We would hope that you would not immediately turn to the appendices or the CDC website to search for clinic-specific results from two to three years ago and choose the center with the highest success rate in the country.

First of all, what happened in a given year can only be used as a guideline because in assisted reproduction two or three years ago is almost ancient history. You will certainly want to try to obtain the most recent statistics reported by any center you are considering. Second, there are many factors other than success rates to be considered. We review these for you in chapter 9, which you should read before making a selection.

8. "Ethics, shmethics! All we want is a baby."

Why are ethics important? It might seem acceptable to do anything you can to achieve your goal. However, following ethical principles protects you from potential harm. In fact, the first medical ethical guideline is, "First, do no harm." The issue of ethics in assisted reproduction has been paramount since its inception. Without ethical principles, doctors could do anything they wanted to achieve results and attract patients.

In November 1994 (with a supplement in May 1997) the Ethics Committee of the American Society for Reproductive Medicine (ASRM) published its latest report, "Ethical Considerations of Assisted Reproductive Technologies." The primary purpose of this report was to "prevent the exploitation for personal gain of procedures that pose significant risk to patients or that may be unethical for other reasons." This report updated previous guidelines to conform to the latest changes in technology and is what ethical physicians in reproduction use as a guide to their practices.

Let's look at one seemingly small issue—the number of embryos to transfer into the uterus. The committee condemned the practice of transferring excessive numbers of embryos. Some centers employed this practice with the intention of using a procedure called selective reduction (removing one or more of the fetuses after pregnancy has been established) when cases of multiple pregnancies with more than two fetuses resulted. For example, the most recent guidelines, released in November 1999, call for no more than two good-quality embryos to be transferred in patients with the most favorable prognosis. Although in the U.S. and Canada doctors are not required to follow these guidelines, they do provide some constraint on those who would engage in what are defined as unethical practices. In Germany and Britain the issue of number of embryos to transfer goes beyond ethics. By law, Germany rigidly limits the number to three. In Britain the Human Fertilisation and Embryology Authority decreased the number to two in August 2001, to reduce the number of women giving birth to twins or triplets after fertility treatment. Multiple births are undesirable because they carry a higher risk of premature birth, low birth weight, stillbirth and infant death, as well as long-term disability.

Ethics provide important protection for you and you should make yourself aware of what constitutes ethical practices in assisted reproduction.

Among the most recent ethical issues to come to the forefront have been facilitating pregnancy in women of advanced age, embryo "cloning" (separating and culturing genetically identical embryos) and the use of fetal eggs from aborted fetuses for assisted reproductive procedures. The issue of cloning resurfaced in February 1997, when a report in the British journal *Nature* announced the first cloning of an adult mammal resulting in the birth of a sheep named Dolly—an exact duplicate of the animal from which the single cell to be cloned was taken. Barely a week after the world said, "Hello, Dolly!" it was revealed that scientists at the Oregon Regional Primate Research Center had successfully produced monkeys from cloned embryos: first sheep, then monkeys. What's next? Are Dolly the sheep and a couple of unnamed monkeys equivalent in cloning to what Louise Brown represented for in vitro fertilization? You would think so when you heard the clamor. It brought ethicists out of the woodwork. Dr. Arthur Caplan, a noted bioethicist at the University of Pennsylvania and director of its

Center for Bioethics, said, "You're probably heading down the path to criminal arrest, not the Nobel Prize, if you try this in people." Even U.S. President Clinton got into the act by banning all federal funds for research into human cloning and asking private institutions to voluntarily avoid this technique in humans. In 2003 the Senate was considering The Human Cloning Ban and Stem Cell Research Protection Act which draws a distinction between reproductive cloning, which was banned in the bill, and therapeutic cloning to develop stem cells to overcome disease, which would have been allowed in a regulated research environment. If passed by Congress, it is still unlikely President Bush will sign it, since in August 2001 he restricted stem-cell research only to those lines already developed by that time and expressed his opposition to using frozen embryos stored in the nation's fertility clinics for stem-cell research.

More is not better; better is better.

The point is that these are not issues which should be decided by a single scientist or physician based on his or her own ethical or moral background. Ethical committees representing a variety of religious, moral and scientific disciplines should decide these issues. Doctors and scientists should follow broadly established guidelines. So, a good question to ask any doctor or clinic you are considering is, "Do you follow the ethical guidelines of the ASRM?" Following broadly established ethical guidelines and avoiding those clinics taking unethical shortcuts protects you.

7. "More is better."

One might assume that if something is good, more of it would be better. This is a misconception when applied to assisted reproductive technology. First, in the selection of a physician or group to do your ART procedure, picking a center because it is larger might be a mistake. When you examine the SART/CDC survey it is apparent that the size of the group or the number of cases they treat does not correlate to success rate. However, it is important that a center does enough cases to make their statistics significant.

Second, in making decisions as you proceed through a cycle there is an inherent tendency to apply the "more is better" rule. For example, we often hear from patients, "If I take more drugs, I'll make more eggs." "If you transfer more embryos I'll have a better chance of pregnancy. If three embryos are good, six would be twice as good." "Having quadruplets would be cool." Of course this is all nonsense.

ART is a science, and decisions should be made on a rational basis designed to achieve an optimal outcome. You really don't want to overshoot the mark. More drugs and more embryos could be disastrous and result in a serious medical problem called hyperstimulation of the ovaries. A high-level multiple pregnancy could result in the loss of the entire pregnancy, or the possibility of the health and cost issues related to prematurity.

We are reminded of a patient who became pregnant with a single fetus. Despite the conservative use of stimulation medications, only a moderate elevation of hormone levels and a modest number of eggs, she developed severe hyperstimulation. She required repeated hospitalizations, time away from work and prolonged recuperation, and during all of this was totally miserable. Although she eventually recovered and went on to have a healthy baby, she was so turned off by her experience that she vowed never to become pregnant again.

Misconceptions can lead to "missed conceptions."

ART can be a risky business. Too much of a good thing can quickly get you into big trouble. As our patient demonstrates, even with conservative treatment protocols, things can go wrong.

6. "Don't worry—this is a 'simple' procedure."

This is an easy misconception to explain because there is no such thing as a simple medical procedure. Even the seemingly simple act of taking an over-the-counter medication such as aspirin can be fraught with danger. A "simple aspirin" can cause havoc if given to the wrong person; for example, it has been associated with the deadly Reye's syndrome when given to children with influenza or chickenpox. If an aspirin can have such profound consequences, you may imagine what taking huge doses of powerful pituitary hormones for many days can do. It can drive the ovary to produce many times the number of eggs and hormones it usually produces. And how about putting a needle into a major body cavity guided by an ultrasound probe just millimeters from other vital organs and major blood vessels?

Now, of course, we are overstating the dangers of assisted reproductive procedures to make a point: it is just as wrong to grossly understate the potential risks of assisted reproduction as it is to overemphasize them. We believe each couple deserves a fair and balanced discussion of potential side effects and complications so they can make informed decisions. And that's not just our belief, it's the standard of care.

There are a few risks inherent to fertility treatments that should be included in any discussion. They include the following:

- Multiple pregnancy. This is the side effect most closely associated with assisted reproduction. In 2001, the multiple birth rate of the general population was 3%. In cycles initiated in 2001, 32% of births resulting from ART were twins. Triplets and higher level multiple pregnancies accounted for an additional 3.8%. Only one in 10,000 pregnancies conceived without fertility drugs represents triplets or greater. These figures are important because multiple pregnancies, especially those with three or more babies, frequently result in premature labor with its attendant costs of newborn care and potential developmental problems in the babies.

Make sure that you are aware of the risks of any medical treatment or procedure you are considering.

- Hyperstimulation. When powerful ovulation-inducing drugs are given in high doses, both in ART and conventional fertility treatment, they increase the risk of overstimulating the ovaries, producing an abundance of eggs and driving the woman's hormone levels into the stratosphere. One consequence of this is the development of a syndrome involving enlargement of the ovaries, retention of fluid, accumulation of fluid in the body cavities, electrolyte imbalances and, in the most severe cases, development of blood clots and even death. Fortunately this degree of hyperstimulation is very rare. But it reminds you to be wary when someone claims "more is better."

- Procedural risks. These are about the same risks you would run with almost any medical procedure or surgery. In this category we would include anything that can happen when you place a needle in the body, such as bleeding, infection or injury to a vital organ adjacent to the intended location for the needle. Even with the most careful technique it is possible to puncture a major blood vessel or the bowel, with serious consequences. Again, in experienced hands, these complications are rare.

- Long-term risks. We frequently hear concerns from patients about potential long-term effects from the powerful drugs used for ovarian stimulation. These fears were heightened when a much publicized report by A.S. Whittemore in the prestigious *New England Journal of Medicine* in 1994 raised the possibility of an association between the use of any type of fertility drug and the subsequent development of ovarian cancer in women who never achieved pregnancy.

It is well known that women who have fewer or no children have a higher risk of ovarian cancer. This protection conferred by childbearing is thought to be due to the effect of the pregnancy on suppression of ovulation. Infertility with its continuous ovulation unbroken by pregnancy or the use of birth control pills is thought to be the mechanism for the association. Therefore it might make sense that the stimulatory effects of fertility medications could increase this risk.

The good news is that reviews and studies subsequent to Whittemore's study conclude that the cause of ovarian cancer is a complex combination of genetic, hormonal, environmental and viral factors, and that the studies which drew the conclusion implicating fertility drugs were flawed. There were a small number of patients in the study and a lack of information regarding the cause of the infertility, the drugs used, dosage and duration of treatment. Additionally, a large Australian study reported in 1996 showed no increase in any gynecologic cancer in over 5,500 women undergoing ovulation induction compared with a similar group of infertile women who were not treated with drugs. In a scholarly review published in *Seminars in Reproductive Medicine*, the complex process of assessing a study's validity, importance and applicability to an individual patient was reviewed and concluded that the data from studies to date do not support a causal relationship between fertility drugs and ovarian cancer. Another 2003 study in *Fertility and Sterility* of almost 10,000 subjects concluded that there was no significant association between infertility drug use and invasive breast cancer.

Of course, very few individuals going through assisted reproduction experience even one of these potentially serious complications. But it's a basic premise that one should be informed about the potential risks of any contemplated medical procedure. So if anyone tells you, "This is a simple procedure," you need to go somewhere else.

5. "Don't put all your eggs in one basket."

If you are talking about investments, you don't want to put all your eggs in one basket. On the other hand, if you are going through assisted reproduction you *will* want all your eggs in one basket. Not only will you want them in one basket, you will want to make sure that it's *your* basket. Furthermore, you want to make sure that someone doesn't take them out of your basket and put them into someone else's without your knowledge or permission.

Do you think that could never happen? Let us tell you a story.

> This is a tale of fertility gods, not the kind you see in collections of primitive art, but the real life variety—several renowned medical idols who let themselves be seduced by ancient mortal frailties.
>
> This is a tale of technology, the application of cutting-edge medical and biotechnology to what today is a virtually unregulated, free-market and burgeoning branch of medicine.
>
> It is also a story of secrets and scandal: secrets that would shake many innocent families and a prestigious university to the core, and one of the biggest medical scandals in United States history.
>
> In May 1995, the University of California, Irvine (UCI) announced it was severing its ties to the renowned Center for Reproductive Health amid allegations that doctors conducted unapproved medical experiments on patients. Three days after breaking this story, the Orange County Register, a local newspaper, reported that the center's director had removed eggs from a woman, had them fertilized, and without the patient's consent had transferred the embryos into another woman. The other woman later gave birth to a boy.
>
> Audits conducted for the university revealed missing patient records and credible evidence of egg and embryo misuse involving many patients. Physicians were also charged with illegally billing insurance companies by using false diagnoses to obtain payment for procedures that were never performed. Top administrators at the UCI Medical Center were fired after it was reported that almost $1 million had been paid to silence former employees.

In June 1995, three UCI fertility specialists came under additional fire for allegedly pocketing tens of thousands of dollars in cash payments in violation of university agreements, and almost $1 million in unreported funds. The fertility center was abruptly shut down.

By November 1995, the number of patients discovered to have been unknowingly involved in illicit egg or embryo transfers by UCI fertility specialists had reached 60. There have been at least 85 lawsuits filed alleging illicit transfers of eggs and embryos.

There were at least seven investigations initiated by the FBI, IRS, U.S. Customs, U.S. Postal Inspectors, the Medical Board of California and the UCI Police Department. At the time, embryo theft was not a crime in California. Subsequently, a bill introduced by Senator Tom Hayden has made it a felony to donate eggs or embryos without the specific written consent of the "donor." Unfortunately, that law applies only in California.

What has happened to the cast of this tale?

Dr. Ricardo Asch, director of the Center for Reproductive Health, was indicted in November 1996 by a federal grand jury in Los Angeles on multiple counts of using the U.S. mails to send insurers more than $66,000 in fraudulent bills. The charges carry a prison term of up to five years per count, or a fine of up to $250,000. In June 1997 additional charges of income tax fraud and conspiracy were added. No charges thus far have been filed regarding allegations of egg and embryo stealing. Dr. Asch is currently practicing in Mexico and has never been tried on these charges.

Dr. Jose Balmaceda was previously indicted on fraud charges and also named in this indictment, facing five new charges. No charges thus far have been filed regarding allegations of egg and embryo stealing. Dr. Balmaceda has returned to his native Chile where he now practices. He, too, has not been tried.

Dr. Sergio Stone, a physician associated with the center, was the only one of the three principals who did not do in vitro procedures. He, like Drs. Asch and Balmaceda, faced multiple fraud, income tax and conspiracy charges. Ironically Dr. Stone, who apparently was not connected to allegations of egg and embryo theft, is the only physician of the three indicted who did not leave the United States. He was convicted of insurance fraud for writing false reports, suggesting that assistant surgeons were present during the surgeries, when *in fact he was the only one present. Stone was also convicted of charging insurance companies for work he claimed to have done, but that was actually performed by medical residents. Following his conviction, Stone was fined $50,000 and was ordered to serve a one-year term of home detention. Based on the conviction the Medical Board of California revoked his license, but stayed the revocation and allowed him to practice on probation for three years. In March 2000 the University of California Regents voted to dismiss Dr. Stone from the UCI faculty.*

As you can see, none of the indictments against any of the three physicians touched the issue of egg stealing. Scores of couples have been left with their lives in limbo. Some do not know if they have a child out there. Others look at a child they have and wonder if he or she is biologically theirs, afraid to do DNA testing to find out the truth. Reactions reported by the *Orange County Register* included that of Barbara and Carlos Parham of Fullerton who, after learning from records that all three of her eggs were stolen, believed their chance at childbirth was lost. Elizabeth Shaw Smith of Tustin told the *Register,* "I don't feel a lot of anger. I feel sick to my stomach. I feel they used me. They manipulated my body and stole my eggs and my money." After Wanda Nagy of Anaheim Hills underwent a GIFT procedure in May 1987, logs showed that 10 of her 34 eggs were given to two other patients. She said, "You know, you put your trust in someone and you have high hopes for them and then all of a sudden—boom—it just drops. You never want to believe it, and you never think it could be you. It's shocking."

Even now, years after the first revelations about the allegations at the University of California were revealed, no other similar allegations at any other fertility clinic have surfaced.

The university at one time was reported to have secretly paid $2 million to at least seven former patients. According to the *Orange County Register* in February 1997, a total of $3 million was paid to settle at least 10 claims that eggs and embryos were taken without patient consent. The first two claims were reportedly settled for $600,000 and $510,000 each. These settlements were reportedly motivated in part by the university's desire to establish a "de facto" ceiling on all the other lawsuits. In July 1997 the California Board of Regents reportedly approved a $10 million settlement between the university and 50 couples whose eggs were allegedly stolen.

This sounds like a storyline for a TV movie of the week. Actually a movie of the week was based on the case, but the lawsuits, indictments and lives ruined were real.

You should put all your eggs into one basket, and you'd better be careful about the sperm, too. A lawsuit has been filed against a Jacksonville, Florida hospital alleging that its in vitro fertilization program used the wrong sperm specimen to impregnate a patient. Elizabeth Higgins gave birth to healthy twins in April 1995, but subsequent DNA tests showed that her husband, Michael, was not the girls' biological father. A former employee testified in a deposition that the sperm collection process was "certainly less than an ideal situation." The couple said that after they learned that Michael was not the biological father, their marriage deteriorated and both sought counseling for depression.

Perhaps the most shocking instance of using sperm not belonging to the infertile woman's partner was the case of Dr. Cecil Jacobson, the South Carolina doctor who used *his own sperm* to inseminate patients, resulting in an estimated 75 pregnancies. Not only was Dr. Jacobson not a fertility specialist, he was not even a gynecologist. Dr. Jacobson received a felony conviction and a sentence of five years in jail.

The message here is to make sure you're armed with all the information you need to be a well-educated consumer, asking lots of detailed questions and being aware of procedures, protocols and the progress of your progeny.

Become a partner with your physician in making these important decisions about your reproductive future.

4. "Let the doctor decide: he/she knows best."

There are many things about which the doctor knows best. But does this mean that you should leave all the decisions to the doctor without any input from you? Of course not.

You should follow the progress of your ART cycle very closely and be aware of numbers of eggs and embryos and their fate, as illustrated in the above story about the University of California, Irvine. We do not mean to say that you need to go into the laboratory and watch every movement by the doctors and embryologists. But a healthy show of interest and involvement in key areas of decision will let your doctor know that you are watching. By reading the rest of this book you will know what those key areas are, but here are the two primary ones.

Probably the most important area in which you should have your say is the number of embryos in IVF or eggs in GIFT to be transferred, being mindful of our warning about "more is better" and fears about high levels of multiple pregnancy. This is a decision that certainly needs your careful consideration. There are some groups which, in conjunction with certain rebate schemes, require that you follow the doctor's advice in regard to numbers to be transferred. In our opinion, this practice is unthinkable. When the doctor has a financial stake in the outcome of the cycle it is likely that your best interest is not of primary consideration when decisions are being made.

The second most important area is the decision of when to move on to ART from conventional infertility treatment. Here, again, your active involvement is vital. You'll be the ones spending your money and, more critically, investing your hopes and dreams in this decision. By being in the position to need ART, you are vulnerable to deception and must be careful. According to ethicist Arthur Caplan, "Patients will do anything to get that biological baby. I've seen lots of desperate people around the hospitals—people who are dying, or with critically ill children—but the infertile couple are among the most desperate." That's why you must be careful and not let your desperation cause you to be victimized.

3. "There is such a thing as a free lunch."

If it sounds too good to be true, it probably is. Since the early days of assisted reproduction, the enthusiasm of some of its practitioners has led to a variety of misleading advertising claims and marketing schemes, some of which have been cited by the U.S. Federal Trade Commission, and others which are currently still being promoted.

The potential for exploitation of infertility patients is manifest in a host of claims from centers throughout the U.S. regarding their success rates that date back prior to, and were the primary reasons for, Representative Wyden's 1989 congressional hearings. Some of the abuses that led to the need for the hearings include:

- The September 1988 issue of *Better Homes & Gardens* featured an attractive advertisement including pictures of babies and the claim that "4 of the first 12 patients have achieved a pregnancy.... Our first test tube baby is due this October.... Our success rate is an impressive 30%, well above the national average." But what does success mean? Stating a percentage is meaningless without defining the group being measured. Presumably the 30% refers to 4 of the first 12 patients who became pregnant. However, no babies had been born yet, and the number of cycles was so small as to be almost meaningless.

- In December 1988 the magazine ad ran again, but without the "Our success rate is an impressive 30%, well above the national average." Why was this sentence deleted? In reviewing the data presented to the subcommittee from this clinic it appeared that 4 of the first 20 became pregnant. That would mean that after the first 12 patients, no pregnancies were achieved. Yet the ad continued to state that the first 4 of 12 became pregnant. Actually, this clinic formally reported for that year one live birth and a continuing pregnancy rate of 11% per cycle stimulated by fertility drugs and 13% per cycle resulting from eggs being retrieved.

- In September 1988, IVF Australia ran an ad in the *Boston Globe* stating that 236 babies had been born as the result of IVF Australia programs. That figure is correct. However, IVF Australia had two programs in the U.S.—and when that ad ran the Boston program was only three months old. Exactly the same techniques were being used by the newer program and the same rate of success was naturally anticipated, but the consumer was not made aware that the Boston program was relatively new.

- An ad described by syndicated columnist Ellen Goodman included a picture of a newborn with the headline, "Before you let go of the dream, talk to us." The text enthused, "There's no other perfume like it, the smell of a newborn: a milk-scent, warm scent, cuddle essence. Her skin a new kind of velvet. Toes more wrinkled than cabbage, yet roselike. Tender, soft, totally trusting; a blessing of your own. …That dream might still come true for you. New techniques can resolve many infertility problems, including some that were previously considered hopeless." Now, this may all be true, but Goodman concluded that such ads play upon the vulnerabilities of the infertile couple. They certainly do not provide important information about the chance of becoming pregnant.

Subsequent to Rep. Wyden's hearings the situation did not immediately change dramatically.

- According to a September 4, 1995 article in *Newsweek,* the U.S. Federal Trade Commission had obtained cease-and-desist orders against 11 fertility clinics over deceptive advertising claims.
- In 1994, a prominent hospital in New York City paid $4 million to hundreds of former infertility patients to settle a suit over false success-rate claims. An investigation by the New York City Department of Consumer Affairs resulted in charges that the hospital exaggerated success rates in a promotional brochure and flyer.
- Advertising claims are not limited to IVF programs, but also include devices intended to improve fertility. An ad for a basal body temperature device called Rabbit, for instance, proclaimed: "'Yes! You Will Become Pregnant' if you use Rabbit." In small type underneath is the disclaimer "and you're medically able to conceive."

Make sure that any statistics you are given conform to the SART Registry standard expressed as percent of deliveries per egg retrieval over a one year period. Frozen cycles should not be included.

ART centers are now becoming more sophisticated in their advertising and marketing. Since it is no longer fashionable to exaggerate success rates, new schemes have emerged.

- A number of centers still refuse to report to the CDC, which provides a uniform format for reporting all the facts and figures. They choose to use a format that will put their statistics in a favorable light. They may even hire a nationally known audit firm to make the report sound credible. But you must remember that when you look at a report from a center that does not participate in the CDC report, you cannot directly compare their success rate with that of a center that does report. It's like comparing apples and oranges. For example, they may include all the pregnancies resulting from frozen embryos with the pregnancies resulting from fresh embryo transfers for a particular group of egg retrievals. This will increase their rate substantially and, if you are not aware of this tactic, it may confuse you.

- Another marketing scheme is to offer refunds, in the form of a "guarantee," for couples who do not get pregnant. They claim that they are doing this to "share the risk" with the infertile couple. On the surface this sounds great.

  But what really happens is that the couple pays more—a lot more—for a cycle of ART. For example, at one clinic, if they did not achieve a viable pregnancy for 12 weeks, they would get a refund of 90% of their money, other than that spent on medications. Key provisions include that the woman must first have a hysteroscopy (not usually required), and the doctor makes the decision as to how many embryos will be transferred. This may not sound too bad.

  However, as we and others see it, there are problems. First of all, remember what Dr. Arthur Caplan said about the desperation of infertile couples. If you add to that desperation the argument, "Don't worry, if you don't get pregnant, you get your money back," you can see how couples potentially could be steered into ART procedures prematurely. The other major problem is that the doctor now has a financial stake in the outcome of the ART cycle. That leads to the potential for the physician to take unreasonable chances to achieve success, which may increase the chance for complications. The most obvious example of this is the issue of numbers of embryos to be transferred. It is very easy for the doctor to apply the "more is better" rule, especially when the couple has no say in the number of embryos to be transferred.
- These marketing schemes are often hyped at "free educational seminars" which, according to Judith Turiel, Ed.D., author of *Beyond Second Opinions: Rethinking Questions about Infertility* (University of California Press, 1997), "often constitute an elaborate sales pitch—with slides or a bound report displaying success statistics, reprints of favorable journal articles, and testimonials from satisfied patients. These presentations may be skewed more toward convincing than informing, and toward downplaying potential for harm rather than helping people understand and assess legitimate concern about risk."

This has led to a great ethical debate. The American Medical Association's Joint Report of the Council on Ethical and Judicial Affairs and Council on

Scientific Affairs concluded that "such publicized 'guarantees' manipulate and unfairly attract patients." In addition, basing payment for medical treatments on outcomes is unethical according to Opinion 6.01, AMA Code of Medical Ethics. In September 1998, the ASRM Ethics Committee issued a report on Shared-Risk and Refund Programs and reached the following conclusions:

> The Committee finds that the shared-risk form of payment for IVF is an option that might be ethically offered to patients without health insurance coverage for IVF if certain conditions that protect patient interests are met. These conditions are that the criterion of success is clearly specified, that patients are fully informed of the financial costs and advantages and disadvantages of such programs, that informed consent materials clearly inform patients of their chances of success if found eligible for the shared risk program, and that the program is not guaranteeing pregnancy and delivery. It should also be clear to patients that they will be paying a higher cost for IVF if they in fact succeed on the first or second cycle than if they had not chosen the shared-risk program, and that, in any event, the costs of screening and drugs are not included.
>
> The Committee was especially concerned about the incentives that shared-risk programs create for providers to take actions that might harm patients in order to achieve success and avoid a refund. For shared-risk programs to be ethical, it is imperative that patients be aware of this potential conflict of interest and that shared-risk programs not over-stimulate patients to obtain a large supply of eggs or transfer more embryos than is safe for the patient, fetus, and prospective offspring. Patients should be fully informed of the risks of multifetal gestation for mother and fetus, and have had ample time to discuss and consider them prior to egg retrieval.

Bob, 42, and Carolyn, 39, attended one of these seminars arranged by a center offering a 90% refund if a 12-week pregnancy is not achieved. They had been trying to become pregnant for only nine months. Bob had a normal semen analysis, and Carolyn a normal tubal dye test. A laparoscopy on Carolyn revealed minimal endometriosis. When they mentioned that Carolyn had a touch of endometriosis, they were told by the doctor running the seminar that trying conventional treatment would be a waste of time. He recommended that they shouldn't "waste any time with other doctors."

"Don't spin your wheels," was his advice. Physicians from that center insisted that they go right into IVF. Bob and Carolyn came to us for a consultation and before we could plan any conventional treatment, Carolyn became pregnant on her own.

So, when you are being offered a "free lunch," be sure to read the fine print on the menu.

2. *"Don't worry. I'm sure our insurance covers this."*

If you live in Canada or the U.S., we would bet that your insurance covers neither the diagnosis nor conventional treatment of infertility, especially assisted reproductive (ART) procedures. If we made that bet, we would be right far more than we would be wrong because most people do not have infertility coverage. Your coverage or lack of coverage depends on what state or province you live in and whether federal, state or provincial laws pertain to your employer. For example, in the U.S., even if you live in a state mandating coverage you will not be covered if your employer is self-insured, because as the result of a federal law known as ERISA (Employee Retirement Income Security Act) self-insured companies do not have to comply with state insurance mandates. Depending on where you live, roughly 40% to 65% of employee insurance plans are self-insured.

Obviously, insurance coverage is important to provide you with the funds to persist through some very costly treatments in your quest for a child. ART procedures are expensive because they involve space-age technology applied to you by doctors and scientists on a one-on-one basis. All of this technology, including the medications, was developed by private institutions without government assistance. The cost of developing, maintaining and utilizing the technology is enormous. One example that comes to mind is the development in our own center of the expertise to inject a single sperm into an egg (intracytoplasmic sperm injection, or ICSI). Not only did we have to buy the expensive micromanipulation equipment, but we also sent our embryologists to Belgium and New York to learn the technique and then brought in embryologists from Cornell in New York to work with our embryologists on the first group of cases.

In countries such as England and France, where ART procedures are included in the national health program, the incidence per capita of ART procedures is five times that of the United States. Are they doing too many, or are we doing too few? In the U.S., the number of clinics in a state roughly corresponds to the state's population; however, state laws requiring insurance coverage exert a tangible influence. For example, Massachusetts, which has one of the most comprehensive state mandates for ART treatment, in 2000 ranked 3rd in the number of procedures performed while it is 13th for the number of female residents of reproductive age. From our vantage point, we feel that there are many couples who would benefit from ART but just can't afford it.

There are several arguments used by opponents of insurance coverage for infertility to justify not covering it.

- "Infertility is neither a medical condition nor a disease." Well, if it's not a medical condition, what is it? Webster's defines a disease as "a condition of the living animal or plant body, or one of its parts that impairs the performance of a vital function." The reproductive system fulfills an important function in the body: reproduction. In 1998 in a 5-4 decision in an HIV discrimination suit, the Supreme Court of the U.S. ruled that reproduction is a major life activity. Perhaps it is not as critical as the cardiovascular system in day-to-day life, but is it so unimportant as to be denied insurance coverage? When it malfunctions in certain ways, such as growing tumors, it is covered. Why should its malfunction in doing what it was meant to do not be covered? Also, when a condition results in the degree of disruption to people's lives that infertility causes, surely it warrants insurance coverage. Ultimately the Supreme Court decision may pave the way for more insurance coverage as well as curbing discrimination in the workplace such as denying time off for treatments.
- "Nobody dies from infertility." This is also a specious argument because insurance covers many conditions of the body that are not fatal.
- "IVF and GIFT are experimental procedures." Not anymore. They have been so well developed and widely practiced that they are considered to be part of the clinical armamentarium.
- "IVF and GIFT are not successful enough." How successful does a treatment have to be to be paid for by insurance? IVF and GIFT are,

on average, achieving success rates better than Mother Nature, and the best centers are achieving success rates of more than double the spontaneous pregnancy rate in a "normally fertile" population. If this argument was valid, treatment for advanced cancer and AIDS should not be covered, and we know that would be nonsense.

Probably the real reason insurance companies don't want to cover infertility and ART goes straight to the bottom line. They want to keep premiums as low as possible to be competitive while maintaining good profitability, although a study calculated that adding IVF coverage would increase the typical annual premium by only $9 to $16 per year, depending on how much the demand increased. What they may really fear is the increased numbers of multiple pregnancies they may have to cover if more of their insureds were covered for ART procedures.

Unlike England and France, Canada does not cover IVF as part of its national health insurance.

There is a small trend for some HMOs to cover ART procedures as a marketing tool to make them more attractive to certain employee groups. But the trend is not a strong one. For example, an HMO that covered GIFT announced a few years ago that it was curtailing that coverage as new contracts came up.

Some states do have a mandate to "cover" infertility and ART, while others have a mandate to "offer" coverage, and the majority of states have no laws governing insurance coverage at all. Mandates to "offer" are much weaker because they only require insurers to let employers know coverage is available, but it does not require that they provide the coverage. This is a fluid situation and we would suggest you contact the American Society for Reproductive Medicine (ASRM), your local Resolve, Inc. chapter, or the Canadian Fertility and Andrology Society (CFAS) or Infertility Awareness Association of Canada (IAAC) to find out the coverage mandated in your state or province. One potential advantage to the insurance companies in mandated states or provinces was demonstrated in a July 2003 study showing that universal coverage had an impact on reducing the numbers of embryos transferred, which ultimately reduces the incidence of very expensive multiple pregnancies.

The insurance situation is changing rapidly as infertility support groups, physicians and other interested parties lobby their state legislatures to have basic infertility and assisted reproductive procedures mandated in health insurance coverage. Court decisions in some states have held that these procedures must be covered if they are not specifically excluded. Of course, many insurance companies have already rewritten their contracts to exclude these services. We suggest you become an active advocate for legislation in your state through Resolve, Inc. in the U.S. or the IAAC in Canada, because insurance coverage will help you persevere financially through enough treatment to be successful.

Even if you are not eligible for infertility services, many tests and procedures can be indirectly covered as they legitimately relate to the treatment of disease. For example, if a laparoscopy done to evaluate infertility uncovers and treats endometriosis, adhesions or tubal disease, you might want to apply for benefits based on the condition found. Legal advice might be useful in determining your rights under your health insurance contract.

To avoid falling prey to the Top 10 Misconceptions, be a good consumer—it will help you find a doctor deserving of your trust.

In Canada the insurance situation is not much different. According to the Canadian Fertility and Andrology Society (CFAS), "Canada does less to assist the medical need of infertile couples than almost all other countries with government-funded health care systems." They further state that infertility in Canada is "treated more as a cosmetic disorder than a disease." According to the Infertility Awareness Association of Canada (IAAC), most Canadians assume that their health care needs will be met through their respective provincial health plans. The health plans are different in each province. All investigations leading up to infertility treatment are covered everywhere. But broadly speaking, infertility treatment is not covered by either the federal or provincial governments or private health insurance plans. The exception is Ontario, where the Ontario Health Insurance Plan (OHIP) will cover the cost of three IVF cycles if both tubes are blocked. Other provinces may cover some consultations and diagnostic tests.

Currently there is no regulation of fertility clinics in Canada, except on the issues of sperm donation, where there are federal regulations. In 1993 the Royal Commission on New Reproductive Technologies released its final report which recorded 18 clinics in Canada offering IVF at that time. There are presently 22 IVF centers in Canada, 21 of which reported their results to a survey organized by the CFAS. Except in Ontario, these centers, as well as general infertility clinics, must be established and funded through private sources. The commission also contended that these private infertility clinics were not properly regulated or accountable and imposed a voluntary moratorium on nine controversial issues including:

- sex selection
- commercial surrogacy arrangements
- buying and selling eggs, sperm and embryos
- human embryo cloning

The good news is that the commission recommended that the provinces, in cooperation with the federal government, fund the delivery of ART procedures that have been "proven" beneficial. The bad news is that they did not consider IVF to be "proven" beneficial in conditions other than blocked tubes. This is despite the fact that IVF in couples with unexplained infertility is more successful than in the average patient, and the success rate per cycle in the average IVF patient is better than the monthly conception rate in unassisted conception in couples with normal fertility. Most studies suggest the unassisted conception rate per cycle in unexplained infertility is only 2% to 3%.

Up to now, there has not been any expansion of insurance coverage in Canada. However, a bill designed to regulate ART procedures, the Human Reproductive and Genetic Technologies Act (C-47), progressed through Parliament in 1997 until it died on the order paper because of an upcoming federal election. Some of the provisions of the bill would have effectively prohibited the same procedures as in the voluntary moratorium, as well as:

- cloning or splitting a zygote (conceptus less than 15 days old), embryo (15–56 days) or fetus (57 or more days)
- gene therapy on ova, sperm, zygote or embryo
- formation of animal-human hybrids
- retrieval of eggs from fetuses and cadavers

It is our hope that the phrase, "Don't worry, I'm sure our insurance covers this," will disappear from our list of misconceptions.

1. "Trust me. I'm a doctor."

If you are considering the possibility of ART, you are going to need to put a great deal of trust in a team of physicians, scientists and other medical personnel. We feel that the vast majority of teams doing this work are deserving of your trust. But unfortunately, you cannot rely on blind trust. You now know that you must conduct a thorough search and investigation to find your Dr. Perfect. The rest of this book gives you the information and tools you will need to make that selection and to successfully try to reach your goal. That's right—a healthy baby.

CHAPTER 3

The Female Partner

EAT YOUR VEGETABLES!

At some time or other as children we all had the experience of an adult telling us, "Eat your vegetables. They're good for you!" Our advice regarding the information in this chapter is similar: Read this chapter. It's good for you.

Actually, it's essential. A discussion of the normal anatomy and reproductive process in the female is not all that exciting and may not be what you want to read about. But in order to understand the complexities of the technology we describe later in the book, you will need to know the basics. Believe us! By the way, it's probably a pretty good idea to eat your vegetables, too.

ANATOMY

We will concentrate on the anatomy of two areas of the body—the base of the brain and the pelvis (see Figure 1).

At the base of the brain lie two important structures, the hypothalamus and the pituitary gland. The hypothalamus regulates many of the cyclic body functions, such as the menstrual cycle. The pituitary gland, often called the master gland of the body, is located near the hypothalamus and receives its instructions from the hypothalamus to perform its many functions.

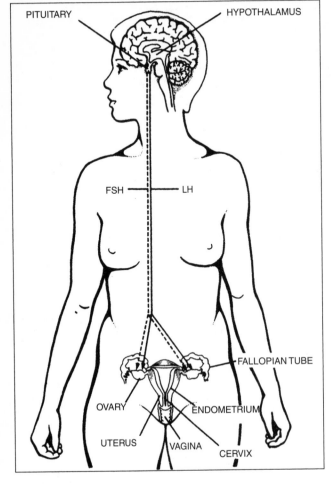

PITUITARY   HYPOTHALAMUS

FSH —— LH

FALLOPIAN TUBE

OVARY   ENDOMETRIUM

UTERUS   VAGINA   CERVIX

Figure 1   Female Reproductive System

In the pelvis, we are concerned with the female reproductive organs that are responsible for the production and transport of eggs and the carrying of a pregnancy. These include:

- *The Vagina*—the canal between the outside of the body and the lower part of the uterus.
- *The Cervix*—the lower part of the uterus, which extends into the upper part of the vagina and is the opening into the upper part of the woman's reproductive tract. The cervix is vulnerable to many different types of infection, which can then travel upward into the upper parts of the reproductive system and cause problems with fertility. (Examples of such infections are gonorrhea and chlamydia.)
- *The Uterus*—a muscular organ normally the size and shape of a pear. Surrounded by the muscular tissue of the uterus is its lining, the endometrium. This lining fluctuates with the menstrual cycle, preparing itself to receive a pregnancy. When a pregnancy is not begun in a particular cycle, the lining breaks down and leaves the body as the menstrual flow. The endometrium connects below to the cervix and above to the fallopian tubes.
- *The Fallopian Tubes*—coming off each side of the top of the uterus, these delicate, thin tubal structures lead from the uterus to the region of the ovaries. Each tube is four to five inches long. At the end of each tube is a particularly delicate structure called the fimbria. The fimbriae sweep across the ovary to pick up the egg.

Proper functioning of the tubes is dependent upon all of their microscopic features working properly, as even small anatomic alterations can result in tubal malfunctioning. This can lead to a pregnancy getting stuck in a particular portion of the tube, as in an ectopic pregnancy. In other cases, partial or complete obstruction may result in infertility (delay in becoming pregnant) or sterility (permanent inability to become pregnant).

- *The Ovaries*—the female's gonads. Gonads are glands that produce gametes, the basic reproductive germ cells (eggs, in the case of the female partner). The ovaries, oval-shaped organs a little over an inch in length, are located along each pelvic wall. At the time of a female's birth the ovaries contain all the germ cells (potential eggs) she will need for her lifetime. During fetal life, it is estimated that there are about six million eggs (oocytes) present in the ovaries. By birth, the number of germ cells has been reduced to approximately one to two million, with a further reduction to around 300,000 to 400,000 by puberty. During a woman's reproductive life, she will average about 500 menstrual cycles, utilizing one egg in each of those cycles. So what happens to all the other eggs before she reaches menopause? Some may start to develop, but when one is "chosen" to become the fully developed egg of that cycle, the others degenerate. Some just never develop. It is a system with an incredible amount of reserve, about a thousand to one at puberty— for every egg that develops, a thousand are discarded.

It's important to first learn the basics in order to understand the complexities of assisted reproductive technology.

PHYSIOLOGY

Physiology is the study of how the body functions and is not much more complex than anatomy. Again, we'll break it down into the same two areas of the body we discussed under anatomy.

At the base of the brain: Beginning at puberty, the hypothalamus starts releasing substances to stimulate the pituitary to secrete a number of hormones that, in turn, stimulate the function of other glands in the body—that's why the pituitary is called the master gland. The glands it stimulates that concern us here are the gonads (ovaries). The substances released by the pituitary gland are gonadotropins (hormones that stimulate the gonads). The substance produced by the hypothalamus that causes release of the gonadotropins is called gonadotropin-releasing hormone (GnRH).

Two different gonadotropins produced by the pituitary mediate the monthly development of an egg. The egg develops in a structure called a follicle—a fluid-filled area surrounded by supporting cells within which the egg develops. The first gonadotropin that stimulates the growth of the follicle is called follicle-stimulating hormone (FSH). When the egg is ripe and ready to come out of the ovary, a second gonadotropin is produced in a large surge to cause release of the egg (ovulation). This also results in a change of the follicle into a structure (corpus luteum) designed to produce hormones that will support implantation of the embryo into the endometrium. This second gonadotropin is called luteinizing hormone (LH). Actually, LH is produced in small amounts throughout the cycle, but it is this surge of LH we are interested in now.

The human reproductive system is very inefficient. It takes millions of eggs and billions of sperm to end up with a few children.

To review: *The hypothalamus produces GnRH, which stimulates the pituitary to produce FSH and LH. The large pulse of LH triggers ovulation.*

In the pelvis: Meanwhile, in the pelvis three organs respond to these cyclic changes in the gonadotropins (see Figure 2).

The ovary both responds to the changes in the gonadotropins and mediates the response of the endometrium. Physicians usually count the day a woman starts her menstrual period as Day 1 of the cycle. At about the time of the menstrual period, increasing secretion of FSH and small amounts of LH lead to the selection of several eggs to start developing. One of these eggs will eventually become the dominant follicle for that month. Under the stimulation of FSH and LH, the process of maturation of the egg cell within that follicle begins. In fact, we can now indirectly observe the development of that follicle with ultrasound. We can monitor the increase in size of the follicle, which is a reflection of the accumulation of follicular fluid and maturation of the egg.

The follicle consists of: (1) the egg cell; (2) the shell (zona pellucida); and (3) the corona and cumulus layers surrounding the egg, consisting of granulosa cells that proliferate and produce the hormone estrogen. So another way we can monitor the development of the follicle is by measuring the level of estradiol, one of the estrogens we can measure in the blood. The number of follicles maturing in any one cycle and the degree of maturity reached by these follicles is directly proportional to the amount of FSH and

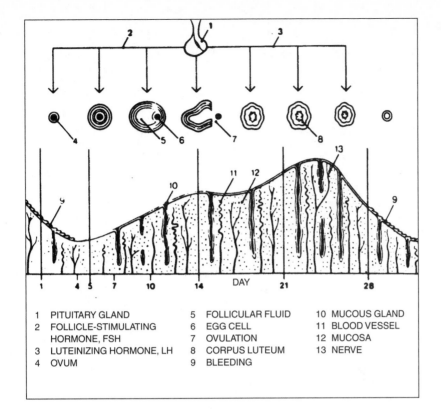

1	PITUITARY GLAND	5	FOLLICULAR FLUID	10 MUCOUS GLAND
2	FOLLICLE-STIMULATING	6	EGG CELL	11 BLOOD VESSEL
	HORMONE, FSH	7	OVULATION	12 MUCOSA
3	LUTEINIZING HORMONE, LH	8	CORPUS LUTEUM	13 NERVE
4	OVUM	9	BLEEDING	

Figure 2   The Menstrual Cycle

You can learn how to detect the surge of LH to determine your most fertile time.

LH present and the sensitivity of the individual's ovary to these gonadotropins. As you might expect, we can cause multiple eggs to develop and mature by giving a woman high doses of gonadotropins.

Of several follicles that begin developing during the menstrual cycle, one will usually progress to maturity by Day 14 in the average woman's cycle. When the follicle reaches maturity, the associated increase of estradiol leads to a surge of LH from the pituitary. This results in the rupture of the follicle and release of the egg (Day 14) and the development of the corpus luteum from the follicle wall after the egg has been released. The corpus luteum produces the hormone progesterone in addition to estrogen. If pregnancy does not occur, the corpus luteum has a natural life of about 12 days and will degenerate on about Day 26.

The endometrium in the uterus is very sensitive to the hormonal changes just described and changes in response to the ovarian hormones.

During the first half of the cycle, as the follicle develops and estrogen is secreted, the endometrium grows and proliferates (proliferative phase). Following ovulation and under the influence of the progesterone produced by the corpus luteum, the endometrium prepares itself for the implantation of the egg (luteal phase). As the corpus luteum degenerates and the levels of estrogen and progesterone decline, the endometrium is broken down and sheds itself as the menstrual period. With the use of an endometrial biopsy we can follow these hormonal changes and the endometrial response very precisely. Alterations in this response can be a cause of infertility.

The mucus-secreting cells in the cervix are also responsive to the ovarian hormones, something that is most apparent just before ovulation—when the levels of estrogen are at their peak and the cervical mucus becomes very abundant, clear and stretchy. (Many women describe mid-cycle mucus as having the consistency of egg white.) This type of mucus is favorable for the transport of sperm. Changes in the mucus are fairly easy to detect, and these observations are the key ingredient in many of the natural family-planning methods that allow avoidance of intercourse while mid-cycle mucus is present. As you have probably guessed, failure of the mucus to respond properly to hormonal changes can also result in infertility.

THE BIRDS AND THE BEES

If intercourse has taken place around the time of ovulation and adequate numbers of sperm are delivered to the cervix, pregnancy may occur. The semen forms a gel following ejaculation that then liquefies in 20 or 30 minutes. Some of the sperm move into the cervical mucus within minutes. Uterine contractions propel the sperm up through the uterus, and sperm can be found in the tube in as little as four minutes. (This extremely rapid movement explains why douching is not an effective contraceptive method.)

The numbers of sperm are dramatically reduced as they ascend the genital tract. Most are lost by simply leaking out of the vagina. However, in the upper genital tract, many get eaten by scavenger cells all along the reproductive tract (a process called phagocytosis). Also, some are lost through the fallopian tube into the pelvic cavity. So the next time someone tells you that all you need is one sperm, you will know what an understatement that is.

As the sperm are making their ascent, the egg, surrounded by its cumulus cells, adheres to the surface of the ovary until the fimbria from the fallopian tube sweeps over the ovary and picks it up. The eggs are quite sticky and will adhere to tissue. Delicate hair-like microscopic structures lining the tube (cilia) move the egg into the tube. Fertilization usually takes place in the outer portion of the tube (the ampulla). The sperm wedge themselves between surrounding cells, and one sperm will penetrate the zona pellucida. The zona then becomes impervious to penetration of a second sperm.

Within 14 to 20 hours fertilization is evidenced by the development of two structures consisting of the genetic material from the sperm and egg (pronuclei), and after about 26 hours the embryo will start dividing. The embryo will continue to divide in the fallopian tube until it is a compact cluster of cells (morula). Then the embryo moves fairly rapidly down the tube, arriving in the uterus three to four days following ovulation.

The natural conception rate is only 20% per cycle if intercourse or insemination takes place around the time of ovulation.

It remains in the uterus, where it continues to divide and finally begins to implant in the endometrium about six days after ovulation. Certain cells of the embryo begin to secrete what we commonly refer to as pregnancy hormone (human chorionic gonadotropin, or hCG). The presence of hCG is sensed by the corpus luteum, which continues to produce progesterone. This prevents the endometrium from breaking down and the menstrual period from occurring. The corpus luteum will continue to function until the pregnancy can produce enough estrogen and progesterone to support itself.

MONITORING YOURSELF

Since much of what we have discussed relates to normal body functions, we want to make you aware of the signs to understand how your own reproductive system is working. All of these observations are safe, fairly simple to do and, except for one, free of cost. In fact, some of the simpler ones are utilized by the natural family-planning methods to try to prevent conception. You can put them to use in helping you get pregnant by optimizing your timing of intercourse.

Monthly cycle

You can calculate your most fertile time based on the history of your previous cycles, especially if your menstrual periods are regular. Ovulation usually occurs about two weeks before the next expected menstrual period. This is because the luteal phase of the cycle usually lasts 12 to 14 days. So if, for example, you have the often-quoted 28-day cycle, your ovulation probably occurs on Day 14 of the cycle. If your cycle is usually 35 days, ovulation will most likely occur on Day 21. If there is a variation of your cycle of never less than 28 or more than 35, you need to take that variation into account—you will probably ovulate between Day 14 and Day 21. It's easy to calculate, but you do need to know the variation of your cycle length. Remember, no woman is absolutely regular. Even some women who thought they were regular found they were actually irregular when cycles were closely observed.

There are now much more sophisticated methods to monitor the cycle than the temperature chart.

Temperature chart

If you've had even the most preliminary infertility workup and treatment, you are probably familiar with the basal body temperature (BBT) chart. The concept is really quite simple. It was observed that one of the effects of progesterone on the woman's body is a slight temperature elevation of about one half of a degree. A woman's temperature has the least variation day-to-day upon awaking, before any physical activity (basal temperature). Therefore the slight shift caused by progesterone is most noticeable at that time.

If you take your temperature first thing in the morning, before you get out of bed even to go to the bathroom, and chart it for one complete menstrual cycle, you should see following ovulation that the temperature rises and stays up until just before the next menstrual period. You don't even need a special thermometer. A good-quality thermometer that you are able to read to one-tenth of a degree will do. If you have difficulty reading a thermometer, try an electronic digital thermometer.

You should not use the temperature chart to time intercourse. The temperature shift from the production of progesterone has a variable relationship to release of the egg and often occurs some time following ovulation, which may be too late! You can sometimes see a slight dip in the temperature before ovulation, but this is not consistent and reliable.

We feel that the BBT is a valuable way for you to understand your cycle and can be used for scheduling and interpreting infertility tests. However, it is not very good for predicting ovulation. Some physicians do not advise its use at all because they feel that it adds to the anxiety and stress already present in the couple experiencing an infertility problem. Some use it on a limited basis (for example, for only three cycles) and then, once it has served its purpose, discontinue it. You should be the judge of its value to you.

Cervical mucus

Like those women learning natural family-planning methods, you can learn to identify the cyclic changes in your cervical mucus. At the time of ovulation, the cervical mucus becomes abundant, clear and stretchy, with the consistency of egg white. Again, you can use this observation along with the regularity of your cycle and the results of previous months' temperature chart to determine your most fertile time of the month. You can check the mucus by observation or, if not enough is visible, you can check it by putting a finger into the vagina and sweeping it across in front of the cervix to obtain some mucus.

We recommend Ovuquick as the most reliable ovulation predictor kit.

Monitoring the LH surge

Now we are getting more scientific. Over the past decade manufacturers have come out with home test kits for various medical conditions. One of the first and most prominent has been the home pregnancy test kit. There are now a number of these on the market; they give the consumer the opportunity of doing her own pregnancy test and obtaining the result privately.

The home testing trend now includes tests for detection of the LH surge. A variety of tests on the market detect the LH surge in the urine, but we find Ovuquick to be the most reliable. Ovuquick usually gives a very clear-cut result. After adding three drops of urine to a Test Cassette, you match a test line, resulting from the concentration of LH, to a reference line. When the test line is darker than the reference line the test is considered positive. The results are accurate and the test takes only a few minutes. However, some women do not get a clear result as Ovuquick seems to be sensitive to increases in fluid intake. So, if the results are not clear, a more definitive result may be obtained if fluids are restricted during the testing period.

We usually recommend that the test be done in the afternoon or evening, starting a few days before anticipated ovulation. We recommend doing the test later in the day because the surge most commonly starts in the early hours of the morning and takes some time to reach levels detectable in the urine. If it is done in the morning, you could miss the surge that day and pick it up the next day, one day late. Remember, we are not detecting the beginning of the surge but detecting evidence that the surge started during the preceding 24 to 36 hours. Since ovulation usually occurs some 36 to 44 hours after the beginning of the surge and we may be detecting it up to 36 hours after the surge has started, we recommend that couples have intercourse that evening or the following morning. If insemination is planned, we time it for the following morning.

PREPARING FOR PREGNANCY

There are some steps you should take before attempting pregnancy.

1. Make sure you want to have a baby. This may sound foolish, but many couples attempt to get pregnant without giving enough thought to the effects on their life of having a child. They say "Let's get pregnant" instead of "Let's have a baby." Creating a baby and being pregnant may sound glamorous, but you must really want to have a baby. Don't get us wrong—we think having a baby is great. But is it great for you? You may think this never happens, but we do see new mothers who say:

"If I had known what this would do to my life…"

"I don't know who is going to watch the baby so I can go back to work…"

"I didn't know how much it was going to cost to have a baby…"

"My husband didn't really want a baby and it's driving us apart…"

Make sure your relationship is strong. It's generally a serious mistake to have a baby to try to patch up a shaky marriage. You just compound your problems and it's certainly not the ideal setting to bring a new life into the world.

2. Learn all you can about your genetic history. If there is any significant history of genetic problems in the family, you may want to investigate it before attempting to get pregnant. This could include a relative with Down syndrome or other mental disability, muscular dystrophy, cystic fibrosis, hemophilia or other inherited diseases. You may belong to a population group that carries an increased risk of diseases specific to that group, such as Tay-Sachs disease in Ashkenazic Jews or certain types of anemia in blacks or in people whose ancestors came from Mediterranean countries. This applies to both wife and husband. Your own doctor can help you with advice in this area, or will refer you to a place where you can get more information. There are now blood tests available to see if you are a carrier of the gene that causes many of these diseases such as Tay-Sachs and cystic fibrosis.

For example, we know of a Jewish couple, one of whom is a physician, who did not come in for care until about 12 weeks into their pregnancy. They had never been tested for Tay-Sachs. They were sent to the local Tay-Sachs testing program and both turned out positive. By this time, she was 17 weeks pregnant.

Since Tay-Sachs is a uniformly fatal disease with progressive neurological deterioration and death by age three, they were sent for genetic counseling. They were told that their offspring would have a 25% chance of having the disease and a 50% chance of being a carrier. Fortunately, it can be detected in the amniotic fluid and an amniocentesis (withdrawing amniotic fluid with a needle) was scheduled immediately. We were all relieved when the amniotic fluid revealed that the baby was not affected. But this should ideally have been known and planned for before the pregnancy. If they had waited any longer and if the result showed an affected baby, they would have had no choice but to continue the pregnancy and subject the baby to the certain fate of Tay-Sachs.

3. *Clean up your act!* Both of you should get into the best physical shape possible. Stop all medically unnecessary drugs, especially recreational drugs, including marijuana. These can have an effect on fertility as well as on the baby. Avoid smoking, alcohol and caffeine, as caffeine and smoking are both implicated in infertility. One study comparing smokers and non-smokers going through in vitro fertilization found that the smokers had lower fertilization rates and lower estrogen levels, required greater amounts of fertility drugs and had lower pregnancy rates. Another study showed that a cup of brewed coffee daily was associated with a 50% reduction in the chance of conceiving each month. A 2002 study on caffeine's effect on outcomes of infertility treatments showed that one cup of coffee a

day was a strong risk factor for not achieving a live birth with IVF or GIFT. For those who did get pregnant, one cup daily decreased the length of the pregnancy by more than three weeks. In addition to coffee, other sources of caffeine include tea, colas and chocolate.

If you are overweight, it is a good idea to lose the weight before you get pregnant and do it in a manner consistent with good nutrition. Then continue on a nutritionally sound weight-maintenance program. If your weight is normal or you are underweight, make sure that you are eating a well-balanced diet. If strenuous exercise has made your periods irregular, you might want to modify your routine while trying to conceive. Check at work for any environmental hazards to conception or pregnancy. Finally, if your level of stress is a problem, you can try to avoid stress or use stress-reduction techniques. Your doctor can help with this type of planning.

4. Take prenatal vitamins daily. In preparation for pregnancy, authorities are recommending the use of vitamins containing the daily requirement for pregnant women. Do they help? Studies have suggested a much lower incidence of neural tube and heart defects in infants whose mothers took vitamins containing 0.4 milligrams (mg) of folic acid before conception. In any event, they can't hurt if taken as directed.

Prenatal vitamins are easily obtained over the counter at any pharmacy and are fairly inexpensive. In order to obtain the dose of 1 mg of folic acid utilized in prescription prenatal vitamins, you will need to get a prescription from your physician. There are many different brands, but all contain about the same formula.

5. Consider existing medical problems. If there is any question of a medical problem, it is a good idea to have this evaluated and treated before getting pregnant. This is especially true if diabetes is present or suspected. Fertility will be greatest, and the chance of fetal abnormalities will be minimized, by starting the pregnancy with normal blood sugars. We recommend that all diabetics be checked and receive an okay from their doctor before even attempting to get pregnant.

You should also be sure that other medical conditions are under control and that medications to control them are appropriate during pregnancy, since some medications could increase the chance of fetal abnormalities.

MAXIMIZING YOUR CHANCES

As we will explain in greater detail later, a young couple with normal fertility who have intercourse at or about the time of ovulation stands about a 20% to 25% chance that a pregnancy will result. In order to reach this level of maximum efficiency of the human reproductive system, be sure that:

- Intercourse occurs as close to the time of ovulation as possible.
- The man's sperm is at optimal levels.
- The environment is suitable.

Intercourse can be timed to occur on the day of ovulation as determined by the calendar, examination of previous BBTS, cervical mucus or (for the more scientifically minded) the urinary LH home test. Precise timing may be more scientific, but it does tend to add stress to the process and can even take the fun out of it. An alternative is to be sure to have intercourse at least every other day around the estimated time of ovulation. Given the life of the sperm and the egg, this would tend to have sperm present during the "life" of the egg no matter when ovulation occurs. Currently no evidence exists that more frequent intercourse impairs fertility. Just don't let more than two days pass without having sexual relations. It is not a good idea to limit sex in order to "save it up" for one prime time, because that may reduce the motility (movement) of the sperm. Motility tends to decrease with longer periods between ejaculations. The best compromise appears to be a two-day interval to maximize your chances of conception.

By environment we do not mean candlelight, music and wine. We are talking about position and the avoidance of practices that might be harmful to sperm. The man-above/woman-below position is best for most couples, with the woman staying on her back for about 20 minutes following ejaculation. The use of artificial lubricants and douching after intercourse should be avoided.

INFERTILITY

So far, almost all we have discussed pertains to normal reproduction and the couple who has no problem conceiving. So how do you know if you have an infertility problem? Infertility is defined as the inability to conceive a baby after one year of fairly regular unprotected intercourse. That's *not* the same as trying to have a baby for a year. For example, we have seen couples come in with a history of unprotected intercourse for several years, but they didn't think they had an infertility problem. We don't know where the notion that you have to be "trying" came from. If the factors controlling your fertility are normal and you are having regular unprotected intercourse, you will get pregnant whether you are "trying" or not.

In some couples, we reduce the period of time of unprotected intercourse to six months before considering them as possibly having an infertility problem. These might be couples who are in their late thirties or forties and who, for that reason, are anxious to conceive quickly. Also included would be those couples in whom we can identify a potential problem. But for most couples the rule of one year of unprotected intercourse applies.

After a review of the basics of male reproduction in chapter 4, we will discuss the causes of infertility in chapter 5. But don't skip chapter 4. There are essentials that you need to know.

It's a good idea to have a pre-conceptional counseling session with your physician, whether you are experiencing a fertility problem or not.

CHAPTER 4

The Male Partner

OH NO! NOT MORE ANATOMY!

Just as we stressed in chapter 3 regarding the female, it is vital to understand the normal reproductive process in the male in order to be able to appreciate the complexities of the technology we describe later in the book.

The male partner is either the sole or a contributing cause of infertility in up to 40% of infertile couples, but his role in the fertility process has generally been understated until recently. Actually, the parameters to establish normal male fertility were not even developed until the 1950s, when normal semen was defined by Dr. J. MacLeod in 1,000 fertile men and in 800 men in infertile marriages. However, with the advent of assisted reproductive technology, there has been renewed interest in the male's role in the fertility process. Much has been learned about male reproduction based on the procedures developed to enhance fertilization in the laboratory, and this knowledge is now being applied to conventional fertility testing and treatments as well as to advanced reproductive technologies.

ANATOMY

As with the female, we will concentrate on the anatomy in two areas of the male body—the base of the brain and the pelvis.

At the base of the brain is the pituitary gland, the master gland of the body, which controls many other glands just as it does in the female. However, in the male we are not concerned with a cyclic function, like the menstrual cycle of the woman controlled by the hypothalamus, but with the continuous production of the pituitary hormones.

In the pelvic and groin areas we find the male reproductive organs (Figure 3) consisting of:

- *The Testicles*—the male's gonads, located in the scrotum. They consist of a compartment that produces sperm, and cells (Leydig cells) that produce male hormone (testosterone).
- *The Epididymis*—a tubular network located at the top of each testicle. It leads sperm away from the testicle and consists of a single long, narrow coiled tube about 12 to 18 feet long attached to each testicle. The epididymis is about 1/300 of an inch in diameter.
- *The Vas Deferens*—the next part of the tubal system. It is connected to the epididymis on each side and travels from the scrotum into the groin and ultimately empties with fluid from other reproductive organs into the urinating channel (urethra).
- *The Seminal Vesicles*—add fluid to the semen, which aids ejaculation.
- *The Urethra*—the urinating channel leading from the bladder to the outside, through the penis. The vas deferens and seminal vesicles empty through the ejaculatory duct into the urethra in the region of the prostate gland.
- *Other Organs*—the prostate gland, Cowper's glands and seminal vesicles all contribute fluid to make up the semen. In fact, sperm cells make up only a small fraction of the total ejaculate.

Many people talk about the "sperm count." But there are other parameters that are important.

PHYSIOLOGY

As in the female, the hypothalamus stimulates the pituitary gland to produce hormones that, in the male, instruct the testicles to produce sperm as well as male hormones, primarily testosterone. The pituitary hormones leave the gland and enter the blood circulation to reach the testicles. Although the pituitary hormones stimulate both sperm development and testosterone production in the testicles, these are independent functions, and it is common for abnormalities to exist in sperm-producing areas of the testicles with normal production of male hormones. The two pituitary hormones are the same as in the female but are not cyclic. Follicle-stimulating hormone (FSH) primarily stimulates the production of sperm, while LH is responsible for stimulating Leydig cells to produce testosterone. This differs from the female, where the hormones must be produced in the proper sequence to cause ovulation.

Sperm begin as very simple cells and go through prolonged phases of development to reach maturity. They are manufactured in tube-like structures called seminiferous tubules. Initially, immature sperm cells are round, but as they mature they elongate and assume the typical tadpole appearance of a mature sperm. The sperm consists of:

- a head, containing all the genetic material;
- a middle part to provide energy needed for movement; and
- a tail that moves to propel it forward.

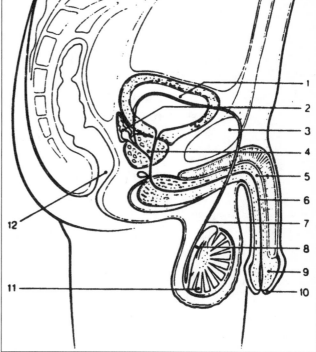

1	bladder	7	spermatic duct
2	seminal vesicle	8	epididymis
3	symphysis pubis	9	glans
4	prostate	10	foreskin
5	erectile tissue	11	testis
6	urethra	12	anus

Figure 3   Male Reproductive Organs

The sperm travel from the testicle through the epididymis into the vas deferens. The vas deferens takes them from the scrotum into the groin and ultimately empties them with secretions from the other reproductive organs into the urethra. The urethra, which usually carries urine from the bladder to the outside, has a muscle at the outlet of the bladder that closes, normally preventing the ejaculatory fluid (semen) from going back into the bladder at the time of ejaculation (retrograde ejaculation). With contraction of these muscles, the fluid in the urethra has only one way to exit—

through the penis. A tiny amount of fluid from the Cowper's glands, located at the base of the penis, is added to the semen and appears at the tip of the penis just prior to ejaculation.

When the sperm leave the testicle, they are fully formed but have no motility (movement). As they travel the entire length of the epididymis, they acquire motility and complete their maturation. It takes about 72 days for the sperm to begin its development and progress through complete maturation. Any abnormality in this complex system can result in subfertility or infertility. Since it takes almost three months for sperm to develop fully and be transported, it stands to reason that any treatment which improves sperm production can take up to three months to be reflected in the ejaculate.

Near the seminiferous tubules are the Leydig cells, which produce testosterone. This hormone is responsible for the development of all the masculine characteristics: deep voice, male hair pattern, heavy musculature. Since different cells produce sperm and hormones and different pituitary hormones stimulate the two different functions, it is common for a man to be fully masculine yet have a problem producing sperm.

WHAT MAKES A GOOD SPERM

There are a number of parameters used to determine the quality of sperm sample. Some of these criteria may not directly relate to sperm function and, despite the fact that a specimen may appear perfectly normal, there may be other factors that could prevent the sperm from fertilizing an egg. Some common parameters used in the complete semen analysis are:

- *Sperm density*—the numbers of sperm in a milliliter (cubic centimeter) of ejaculate (over 20 million per milliliter is considered normal).
- *Morphology*—categorizing sperm by their shape. Every man has some abnormally shaped sperm in the ejaculate. In fact, it is considered normal for up to 70% of the sperm to be shaped abnormally. There is no evidence that these abnormal forms increase the chance of birth defects. They are simply less able to fertilize an egg. "Strict morphology" assesses whether sperm shape satisfies more stringent criteria (14% of sperm or more are strictly normal). This parameter is more predictive, particularly for IVF success.

- *Motility*—represents the percentage of sperm that are moving. The degree of motility is assessed and varies between grade C (moving in place) and grade A (rapid progression). Greater than 25% grade A or greater than 50% grade A and B is normal. Newer computer-assisted semen analysis actually measures their velocities and even the quality of motion, although this is used mostly in research.
- *Viscosity*—an evaluation of the thickness of the semen after a period of time following ejaculation, when the semen should become more fluid, or liquefied. If the semen fails to liquefy, the sperm may not migrate well into the cervical mucus.
- *Volume*—the total amount of the ejaculate (varies from one to five milliliters). If the volume is too low, the sperm may not reach the cervix.

MAXIMIZING YOUR CHANCES

In chapter 3 we discussed many of the ways a woman can monitor her menstrual cycles and advised methods to maximize the couple's chances of conceiving. There is no such advice directly applicable to men with the exception of general advice, such as avoiding X-rays, or excessive heat to the scrotum; avoiding medications and drugs (especially recreational drugs); avoiding smoking, excess alcohol, excessive stress and toxic agents such as pesticides and industrial chemicals. The combination of heavy caffeine intake (four cups of coffee a day) with heavy smoking (more than 20 cigarettes a day) has been shown to cause significant decreases in sperm motility and increases in numbers of dead sperm. Excessive and chronic alcohol use also has a harmful influence on sperm development.

Excessive heat to the testicles can be prevented by not using heated spa-type baths or tight-fitting clothing such as briefs. However, changing underwear from briefs to boxer shorts has never been proven to improve fertility, and if a man is uncomfortable with looser-fitting shorts most experts in male fertility would not recommend a change.

INFERTILITY

Just because a man is sent for a reproductive evaluation does not mean that he has an abnormality. He is simply a partner in a couple with reproductive delay. In a later chapter, we will describe the evaluation of the semen by various other techniques that further clarify the likelihood of his being a contributor to the reproductive problem.

It is normal for a man's semen to be quite variable even on a day-to-day basis. For this reason, when a man is evaluated for reduced semen quality, three specimens may be obtained before drawing any conclusions. Also, it is necessary to wait at least three months between collecting groups of samples in order to see a real change resulting from treatment because of the time required for maturation and transportation of sperm.

Now that you have the basic knowledge needed to understand the information in the rest of the book, you can move on to chapter 5, where we consider what types of problems can cause a delay or inability of a couple to conceive.

CHAPTER 5

When It Doesn't Work

It's as American as Motherhood, Apple Pie, The Flag and Baseball.

You grow up, go to school, get married and start a family.

Not necessarily. At least not for the approximately 15% of American couples for whom motherhood or, more correctly, parenthood does not come so easily. These are the couples plagued by infertility. For many reasons, the least of which may be that the couple does not meet the expectations of well-meaning friends and relatives, trying to solve an infertility problem can be a humiliating, demeaning and totally frustrating experience. It can even lead to the end of a relationship.

A common perception among infertile couples is that everyone else they know is getting pregnant. But this is probably a misconception. It seemed a cruel irony that in 1988, just as the birthrate for the United States climbed to its highest point since 1964, the Office of Technology Assessment (OTA) reported that an estimated billion dollars was spent the preceding year on the treatment of infertility. So, not everyone else is really getting pregnant, even if it may look that way.

Provisional data released by the National Center for Health Statistics show that an estimated 3.9 million babies were born in the United States in 1988. That figure increased to 4.2 million in 1990, then decreased back to 4.0

million by 2002 which still puts us in the midst of a minor baby boom compared to the late 1980s. In 1988 the OTA was reporting that 2.4 million couples were plagued by infertility and that the number of visits to physicians for infertility had doubled, going from 1 to 2 million in the past several years. Infertility is now estimated to affect over 4 million American couples. In 1996 the National Center for Health Statistics estimated that the age structure of the population will cause the number of women with impaired fertility to rise to 4.8 to 5.9 million by 2020. Are we, therefore, in the midst of a baby boom and an infertility epidemic at the same time?

It looks like we are in the midst of a minor baby boom and an infertility epidemic at the same time.

If we add the 4.0 million babies born in 2002 to the Centers for Disease Control (CDC) estimate of 1.3 million abortions being performed every year, we can get a fairly accurate count of how many women are getting pregnant. However, we cannot determine with absolute accuracy if there is an infertility epidemic because we can only roughly estimate how many couples are currently infertile in the United States. We do know there is an increasing demand for infertility services. But is it because more couples are actually infertile or more women are starting to try at older ages, or has more awareness of the availability of new reproductive technologies brought more infertile couples in for treatment?

Many experts feel that, instead of an infertility "epidemic," there's merely greater demand for services based on more effective treatment and the recognition of infertility as an acceptable problem. We actually may be witnessing both an increase in the incidence of infertility and an increased demand for services.

SOCIAL FACTORS THAT INCREASE INFERTILITY

It makes sense to postulate a true increase in infertility when you examine the social forces that tend to result in more infertility.

Delayed childbearing—the chronological age factor

This is perhaps the most frequently quoted reason for our "infertility epidemic." Anyone who has been practicing obstetrics during the past 30 years cannot help noticing a dramatic change. The norm 30 or more years ago was for women to finish their secondary education, get married, and have a baby in their late teens or early twenties. Now that situation is far less commonplace and we are seeing many women finishing advanced education, developing a career and becoming financially stable before thinking of having a baby. By the time they accomplish all this they are often in their mid-thirties or early forties. Suddenly, it seems, they realize that it is time to start a family before time passes them by. The change in the birth rate in the U.S. supports this observation. In 2002 the birth rate in teenagers was down to 42.9 per 1000 from 47.7 in 2000, while for women 35 to 39 and 40 to 44 the birth rates edged up from 40.6 to 41.4 for the former, and 8.1 to 8.3 for the latter. Note the large disparity in these two age groups, reflecting not only fewer couples trying to conceive in the 40 to 44 age group, but also the more important factor of sharply reduced fertility potential in the older age group.

A widely accepted notion is that age is the most critically important factor in a woman's ability to become pregnant. A 1982 French study led to the perception that all women in their early to mid-thirties are at risk for infertility if they delay childbearing. The study reported that fertility rates (the ability to become pregnant) in women who were never previously pregnant declined from 74% before age 30 to 62% between ages 31 and 35 and down to 54% by age 36. According to these data, by ages 31 to 35 fully one-third of women would not get pregnant. And, by age 36, almost half would be barren. That's pretty scary if you're over age 35 and trying to conceive. But there's a problem with these results. They were obtained only in women who were never previously pregnant and then were applied to all women. This invalidates the study, since a group of women who have never gotten pregnant may be infertile for reasons other than age.

Another problem with this French study is that it was conducted only in women undergoing 12 cycles of artificial insemination by a donor. That eliminated any fertility effects due to frequency of intercourse or husband's fertility. Even though the donors were all assumed to be fertile, it is believed that 12 cycles of artificial insemination would not yield as many pregnancies as one year of intercourse.

An English study of women who have previously had babies and thus have proven fertility found that age alone does not significantly increase the risk of infertility until age 38. This is in general agreement with the 1982 U.S. National Family Growth Survey, which showed increases in infertility rising from 10.6% at ages 20 to 24, 13.6% at 30 to 34, and only dramatically rising to 24.4% at ages 35 to 39 and then to 27.2% at 40 to 44. Again, this study was of women who had previously been pregnant. For those women who are trying to decide whether they can space their children, it is reassuring that the effects of age alone are not so dramatic as to deny them that luxury.

What is the sum total of the effects of age on fertility? The studies quoted above looked only at the effect of age in women without a known fertility or other problem when they first attempted pregnancy and did not indicate the chance of the older woman with a fertility problem becoming pregnant. In studies of infertile older women who have failed to conceive even with treatment, the effects of age have been fairly dramatic, often reducing success rates by more than 50%.

It seems that having that first child confers some protection against future infertility.

Delayed childbearing—other factors

It would stand to reason that delaying childbearing would allow other conditions, such as gynecologic disease and numerous medical conditions which might afflict an individual, to occur. By far the most important would be gynecologic disease, primarily pelvic endometriosis, and to a lesser extent tubal disease and adhesions as the result of pelvic infection from sexually transmitted diseases. We'll discuss these conditions in greater detail later in this chapter. But first, let's take a brief look at them as they relate to delay in childbearing.

THE DELAY ITSELF

A delay in childbearing itself would appear to lead to infertility since previous childbearing confers protection against infertility. Over the 20 years studied, the National Family Growth Survey found a *decrease* in the infertility rate from 19% to 13% in women who became infertile after having one child. In contrast, they found an *increase* from 16% to 22% among those women who had never had a child. The rate in women with two or more children remained constant at a low 10%. We do not know why there was this apparent decrease in infertility in couples who already had at least one child. It may have been because these couples are monogamous and therefore less likely to contract a sexually transmitted disease. It is possible that childbearing protects against gynecologic disease, or perhaps there may be some as-yet-undiscovered factor.

SEXUALLY TRANSMITTED DISEASES

We have certainly witnessed a change in sexual mores over the last three decades, with a resultant epidemic of sexually transmitted diseases. The CDC reported that in 1999 the rate of infection with gonorrhea in the U.S. was 128 women per 100,000. Total hospitalizations for pelvic inflammatory disease, reflecting serious infections, numbered about 100,000 during the same period. Studies have shown that 11% to 12% of women will be left infertile after one episode of tubal infection. The figure rises to 23% after two episodes and goes above 50% after a third. The number of hospitalizations does not take into account patients who are treated in doctors' offices or those left untreated. In addition, some infections, particularly chlamydia, may silently damage the tubes. In fact, about half the women we see with tubal occlusion (blocked tubes) have no known history of any infection in the past.

IUD USE

In the late 1960s and early 1970s the IUD—intrauterine device—enjoyed increasing popularity. The newer devices were made from plastic instead of metal, as were the earliest devices designed in the 1930s. They were relatively inexpensive and came into wide use. By the time it was alleged that they predisposed the wearer to pelvic infection, many women had suffered irreparable damage to their tubes, especially from the Dalkon Shield IUD.

ENDOMETRIOSIS

Endometriosis is a disease that is most likely caused by chronic reverse flow of menstrual blood back through the tubes. In some predisposed women, fragments of endometrium may implant and grow around the tubes and ovaries. These implants are stimulated by the normal monthly fluctuation of hormones to undergo cyclic changes. Over time the disease creates enough inflammation and scarring to interfere with fertility. Early occurrence of a pregnancy and birth interrupts this process, probably by decreasing retrograde menstrual flow as the result of widening the cervical opening. In addition, the pregnancy treats any areas of the disease already present. Endometriosis is called "the career woman's disease"; women who have a child early in their reproductive years are less often afflicted.

UTERINE FIBROIDS

With age, these benign muscle tumors of the uterus increase markedly in frequency and size. Depending upon their location, they can reduce the chance of conception, increase fetal loss or require surgery—which can cause scarring. A fibroid growing under the lining of the uterus can make the environment less receptive for implantation or, as it may grow rapidly during the pregnancy, can put pressure on the expanding pregnancy and cause miscarriage or premature birth.

GYNECOLOGIC SURGERY, ECTOPIC PREGNANCY, THERAPEUTIC ABORTION

As time passes, there is more chance for the development of an ovarian cyst or other problem that could require surgery. Incisions in the ovary tend to cause adhesions around the tube and ovary that can impair fertility.

If an unwanted pregnancy occurs, the rare complications of an abortion can impair future fertility. In addition, a future pregnancy could lodge in the fallopian tube, resulting in loss or damage to that side. Since ovulation normally only occurs half the time next to a healthy tube, obviously the chance of a normal pregnancy occurring in any one month is decreased markedly.

PREMATURE OVARIAN FAILURE

The ovaries can start to fail many years before the average age of menopause (51). If this occurs, the chance of stimulating residual eggs in the woman's ovaries is small. In smokers, the average age of menopause is four years earlier, and since the ovaries can show signs of impaired function years before the menses cease we can safely say that "smoking and delayed childbearing don't mix!"

How should these complex factors affect your decision of when to start a family? We advise that you not delay unless there is a strong reason, particularly if a fertility problem has already been identified. We have seen too many couples who have waited until "everything is perfect" only to find that the one thing most important to them forever eludes their grasp.

In any event, what we are seeing clinically is more women in their thirties and forties who want a child but are unable to get pregnant. But if there are so many couples dealing with infertility, why do you feel alone?

YOU ARE NOT ALONE!

While there may be another 4 to 5 million couples struggling with infertility, that is little solace for the individual couple facing this problem. First, it is small relief to know that others are suffering with you. Second, couples with infertility do not usually share their problem with others, so we might think of these couples as a "silent minority." The highly visible majority are the people who have gotten pregnant. An example of their high visibility is something we all have experienced, standing in a supermarket line behind a woman with a newborn baby. As you may or may not be admiring her new offspring, her eyes meet yours and you feel compelled to say, "My, what a cute baby." They seem to be everywhere!

She may use your statement as a cue to tell you about her labor and delivery and tell you how smart her baby is. But then are you going to say, "Did you know that I really want to have a baby, but I can't? My tubes are blocked." Probably not. When it doesn't work and you have not met the expectations of friends, family and society in general it is something you, and others like you, do not often go public with.

Not too many years ago, at public health forums in local hospitals, subjects such as heart disease, cataracts, breast cancer and even sexual problems would draw participants in droves. But when the subject was infertility, only a handful of people showed up. They would listen intently, not asking many individual questions. When asked why attendance was not better, many said that their friends who were also having difficulty conceiving would not come because they did not want the world to know that they had this problem. The more recent and healthier trend is for more couples to "come out of the closet" with their infertility, as evidenced by the development and growth of support groups such as Resolve. Sharing any medical problem with family, friends and others with similar problems is more productive because it allows you to get important emotional support.

WHY IS THERE SO MUCH INFERTILITY?

Human reproduction in its unassisted form is remarkably inefficient. Substantial embryonic loss is a routine part of the life cycle among humans and in fact among all mammals. Most eggs are never fertilized and, if fertilization occurs, as many as one-fourth to one-third of human conceptions end in miscarriage, for reasons that are poorly understood.

—Testimony of Gary B. Ellis, Ph.D., senior analyst, Office of Technology Assessment, at U.S. Congressional subcommittee hearing on Consumer Protection Issues Involving In Vitro Fertilization Clinics, March 9, 1989

Most people do not understand the complexities of the human reproductive system and therefore why it's so inefficient.

Reproduction is basically a very inefficient system. After all, it takes millions of eggs in the woman and billions of sperm in the man to create perhaps a handful of offspring during their lifetimes. Consider for a minute what would happen if General Motors did business this way. If it took millions of engines and billions of bodies to create a few automobiles, it would not be long before GM was out of business.

The human reproductive system is a dichotomy. Portions of the system have a fantastic amount of reserve and margin for error. At the same time, portions of the system rely on the successful completion of minute details, any one of which can prevent the system from working. There is not one ovary, but two, and in these two ovaries are not only the 500 or so eggs a woman will need for her reproductive life, but hundreds of thousands at puberty. On the other hand, the portion of the system that controls implantation of the embryo into an adequately prepared endometrium relies on:

- a precise sequence of hormones to prepare the endometrium
- receptors in the cells of the endometrium to accept the proper hormones
- cellular functions controlled by complex codes

Thus we are slaves to a system that contains gross excesses and at the same time precise mechanisms which can be foiled by the slightest alteration in function.

WHAT CAUSES INFERTILITY?

There is a great deal of variation in the incidence of the major causes of infertility among centers in different parts of the continent, and, in fact, even in areas of the same city serving different populations. Although these figures may vary from those in your area, it will be useful as an example to look at the primary factors responsible for infertility in one large study reported in 1980, reviewing over 600 cases. It's important to go this far back in time because making an accurate diagnosis was more important then as ART technology had not yet been developed and only diagnosis-specific conventional treatments were available. Figures in other studies may vary considerably. But this study found the primary causes to be:

	Percent
Endometriosis	25
Male factor	18
Lack of ovulation	15
Tubal problem	12
Luteal phase problem	7
Cervix or mucus problem	5
Uterus problem	2
Other problems and unexplained	16

Premature ovarian failure can only be detected by lab tests; it has no symptoms.

Lack of ovulation

The first requirement for a successful conception is the meeting of two germ cells. A woman's lack of ovulation (anovulation) deprives the system of the female germ cell and foils attempts at conception at the most basic level. Treatment directed at the specific cause of the anovulation can promptly lead to pregnancy.

We can look at anovulation as occurring at three basic levels in the female reproductive system. It can occur as the result of failure of:

- the ovaries
- the reproductive centers in the brain and pituitary
- malfunction in the interactions among parts of the reproductive system resulting in a disruption in the orderly sequence of hormonal changes which controls the maturation and release of the egg

OVARIAN FAILURE

Failure of the ovaries prior to the usual age for menopause is termed premature ovarian failure. This is relatively easy to diagnose by measuring the level of gonadotropins. In premature ovarian failure these are very high, perhaps two or three times the normal level. This results from the hypothalamus and pituitary gland overreacting to a lack of feedback signals from the ovaries. When the hypothalamus senses that the ovaries are not responding, it reacts by stimulating more and more gonadotropin to try to make the ovaries respond. Thus we find the gonadotropins markedly elevated. Occasionally the ovary can be made to respond by first suppressing the level of gonadotropins, which may restore a degree of response of the follicles. This would then be followed by administration of gonadotropins to try to evoke a normal ovarian response. If this is not effective, the difficult decision to consider donation of eggs from another woman may be suggested.

An elevated prolactin level is something to look for if conventional treatments are not working, before going on to advanced treatments.

BRAIN AND PITUITARY PROBLEMS

In patients with failure of the reproductive centers in the brain or pituitary, we find that despite adequate and properly timed signals, the hypothalamic-pituitary axis is unable to respond. This would occur, for example, in the patient who has a pituitary tumor interfering with pituitary function. Such a tumor (or simply an overactive pituitary) can secrete excess amounts of the hormone prolactin, which then suppresses the hypothalamus. Prolactin also stimulates the breasts to secrete milk, a symptom called galactorrhea. Prolactin levels can be elevated with no galactorrhea or only some minor menstrual irregularity. It is possible that small increased amounts of prolactin can prevent conception even without any measurable effect on the ovulatory process.

Sally, 37, and John, 38, went through the usual workup for infertility, including a laparoscopy. Then they switched to a local infertility clinic with a good reputation, and went into higher-level tests without finding any problem whatsoever. Despite the fact that she was ovulating normally, Sally was tried on a course of fertility drugs combined with artificial insemination. As a last resort before going into one of the high-tech procedures, her physician recommended a thorough evaluation of her hormones even though her ovulatory function appeared normal. Sure enough, her prolactin was mildly elevated, about 50% above normal levels. Since a proportion of women with elevated prolactin have a small pituitary tumor called a microadenoma, her doctor ordered a special scan to examine the pituitary gland. They found a small microadenoma of her pituitary gland. The drug bromocriptine (Parlodel) was administered to shrink the tumor and suppress the elevated levels of prolactin. Two months after starting treatment, her prolactin was normal and she became pregnant on her own without any further treatment.

The other common central defect is malfunction of the hypothalamus, the area in the base of the brain that sends out the signals that control the pituitary gland. Reduced function of the hypothalamus, resulting in reduced secretion of gonadotropin-releasing hormone, may be due to stress, anxiety, excessive exercise, crash dieting and anorexia nervosa. Gonadotropin levels may be normal or reduced and menstruation can be infrequent or absent.

FAILURE OF NORMAL INTERACTIONS

The most common problem of signal interaction is polycystic ovarian syndrome (PCO), sometimes called Stein-Leventhal syndrome. In PCO, the problem is now thought to be the result of increased insulin levels in the blood as a response to increased resistance to insulin. As a result, the adrenal gland and the ovaries produce increased male hormones. The fat tissue in the body converts these to female hormones at an increased rate. This constant increase of estrogen disturbs the functions of the pituitary, which secretes increased levels of LH. This increased LH causes the ovary, in turn, to secrete increased amounts of male hormones. Follicles develop only partially. This results in numerous small cystic follicles within the ovary, giving the syndrome its name. PCO can be suspected by a lifelong history of infrequent or absent periods, with or without increased hair growth or excess body weight.

A group of symptoms that may signal an ovulatory problem includes:

- lack of a period (amenorrhea)
- irregular periods, especially less than a 21-day or more than a 35-day cycle

- abnormal hair growth
- lack of menstrual and premenstrual symptoms
- severe acne
- breast secretions

Needless to say, it is very important to relate any of these symptoms to your physician when he or she takes your history. Given modern medicine, except for premature ovarian failure most women with anovulation can be treated successfully with conventional measures.

Male factor

With advanced techniques we can now treat almost all male problems effectively.

The other gamete (germ cell) necessary for conception is the sperm. In general, problems in the male have been thought to contribute to infertility in up to 40% of infertile couples. In the large study mentioned above, male factor accounted for 18%. Despite the significant percentage of couples in which the male factor is important, until recently the male had been relatively ignored in the workup. With the development of a subgroup of physicians interested in the study and treatment of male reproduction (andrology) in conjunction with the use of new assisted reproductive technologies, new developments in the conventional workup and treatment of the male have occurred.

The most important principle when the male factor is evaluated is that it be done with an eye toward making a specific diagnosis in order to be able to implement specific therapy. Unfortunately, there are circumstances when a specific diagnosis is not achievable. When this situation occurs it should be discussed openly and frankly and the choices for nonspecific therapy evaluated.

The conditions most frequently associated with male infertility were studied among 425 men in a male infertility clinic. The following conditions were found in this group of infertile patients:

	Percent
Varicocele (enlarged veins in the scrotum)	37.4
Low sperm count—no apparent reason	25.4
Failure of testicles	9.4
Blockage of the ducts leading from the testicles	6.1
Undescended testicles	6.1

Inadequate semen volume	4.7
Agglutination (clumping together of sperm)	3.1
Sexual problem	2.8
Semen too viscous (thick)	1.9
Could not ejaculate	1.2

Each of the other problems (in the unexplained 1.2%) occurred in less than 1% of the men. We cannot be sure that some of these conditions are the precise cause of the infertility in a particular couple. For example, there is some controversy over the importance of a varicocele in causing infertility in certain couples.

The urologist may categorize the male partner by the results of the semen analysis. He or she will find men falling into one of three categories:

- Semen analysis is normal.
- Semen analysis is abnormal.
- Not sure whether there is a significant abnormality.

NORMAL SEMEN ANALYSIS

The man with normal semen analysis is unlikely to be the sole cause of the couple's infertility. Additional tests may be necessary, because the normal semen analysis eliminates only the possibility that a drastic problem exists. More subtle problems regarding the sperm's ability to travel through cervical mucus and penetrate an egg may still be present in the face of an apparently normal semen analysis. Therefore the specialist may not end the evaluation here, but rather go on to some of the newer tests of sperm function, most of which are unrelated to any specific cause we can yet identify.

ABNORMAL SEMEN ANALYSIS

Azoospermia If there are no sperm present whatsoever, the physician must consider hormone tests to differentiate between an obstruction of the duct system, testicular failure and pituitary malfunction.

Other abnormalities The man with one or many abnormalities in the semen analysis might have one of the conditions mentioned above such as a varicocele, which is an engorgement of the veins surrounding the testicles in the scrotum. These dilated veins in the scrotum can cause impaired sperm function by mechanisms not yet completely understood. Less common causes of abnormalities in the semen may be external environmental factors. One of the most common single abnormalities we see is asthenospermia, a reduction in the motility of sperm below 40% to 50% of the sperm present. If this, for example, is combined with some clumping of the sperm, the physician might suspect the presence of sperm antibodies.

Not sure   Normal men can have significant variability in the results of their semen analysis from day to day. Most urologists will not hang their hat on one result and will want two to three analyses to compare. Even after looking at the results of multiple specimens, they may not be sure if there is an abnormality and will want to test further.

Tubal infertility

Now that we have considered the production of the two germ cells, we have to get them together. The fallopian tube is where the two gametes normally meet. Diseases that cause tubal blockage can prevent conception for mechanical reasons. These tubal problems are important because of the large numbers of patients affected, numbers that seem to be increasing. In the 1980 study cited above, tubal factors accounted for 12% of infertile couples. With the sexually transmitted disease (STD) epidemic of the last few decades, we are seeing a rise in this problem to where it is now thought to be a factor in up to 20% of couples experiencing infertility.

The "classic" STD that causes tubal damage is gonorrhea. The organism spreads through the cervix and endometrium to the fallopian tube, where it causes salpingitis (infection in the tube), often referred to as PID (pelvic inflammatory disease). If untreated or inadequately treated, PID can frequently progress to form an abscess. These processes can damage tubal function, result in partial or complete obstruction and lead to infertility or tubal pregnancy. The final stage of the pathologic process is the development of a hydrosalpinx. That's where the tube becomes a distended, fluid-filled sac that is often not amenable to successful surgical repair because even if the tube can be opened, it may not function properly.

More recently, with the advent of better culture techniques, we have learned that an organism called chlamydia is very frequently associated with the occurrence of milder degrees of salpingitis. One of the most dangerous features of chlamydia is the fact that this organism causes an insidious type of infection that is frequently unrecognized and does its damage silently. Many women with tubal damage from chlamydia cannot recall a distinct episode of tubal infection in their history. In addition to tubal obstruction, these infections can cause adhesions to form in the pelvis around the tubes and ovaries. In some cases the tubes may appear open on X-ray dye tests, but scar tissue surrounding the tubes and ovaries may prevent the egg from reaching the tube.

One of the more recent important causes of pelvic adhesions was the resurgence of the use of IUDs in the late 1960s and early 1970s. Of particular note is the story of the Dalkon Shield IUD, a device released by the A.H. Robins company with the claim that its unusual shape would prevent one of the more common problems with other IUDs, expulsion from the uterus.

To prevent it from being pushed out of the uterus, it was shaped something like a crab, with several small "claws" on its side to help retain its position in the uterus. These claws prevented its expulsion but also made it more difficult to remove. Most IUDs were attached to a string that hung down through the cervix into the vagina to facilitate removal. These were usually made of monofilament nylon similar to fishing line. Because a stronger string was needed due to its shape, the Dalkon Shield had a string made of multifilament nylon rather than the usual monofilament nylon. It is now thought that the multifilament nylon string caused the infections seen with this device. The string acted as a wick, bringing bacteria from the vagina into the upper genital tract.

A self-imposed cause of tubal factor is a previous tubal ligation. It is not unusual for a woman to feel she has completed her family and have a tubal ligation performed as a permanent means of birth control, only to have an unexpected change in her marital status resulting in the desire to have a child with another partner.

An example of how previously "hopeless" tubal damage can be overcome by assisted reproductive technology is well illustrated in the story of Cheryl and Jeff Scruggs. Cheryl, 27, and Jeff, 28, came in with a history of nine months of infertility. Their history was unremarkable, but Cheryl was anxious to the point that she was convinced that something had to be wrong. Although we usually advise a young couple to try for a year before starting any tests, Cheryl didn't want to wait that long. So a workup was started including a tubal dye X-ray test. In view of her negative history it was surprising to find that her tubes were not only blocked but were also distended with fluid. When this was confirmed by laparoscopy, it was determined that her tubes were damaged beyond repair. Because of the poor chance of success afforded by tubal surgery, Cheryl and Jeff elected immediately to try in vitro fertilization, which would bypass the need for tubal function. Their first cycle was not completed due to scheduling problems, but in their second try they had twin girls.

Cheryl and Jeff were fortunate, since we now recognize that the presence of a hydrosalpinx is associated with a 50% reduction in IVF success. We now advise laparoscopic removal or tying off of an abnormal tube, which prevents the hydrosalpinx fluid from washing back through the uterus, and restores a normal prognosis with IVF. (More about the details of these procedures appear in chapter 8 and there is more about Cheryl and Jeff in chapter 10, where we follow them through their IVF cycle.)

Endometriosis is the leading cause of infertility and is often missed.

Endometriosis

Endometriosis was the most common cause of infertility in the study cited above, possibly because it is one of the most common gynecologic disorders seen in women of reproductive age. Even before the advent of sophisticated tests and procedures to determine the causes of infertility, this condition was clinically associated with impaired fertility (subfertility).

Endometriosis is the presence of endometrium, the normal lining tissue in the uterine cavity, growing anywhere outside the uterus. It is normal-appearing tissue that belongs in the cavity of the uterus and is simply somewhere else. Most often, that somewhere else is the ovary or the lining of the pelvic cavity, but it could (and does) occur anywhere in the body. That may include the bowel, appendix or even the elbow! But it is the presence of endometriosis on the organs of the pelvis that results in infertility.

Endometriosis can either be a silent disease or cause severe symptoms. The most common symptoms are worsening menstrual cramps or pain, particularly starting before menstruation, and pain with intercourse. In some cases, there are no symptoms whatsoever except otherwise unexplained infertility. One of the most interesting aspects of this condition is that the amount of endometriosis present does not correlate with the degree of symptoms. For example, it is common to see women with no symptoms turn out to have a pelvis filled with endometriosis. It is just as likely to find a person with severe menstrual cramps and pain having only a tiny bit of endometriosis present and to have those symptoms relieved when the condition is treated.

Typically, small amounts of endometriosis look like burn marks on the affected tissue, almost as if someone had burned the tissue with the head of a match. Larger degrees of the disease will look like brown, raised areas, or when it affects the ovary a "chocolate cyst" (endometrioma) will result. This will be a variably sized fluid-filled sac replacing all or part of the ovary, and it oozes a brown, chocolate-like material when the cyst is opened. All of these manifestations occur because the endometrial tissue bleeds, just as it does in its normal location in the uterus, and the old blood in the tissues turns a dark red-brown.

Endometriosis tends to run in families, as evidenced by the fact that in one study siblings of patients with endometriosis had a 7% incidence of the disease. It is thought to develop primarily in women who have delayed childbearing. It is the second most common gynecologic disease, only surpassed by fibroids.

Various theories have been proposed to explain how the endometrial tissue gets where it's not supposed to be; the most likely is the back-up of menstrual fluid and tissue. Another possible explanation is that some cells in the body have the potential to turn (differentiate) into endometrium. What we do know is that when the endometrial tissue grows elsewhere it mimics the same hormonal pattern of the endometrium in the uterus. These endometrial implants grow as the cycle progresses and then "menstruate" at the end of the cycle. As the implants break down and bleed, you can see how they could cause pain. Since they damage the ovary, they can impair ovarian function and cause menstrual disorders. Also, in cases of severe endometriosis, the presence of large endometriomas and scarring can literally block the pickup of the eggs by the fallopian tube. But even small amounts of endometriosis can inhibit fertility.

Recent research has proposed a number of possibilities of how the disease interferes with fertility. One possible mechanism is a greater number of cells (scavenger cells) that pick up debris in the pelvic cavity. In a patient with endometriosis, the scavenger cells are more active in scavenging sperm as well as those having more cells. Since the number of sperm gathering around the egg is a balance between the number succeeding in reaching the tube and the number being removed, this increased scavenging of sperm reduces the chance of the sperm and egg meeting. Other possible mechanisms include inflammatory substances that injure the sperm or embryos or that can interfere with the development and release of the egg, or an allergic-type response to the endometrial tissue that may interfere with the normal uterine lining. Endometriosis can also be associated with ovulation disturbances, tubal dysfunction and a decrease in implantation.

Luteal phase defect (LPD)

The second half of the menstrual cycle following ovulation, the luteal phase, is critical to the success of the process. The egg can meet the sperm, fertilization can take place and the resulting embryo can be transported down the fallopian tube and into the uterus. But if the endometrium is not prepared to receive the embryo for implantation, the whole process will be aborted.

Following ovulation, progesterone must be secreted in adequate amounts and the endometrium must be capable of responding. If the hormones are not correct, the luteal phase could be shorter than necessary, so that the menstrual period begins shortly after the embryo is ready to implant. Another problem occurs when the amount of progesterone is inadequate to produce an orderly maturation of the endometrium coordinated with the arrival of the embryo. In turn, the embryo must implant adequately to secrete pregnancy hormone (human chorionic gonadotropin or hCG), which will "rescue" the corpus luteum from its normal demise so that it continues to produce estrogen and progesterone, which in turn support the pregnancy.

Although the number of patients with this problem is not large, it is impressive that treatment often works and is generally neither risky nor expensive. In these patients we also look for some other subtle hormone problem, such as an elevated prolactin level.

Cervix or mucus problem

Another less common but treatable cause of infertility is a problem with the functioning of the cervix. It may involve blockage of the cervical canal or deficiencies in the production of the all-important cervical mucus necessary to transport the sperm across the cervix, or both. In addition, the mucus has a function in preparing the sperm for fertilization (capacitation). Infections of the cervix, congenital abnormalities or the presence of sperm antibodies are all factors that can reduce the ability of the mucus to transport the sperm. Another less frequent cause of the cervical factor is previous surgery on the cervix, such as a cone biopsy done to evaluate an abnormal Pap smear. This surgery can result in scarring that can reduce the production of cervical mucus and/or cause a stricture (stenosis) of the canal. Finally, women who were exposed to DES (see discussion under Uterine factor, below) in utero and develop infertility are more likely to have poor cervical mucus.

To fully assess the cervical factor, it is helpful to evaluate the interaction between the mucus and the sperm. The couple is therefore asked to have intercourse the night before or on the morning of the test. (If having to perform on schedule makes you unable to complete this part, that's a normal reaction; simply tell your doctor. He or she can still evaluate the mucus.) If you do have intercourse, male fertility factors can influence the results. (For example, impotence, inability to ejaculate normally and certain anatomical abnormalities of the penis, such as having a urethral opening on the shaft instead of at the tip (hypospadius), may give a bad result. Other male factors previously discussed can also result in a poor outcome on the mucus test.) Most often, however, deficiencies in the amount and viscosity of cervical mucus, as well as the presence of infection or antibodies in the mucus, account for problems related to the cervix.

The timing of the test for cervical mucus problems is crucial

One of the most common causes of an abnormal mucus test is simply poor timing. Timing this test is not easy, since women are generally less regular than they realize. In order to assure that the test is timed to coincide with peak mucus quality, we now recommend the use of simple and accurate self-tests for urinary LH (Ovuquick).

Uterine factor

The uterine factor is relatively rare as a cause of infertility, but in some cases it is treatable. For example, fibroids can be treated by surgery. These are exceedingly common benign tumors of the uterine muscle. In fact, it is estimated that by age 35 about one-third of women will have clinically detectable fibroids. For the vast majority of women, these fibroids have no effect on their ability to become pregnant or carry a pregnancy to term. But fibroids that are large or classified as submucous can cause problems as they push into and distort the uterine cavity. They can interfere with sperm transport and with the blood supply of the endometrium, and can prevent implantation, as well as put pressure on an expanding pregnancy. It is thought that they may also act as a foreign body in the endometrium, which can prevent pregnancy in ways we do not fully understand. In this regard they may act in the same manner as an IUD.

But we must be careful not to accept fibroids as the only cause of infertility until all other causes have been eliminated. Distortions of the uterine cavity have been associated more with early pregnancy loss and late miscarriage than with infertility.

The most severe uterine problems can now be overcome through the use of a surrogate to carry the pregnancy.

The second treatable uterine condition that is occurring more frequently is the development of adhesions in the endometrial cavity. These are usually the result of previous surgery, specifically a D&C (dilation and curettage) related to the termination of a pregnancy. Adhesions can occur if termination of the pregnancy was induced by therapeutic abortion, or they can arise spontaneously after a D&C following a natural miscarriage. It can also happen after a D&C unrelated to pregnancy. Suspicion of this condition would arise if a menstrual period did not occur after such an operation, or if the menstrual periods became scanty following a D&C. At times, enough adhesions can exist to prevent pregnancy but allow normal menstruation. These adhesions can be treated surgically by operating through a telescopic device (hysteroscope) placed into the uterus through the cervix.

Certain malformations of the uterus, such as the presence of a septum dividing the endometrium, could be included in this category and can also be removed through the hysteroscope. These malformations are more likely to result in recurrent pregnancy loss than in infertility.

Infections are the third treatable uterine condition that can lead to infertility. But these are not the usual infections we see that lead to tubal scarring. They include less common organisms such as ureaplasma and even tuberculosis, and can cause a long-standing (chronic) infection in the endometrium. Ureaplasma infections are treatable with common antibiotics. Tuberculosis as a cause of infertility, rare in the United States except in immigrant populations, is more common in developing countries. Medical treatment of the infection will not resolve the problem and the tubal scarring caused by the infection is not correctable by surgery, leaving IVF as the only option.

The one uterine factor that, unfortunately, is not treatable is prenatal exposure to diethylstilbestrol (DES). DES is a synthetic estrogenic hormone but it has a different chemical structure from estrogen. It was a popular practice among obstetricians over 30 years ago to give large doses of DES to women who were threatening to miscarry or who had a history of previous miscarriage, in the belief that the extra estrogen would help the woman retain the pregnancy.

However, it became clear by the early 1970s that the female offspring of women who took DES in pregnancy were experiencing certain specific problems. The first problem to be recognized was a dramatic increase in a rare type of vaginal cancer in a group of young women. As the story unfolded, it was noted that these offspring also had specific changes in their vagina, cervix, uterus and fallopian tubes. The changes in the uterus and tubes are the ones most pertinent to fertility and pregnancy loss. These uteri often have a narrowed, irregular, T-shaped cavity that does not accommodate a pregnancy well and can lead to miscarriage or premature labor. The tubes may also be malformed. Except for documented obstruction of the tubes, it is not known if such DES changes are a direct cause of infertility, except that tubal pregnancy is more common. As mentioned, there is no specific treatment for these DES changes, so patients with this problem need to have all the other aspects of the fertility process studied and treated. They can frequently achieve successful pregnancies, but should be made aware of the problems they may experience in carrying a pregnancy. Because of this, we tend to be more conservative in progressing to treatments that increase the risk of a multiple pregnancy.

As we learn more about the human reproductive system, the percentage of patients in the "unexplained" category will decrease.

Unexplained infertility

As our knowledge of the fertility process improves, the number of couples in this category decreases. Currently about 5% of couples fall into this category, given our present level of knowledge. These are the couples who have been completely worked up medically and in whom all tests are normal.

Perhaps as we continue to increase our knowledge, unexplained infertility will finally disappear. For example, many women whose infertility has been classified as unexplained have an increased population of scavenger cells in the abdomen near the tubes and ovaries, presumably resulting in fewer sperm available to fertilize the egg. Currently the only way we can clinically recognize this factor in a woman with unexplained infertility is if she conceives readily after a tubal X-ray using an oil-based dye that inhibits those scavenger cells.

Psychological and emotional factors

The significance of an emotional factor is controversial. We have all heard of the couple who achieved a pregnancy after adopting a baby or, like the Meldrums, after going away on a long vacation. This is the common advice given infertility patients: "Just relax! When the pressure is off, it'll work." Often it is given by well-meaning friends and relatives. Sometimes it may be given by health care professionals before a full evaluation has been performed. And, at times it is given following a complete evaluation that has shown no apparent cause of the problem. But does the desire to become pregnant along with the seeming inability to achieve this goal result in sufficient emotional and psychological upheaval to prevent pregnancy?

The answer is a definite maybe. We all know that having difficulty in conceiving a baby and going through the process of evaluation and treatment are tremendous stresses for each individual and for the couple together. They have to confront feelings of failure, inadequacy, guilt and loss of self-esteem that may lead to marital and family conflict. Some of the evaluations and treatment may even make matters worse. The couple's sex life may be strained by the demands of "sex by the calendar." The man, who may not have been too pleased about having to go through it all just to have a baby, may become fed up with the necessity of coming to the doctor's office, being handed a plastic cup and being told to perform. He may even tire of wearing boxer shorts to cool his testicles. And so, by the time the couple is many months or even years into the process, infertility becomes an obsession that may truly impair their lives and their relationship.

But can that stress affect and prolong the infertility? There is only anecdotal evidence that it can. For some couples, abandonment of the attempt to become pregnant has quickly resulted in a successful pregnancy. Most reproductive experts know of such cases. But there is no scientifically valid data to support this specific occurrence. A program such as the Mind-Body Connection, which uses relaxation techniques, stress reduction and cognitive realignment to achieve a statistically significant improvement in fertility treatments, lends credibility to this observation. On the contrary, the positive effect of adoption was refuted in a 14-year study at Stanford. They followed 895 infertile couples and found that the ultimate pregnancy rate was not statistically different between couples who eventually adopted and those who didn't.

A TYPICAL PATIENT

A profile of a typical patient struggling to get pregnant with multiple factors (endometriosis, luteal phase defect, cervical factor and perhaps psychological factors) is exemplified by Penny. She and Roger were married for seven years before she first tried to become pregnant at age 36. Tests by a doctor in another city showed evidence of endometriosis with fairly large cysts on the ovaries (endometriomas). An operation removed her left tube and ovary, which were beyond repair, and all but a sliver of her right ovary. She then moved into our area and wanted to continue her quest. This was before assisted reproductive techniques were readily available. So her treatment was geared toward monitoring her cycles for ovulation, treating her luteal phase defect with fertility drugs, promoting better cervical mucus with small doses of estrogen and checking by means of laparoscopy to be sure her endometriosis had not returned. But by age 41 she felt that she had had enough of temperature charts, fertility drugs and sex-by-the-calendar, and she decided to stop trying. Her son, Brett, was born just short of her 42nd birthday.

Which factor was actually preventing her from becoming pregnant? Age? Endometriosis? Cervical factor? Luteal phase defect? Psychological pressures? Did her giving up have anything to do with her conceiving? We will never know. Therefore our advice is not to abandon testing and treatment with the hope that adoption or other change in lifestyle will work. Pursue both at the same time and you will have your maximum chance of success.

FINDING THE PROBLEM

Now that you understand the major causes for a couple not being able to achieve a pregnancy within a reasonable period of time, we will move on to the process for finding the problem in an individual couple: "So, first we have to do some tests."

CHAPTER 6

First, We Have To Do Some Tests

Patient: *We have been trying to have a baby for a year and nothing has happened.*

Doctor: *First, we have to do some tests.*

What a scary statement. No matter what the medical problem, the prospect of having to undergo tests that could be painful, expensive and possibly dangerous strikes fear into the hearts of the bravest among us. The fear surrounding the tests themselves does not even take into account the dread of what those tests might reveal.

"Maybe I can never have a baby."

"Perhaps the test will show that it's my fault and my husband/wife will resent me…or even leave me, and I'll be all alone."

"If they find that I have no sperm, maybe I'm not really a man."

All too often the need for testing in this very sensitive area can bring out underlying marital and psychological problems. For example, Stephanie, 34, came into the office with the concern that she and David, 36, had been trying to have a baby on and off for about two years. She appeared quite anxious about this problem. Her medical and reproductive history did not reveal an obvious cause for their difficulty. The physical examination was equally unrevealing. Only when the process got to the point of outlining which tests would be suggested for the initial part of the workup did we appear to hit upon the source of her anxiety.

When we mentioned the need of a semen specimen from David, she tearfully recounted that David did not really want a child. He agreed to have a child if she wanted to, but now that they were having trouble, he would not cooperate in any way with the infertility workup. He told her that it was probably her problem, anyway. Further discussion led to the discovery of significant marital problems. Shortly after they were referred to a psychologist for marital counseling, they separated. According to the psychologist, their difficulty surrounding the decision to have a family was merely an indication of deeper troubles in the marriage.

Today their friends believe that their breakup was due to the stress caused by the infertility, when in fact the marriage was on shaky ground before the infertility problem surfaced. Happily for her, Stephanie remarried and had no difficulty conceiving. David remarried, to a woman who shared his feelings about not having a family.

We feel that one can learn a lot about a couple by watching their interaction as various tests and procedures are suggested. Excuses and delays by either party or the couple together may indicate a less than enthusiastic commitment to starting or expanding a family.

BEFORE THE TESTS

Actually, tests are not the first step the doctor takes. The first step should be a thorough medical history of the couple as well as an in-depth review of their reproductive history. If you go to see a doctor who, after hearing that you have difficulty getting pregnant, immediately suggests a laparoscopy to see if your tubes are open, this is not the doctor for you. And, even worse, if he or she immediately recommends one of the assisted reproductive technology (ART) procedures at this point, head for the exit!

Most doctors have their own order for scheduling tests. The common thread through all their regimens will be that the safer, simpler, less invasive and less expensive tests should be done first. This reserves the more invasive, expensive and risky tests for later. And later may never come. You may get pregnant before later arrives. The safest, simplest and least expensive part of the evaluation will be the history—which is where all doctors should start.

PREPARING FOR THE FIRST VISIT

In the next section we will give you some of the topics about which you will be asked, so that you can search out the answers you may not know off the top of your head. Also, if this is not your first visit to a doctor for this problem, bring with you any documentation you have regarding previous tests and procedures. If your previous treatment has been extensive, a written chronology of your treatments may be helpful along with the medical records. Actual X-ray films are better than descriptive reports. If an operation has been done, bring a copy of the operative report. Laboratory values for hormone tests are infinitely better than "My thyroid was normal, I think." Seeing semen analysis results will help the doctor determine if it was done properly and thoroughly. If, for example, you had a laparoscopy with video or photographs, ask your previous doctor to loan you the video and photos or copy them for you. A picture is worth...well, you get the point!

TOPICS AND QUESTIONS

Either the doctor or nurse-practitioner-coordinator may ask the questions. In addition to the usual medical and surgical history from both of you, they will want to know about routine medications you take and any allergies you may have. Now, medications will include drugs, and drugs include anything you put into any part of your body that cannot be classified as food. It is very important to reveal any recreational drug use, since some of these compounds can have an effect on your reproductive system. The doctor may not ask about these drugs in so many words, but realize that it may be important, so offer the information even if not specifically asked. This also goes for significant medication you may have taken in the past. This is a good question to ask your mother before the visit, since you might not have been told what you were given as a child. These medications could also include chemotherapy for cancer, or DES or other drugs given to your mother while you were in utero, either of which could have significant implications for your fertility.

For example, Lorraine, 24, and Steve, 32, were concerned about their ability to have a child because Steve had received chemotherapy for an early cancer in a testicle several years before. When tests confirmed that he was indeed sterile, they decided to try artificial insemination with a donor's sperm. They carefully selected a donor who matched Steve's physical and educational characteristics from a list supplied by the regional sperm bank. The first insemination resulted in a pregnancy and the birth of a healthy boy about six weeks before term. Their story is discussed in more detail in chapter 12.

Occupational history may be very important, too; some occupations involve contact with environmental factors that can affect reproduction. An office worker is less likely to run into this type of problem than is an engineer at a toxic waste dump. But if you do come into contact with noxious chemicals in your job, find out what they are before the appointment and present the physician with a list of them so he or she can check them out for you.

It is a good idea to have information written down so you don't forget to tell the doctor any important facts.

Social habits may provide some clues to the cause of a couple's fertility problem. For example, unusual amounts of exercise can have a profound effect on the female reproductive system to the point that marathon-level runners frequently may not even menstruate. Other runners and aerobic exercisers of lesser magnitude may experience less dramatic, but potent, effects on their fertility. In men, practices such as cycling, using spas or wearing tight-fitting underwear that can lead to heating of the testicles are thought by some to diminish fertility.

Unfortunately, smoking is a very common social habit that can not only significantly delay fertility in female smokers, but also reduce the overall fertility rate by 30%. A study reported from the University of North Carolina showed that for men, drinking four or more cups of coffee and smoking more than a pack of cigarettes a day had a deleterious effect on sperm motility and increased the percentage of dead sperm.

Previous reproductive history for both individuals is important. This includes not only previous pregnancies including those with other partners, but also prior contraceptive history. For example, the use of an IUD may be a clue to unrecognized tubal problems. The history can sometimes get a little sticky since there may be something that one of the parties does not want revealed to the other—a child with another partner or, more often, an abortion. Whereas we usually encourage candor with one's partner, you can divulge anything in confidence to the doctor, even if you do not feel able to share it with your spouse. The Health Insurance Portability and Accountability Act of 1996 (HIPAA) regulations, which went into effect in April 2003, specifically prohibit a physician from sharing one's medical information even with a spouse without specific written authorization. If you are worried that your spouse may see copies of the chart, ask the doctor not to write it in the record.

For the female, there will be specific questions relating to menstrual cycle. These will include age of onset, interval between periods, length of periods and associated menstrual symptoms such as cramps and premenstrual symptoms. Other questions relating to the pelvic organs may include whether she has the common physical signs of ovulation, or pain with intercourse.

The sexual history of the couple will be explored. This may include inquiries regarding frequency and position of intercourse, the use of artificial lubricants and douching after intercourse. Many physicians have had the experience of solving an infertility problem at this point merely by teaching the couple proper timing or eliminating the use of a sperm-toxic lubricant or douche.

THE PHYSICAL EXAMINATION

Once the history has been obtained, the next safest and most cost-effective part of the workup is the physical examination. At this time, it is the woman who gets examined first. In fact, most of the time it is the female partner who comes in for the initial visits. We encourage the male partner to come in for the first visit, help provide the history and be there to support his wife through these tests and procedures.

The physical exam is not unlike the complete physical you may get every year from your family doctor, internist or gynecologist. There will be more emphasis on the pelvic examination, of course. The physician will be looking for signs of infection in the cervix that might give a clue to infection in the tubes, evidence of endometriosis or any of the various problems discussed in chapter 5.

THE TESTS

At this time, we would expect that the doctor would sit down with you in the consultation room and explain the series of tests. We like to think of these tests as being done in phases. Again, the tests with the least risk and cost will usually come first; if necessary, the more expensive and invasive tests will be done later. Since not all infertility specialists recommend the tests in exactly the same order, you can expect some variation. Just keep in mind that safer, simpler, less expensive should come first.

We will rate them against each other as to risk, pain and cost from none to low, medium and high. It is not possible for us to give specific and accurate estimates of costs for all these tests and procedures because there is tremendous regional variation; it would be best for you to determine average costs of key procedures when you make your initial search for a provider.

The principle is to do the safer, simpler and less expensive tests first.

In general, for patients without any significant history, our testing would be phased as follows:

PHASE I
Basal body temperature chart or ovulation detection kit
Semen analysis

PHASE 2
Postcoital test
Endometrial biopsy (not routinely done for infertility but may be
    done if recurrent early pregnancy loss is a problem)
Serum progesterone
Tubal dye test (hysterosalpingogram)

PHASE 3
Laparoscopy
Other tests

Phase 1

BASAL BODY TEMPERATURE CHART (BBT)
Most of the fertility tests will be timed to your menstrual cycle; in order to do this we have to monitor your cycle. One of the simplest ways is to utilize

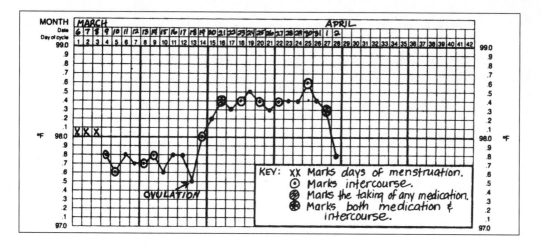

Figure 4   Basal Body Temperature Chart

the basal body temperature chart (BBT) (Figure 4). The basal temperature, the lowest temperature of the day, is fairly constant. Once you get up and engage in any activity, there will be a significant and variable increase in your body temperature. The BBT takes advantage of the principle that after ovulation the secretion of progesterone causes a half- to one-degree rise in your temperature, most evident in your basal temperature. Thus the BBT can estimate if and when you are ovulating and the length of each phase of the cycle. All you need is a good-quality thermometer that you can read to a tenth of a degree (for example, 98.7°F). You can use a digital-readout thermometer if that is easier for you, but you do not need to invest in a special "basal thermometer."

You can make up a chart starting with the first day of your period as Day 1. You then take your temperature each morning, as soon as you wake up, *before* you get out of bed, when it reflects a true basal reading. Have the thermometer at the bedside, take your temperature immediately upon awaking and record it on the chart in the column next to the appropriate date. If you can't wait to empty your bladder, keep the thermometer in a Styrofoam cup in the bathroom and urinate into the cup. The temperature of the urine will be the same as your body temperature.

After you have done this for one or two months, the doctor can review the chart and probably tell if and when you ovulated, whether you had intercourse at the correct time of the cycle to maximize your chance of getting pregnant and whether there was adequate time following ovulation for an embryo to implant in the endometrium before your period.

Some physicians do not use the BBT at all since they feel that the daily gathering and recording of this information may increase stress and that the information can be obtained in other ways. Others use it on a limited basis, for just a few months, and then discontinue its use once ovulation has been established and the patient has learned about the timing of her menstrual cycle. A further alternative is to monitor the LH surge with an ovulation detection kit, which gives similar information as to timing, the consistency of ovulation and the length of the luteal phase. (RISK—NONE; PAIN—NONE; COST—NONE)

SEMEN ANALYSIS

The semen analysis is much more than a simple "count." Make sure the lab does a full evaluation of all the parameters. A lab specializing in reproductive testing is best.

Just as we need to learn that the woman is producing eggs, it is equally important to find out if the man is producing adequate sperm to achieve a pregnancy. To determine the man's status, a complete semen analysis will be obtained. If the doctor does not have his own reproductive laboratory, the male partner will usually be referred to a specific laboratory to have this done. At the lab or at home, he will masturbate a specimen into a special collection cup. It is best to have adequate sexual arousal before and during collection, otherwise a poor specimen could merely be an artifact of the collection procedure. One study showed that many male factors disappeared when the specimen was collected in a special sheath during intercourse. Another study showed similar improvements using sexually explicit videos. The laboratory should provide reading materials or videos and an unhurried atmosphere. At home the wife may help with the collection.

It is advisable to abstain from ejaculation for two to three days before the test in order to get his best specimen. This is because with a shorter interval the sperm density may be lower. But more importantly, it will enable us to standardize the collection interval in order to compare results more accurately. With a longer period of abstinence the sperm may have lower motility. We usually recommend he give the specimen around the time of his wife's menstrual period since it is unlikely that she would get pregnant at that time.

We find that up to 40% of couples with an infertility problem have some male factor contributing to the couple's infertility. It does not make sense for the wife to go through tests that may involve some risk, discomfort and expense if we don't at least find out if her partner's semen is adequate. In fact, physicians usually obtain several samples since health and environmental factors such as fatigue, smoking, stress and use of caffeine or drugs can affect the results. Variation is expected, and only with repeated specimens is a full evaluation obtained.

A semen analysis is not just a sperm count (quantity) but also an assessment of sperm quality. In addition to the number of sperm present in a certain volume (count), we need to know the total amount of the semen (volume), how viscous or liquid it is (liquefaction), the number of sperm moving at various rates at different times (motility) and the shape of the sperm (morphology). (RISK—NONE; PAIN—NONE; COST—LOW)

The results of the semen analysis will be placed into one of three categories:

The postcoital test is completely painless.

1. *Normal.* This result most frequently represents reproductively normal men, but a small group of men whose semen appears reproductively normal have abnormalities of sperm function detectable only with more sophisticated testing.
2. *No sperm found (azoospermia).* This result should not only be confirmed with three specimens but also should be checked by two specimens that have been centrifuged, since azoospermia can be confused with a specimen with only a few sperm (marked oligospermia) if they have not been carefully evaluated.
3. *Abnormal, but with sperm present.* These men will have to be evaluated, as we discuss later in this chapter.

Phase 2
(about 1 month later)

POSTCOITAL TEST (PCT)

We now move on to slightly more sophisticated tests. The postcoital test involves the examination of cervical mucus under the microscope for the presence of moving sperm after the couple has had intercourse just before or at the time of ovulation. The timing of this test is most crucial to its accurate determination of the quality of the sperm-mucus interaction.

Since proper timing is so vital, in addition to the BBT we often have the patient use a urine test to determine the LH surge as the means for assuring precise scheduling of this test. Otherwise repeated visits may be necessary, since often a poor test is simply due to poor timing. The LH surge will occur the day before ovulation, when the cervical mucus should be most favorable for sperm transit.

There are a number of test kits available both from doctors' offices and in drug stores. Research has shown Ovuquick to be the most accurate. The most important instruction regarding this test is that the urine be tested in the afternoon or early evening. This is because the surge most often begins in the early morning; if you do the test too early you might not pick up the surge until the next day because it takes time for the hormone to build up in the urine. After adding three drops of urine to a Test Cassette, you match a test line, resulting from the concentration of LH, to a reference line. When the test line is darker than the reference line the test is considered positive and indicates that the surge took place that day and that ovulation should take place the next day.

The endometrial biopsy is now less painful than it used to be because of the development of smaller plastic instruments.

The couple would generally have intercourse late in the evening of or in the morning following the detection of the surge and then the woman will come into the office for an examination of the cervical mucus for the presence of sperm. This test can be helpful because it shows whether there is enough mucus, the quality of the mucus and if her spouse's sperm can get into and survive in the cervical mucus. Some experts have questioned the accuracy and therefore the usefulness of this test, but since it is simple and inexpensive, we feel it is worthwhile.

Many couples ask if they should have intercourse any special way in order to have a better result on their PCT. The answer is no, because we want to be able to tell whether there are enough motile sperm in the cervical mucus based on their usual coital technique. (RISK—NONE; PAIN—NONE; COST—LOW)

ENDOMETRIAL BIOPSY

Another test which may be obtained in this phase, especially if one has experienced recurrent early pregnancy loss, is the endometrial biopsy. This test can tell if a woman is ovulating, the level of hormones in the second half of the cycle and the response of the lining of the uterus to these hormones as it prepares to accept an embryo for implantation. A normal result indicates that the whole system is functioning properly from the hormonal point of view.

FIRST, WE HAVE TO DO SOME TESTS

The test is usually done 12 days after the surge is detected. (If the menstrual period occurs before the 12th day, the cycle is too short and a problem exists.) The patient is positioned as for a pelvic examination. A thin plastic tube is placed into the uterus and suction is applied to draw in a small amount of endometrial tissue. The main concern with this test is that if the patient is pregnant at the time, the pregnancy could theoretically be interrupted if the biopsy disturbed the implanting pregnancy tissue. Fortunately, this almost never occurs and may be avoided by obtaining a quantitative test for pregnancy hormone the day before the scheduled biopsy. But even if one were pregnant it is reassuring to know that the rate of miscarriages in cycles in which an endometrial biopsy was done is no greater than the average miscarriage rate.

The biopsy sometimes results in cramping, but we now use a smaller and more flexible instrument, which reduces the discomfort. Some physicians routinely use premedication or inject a local anesthetic beside the cervix. Prophylactic antibiotics may be used to prevent infection. Since there can be some variation in any woman's cycle, this test may have to be done more than once to insure consistency, especially if the result is not perfectly normal.

Some specialists reserve this test for couples with unexplained infertility; others for those experiencing recurrent early pregnancy loss. Also, because of controversy over its accuracy and the effectiveness of treatment for luteal phase defect, many do not recommend it. (RISK—LOW; PAIN—LOW TO MODERATE; COST—LOW TO MODERATE)

The HSG can be uncomfortable, so ask for a mild sedative and take an ibuprofen-type pain reliever an hour before the test.

SERUM PROGESTERONE

Some doctors obtain a blood level of the hormone progesterone instead of the biopsy. It is easier than the biopsy since it only requires obtaining a sample of blood, but yields much less information. (RISK—NONE; PAIN—NONE; COST—LOW)

TUBAL DYE TEST (HYSTEROSALPINGOGRAM OR HSG)

We usually obtain a tubal dye test (hysterosalpingogram) just after a menstrual period is over. You will generally be referred to a radiologist since this test involves X-rays, although some gynecologists do their own HSGs in conjunction with an X-ray department in a hospital.

This test involves a pelvic examination similar to a Pap smear. But this time a small instrument is placed through the cervix into the lower part of the uterus and some dye is injected. The radiologist will follow the dye with a fluoroscope and take pictures as he or she sees the dye go through and out the end of the tubes. This will allow visualization of the contours of the endometrial cavity to determine if there might be an abnormally shaped uterus, polyps or fibroids. The radiologist can see not only if the tubes are open and look healthy but also if the pattern of the spill indicates there may be adhesions in the pelvis. Another potential benefit is that if your tubes are open, the doctor can inject a small amount of a special oil-based dye. According to a UCLA study, the oil-based dye may help you get pregnant during the six months following the test by inhibiting the ability of scavenger cells in the pelvis to engulf sperm.

With video documentation and the ability to do surgery through the scope, many physicians now refer to laparoscopy as pelviscopy.

Cramping is fairly common with the injection of the dye, but you can be premedicated with a mild tranquilizer and given a prophylactic dose of a pain medication to help prevent or minimize the pain. If you are particularly concerned, you can also simply take two ibuprofen tablets (Advil, Motrin) one hour before the procedure. Prior to having this test some physicians order a sedimentation rate blood test to look for evidence of a previous pelvic infection, indicating the possible need for antibiotic treatment before evaluating the tubes. It is our routine to recommend the antibiotic doxycycline as a prophylactic so that even rare infections in women with normal tubes will usually be prevented. (RISK—LOW; PAIN—MODERATE; COST—LOW TO MODERATE)

Phase 3
(4 to 6 months later)

LAPAROSCOPY

This phase consists of a thorough look at the woman's reproductive organs by means of an operative procedure called laparoscopy. Before going on to this procedure, we usually wait four to six months after the HSG to allow for its therapeutic effect by reducing the activity of pelvic scavenger cells in patients with unexplained infertility and endometriosis.

The woman is usually admitted to an outpatient surgical center or the outpatient surgery department of a hospital. The procedure is usually done under general anesthesia but can also be performed with a spinal, epidural or even local anesthetic. A small incision is made in the navel and a telescopic device is placed through this incision to look at all the internal reproductive organs. A small cut is made in the pubic hairline to insert another instrument to move the organs around so all aspects can be visualized. A dilute solution of dye will be flushed through the fallopian tubes by means of a small tube placed into the uterus through the cervix. This way the doctor can see not only if dye comes through the tubes but also that there is no scar tissue around the ovaries and tubes. With the anesthetic there is no pain felt during the operation, but there may be some minor discomfort afterward. Carbon dioxide gas is used to expand the abdomen to enable visualization of the organs. Although as much CO_2 as possible is removed, a small amount may remain and for a few days cause a bloated feeling and shoulder pain from irritation of the diaphragm by retained gas.

Although the HSG evaluates the inside of the tubes, there are other conditions that may be preventing pregnancy, such as adhesions or endometriosis, conditions which we have no way of finding except by looking directly in the pelvis. The tubes can be open and yet adhesions around the ovary can block the egg from getting to the tube. Also, if adhesions or endometriosis are found at laparoscopy, there is a good chance that they can be corrected through laparoscopic surgery at the same time. As in any operation, there are rare surgical risks, such as bleeding or injury to bowel or bladder as the instruments are inserted and the organs manipulated. But the risk is small and the recovery period usually only a few days. It is often recommended that the laparoscopy be performed before going on to even more sophisticated tests or treatments.

Some doctors now combine the laparoscopy with hysteroscopy. That is, at the same time they insert a telescope into the uterus through the cervix to make sure there are no congenital abnormalities, polyps, fibroids pushing on the cavity or scarring. There is controversy over whether this adds any information to a normal HSG.

Laparoscopy is one of the most common operations performed by gynecologists. Many insurance plans will cover the procedure even if it is done to evaluate infertility. But be careful; some insurance policies specifically exclude procedures done to evaluate or treat infertility. If an insurance policy does exclude infertility but some other condition such as endometriosis or pelvic adhesions is discovered, the insurance may cover the procedure on that basis. Nowadays many plans require precertification, or even a second opinion, and may even provide higher benefits in a particular hospital or surgical center. We recommend that patients contact their insurance company before having the operation to make sure they are eligible for the best benefits. (RISK—MODERATE; PAIN—MODERATE: COST—HIGH)

"WE FOUND A PROBLEM"

There are a number of areas in which problems may be found during the workup. The most common conditions encountered include:

Finding a problem that is easy to resolve often leads to a quick solution.

- problems with ovulation
- problems with the semen
- fallopian tube obstruction
- pelvic adhesions
- endometriosis

Ovulation defect

About 10% of patients demonstrate some defect in the ovulatory cycle. This could range from a history of lack of or infrequent menstrual periods, irregular cycles, evidence of lack of ovulation or short luteal phase on the temperature chart, or suggestion of a luteal phase defect on the endometrial biopsy.

For these patients the physician will probably initiate a series of blood tests to determine the source of the problem. These may include:

- Serum FSH
- Serum LH
- Prolactin
- Testosterone
- DHEA-sulphate

Specific combinations of results from these tests can indicate the probable cause of the ovulatory problem and can help suggest therapy tailored to overcome the problem at its root. It is seldom necessary to do all of these tests. Depending on the clinical setting, usually one or two will suffice. (RISK——NONE; PAIN——NONE; COST——LOW TO MODERATE)

Semen problems (male factor)

Whether the semen analysis is normal or abnormal in any or several of its parameters, it needs to be repeated several times to determine if the results are consistent, realizing that it is normal for the semen analysis to show some variability. If the abnormality does show up repeatedly, referral to a urologist or an andrologist (a physician specializing in male reproductive problems) will be a likely next step.

The specialist in male infertility will begin, as for the female, by taking a history—including a sexual and reproductive as well as a general medical history. Of particular interest will be:

Do not withhold information regarding recreational drugs and especially steroid use from the doctor; it is very important information.

REPRODUCTIVE
- previous pregnancies fathered
- history of undescended testicles
- operations performed on the testicles
- genital trauma
- mumps after puberty
- hernia operations
- bladder surgery
- delayed puberty treated with hormones

MEDICAL
- diabetes mellitus
- urinary tract infections
- environmental exposures to chemicals, radiation or heat, including high fevers within three months of semen collections
- current and past drug use, including chemotherapeutic agents, recreational drugs, anabolic steroids and all prescribed drugs

SEXUAL
- venereal disease
- other infection
- prostate gland infection

- trauma to or infection of the scrotum
- sexual dysfunction such as impotence
- exposure to diethylstilbestrol (DES) as a fetus

In addition, special questions that help to assess any hormone abnormality focus on:

- visual problems, particularly blind spots
- change in frequency of shaving
- abnormal sexual hair pattern
- whether a normal sense of smell is present
- change in physical strength

Again, as with the female partner, the next step will be the physical examination, with special attention to signs of a hormone problem or genital abnormality. The examination will focus specifically on:

- physical proportions
- male hair distribution
- presence of abnormal amounts of breast tissue
- abnormalities of epididymis, vas deferens or prostate
- size and consistency of testicles
- signs of enlarged veins in the scrotum (varicocele)
  (RISK—NONE; PAIN—NONE; COST—LOW TO MODERATE)

The remainder of the tests to be done depend upon which parameters of the semen analysis are abnormal. Absence (azoospermia) or almost total lack of sperm (marked oligospermia) can result from obstruction of the ductal system in the testicle or a significant chromosomal, developmental or hormonal problem. If one or several parameters—count, motility and/or morphology—are abnormal, a less serious hormone problem, environmental cause or stress would be suspected.

Hormone tests similar to those done in the female partner would be indicated in the case of azoospermia. Since azoospermia may occur because of lack of pituitary stimulation, tests may include blood tests for levels of

FSH, LH, testosterone or occasionally prolactin. Again, as in the female partner, the combination of results will give the doctor a clue to the cause of the abnormality. For example, if a man has an elevated FSH and LH and a low level of testosterone his problem may be failure of the testicles. (RISK—NONE; PAIN—NONE; COST—LOW TO MODERATE)

With azoospermia a biopsy of the testicle may be recommended. The biopsy is an outpatient surgical procedure with minimal recuperation required. (RISK—LOW; PAIN—LOW; COST—LOW TO MODERATE) Unfortunately, if the biopsy confirms that no sperm are being produced, no treatment may be possible and the couple may have to consider either donor insemination or adoption. The exception here is that in some circumstances more extensive biopsies may find enough sperm to perform intracytoplasmic sperm injection (ICSI). Azoospermia may arise because of chromosomal problems, absence of sperm-producing cells, trauma, mumps after puberty or exposure to toxic agents.

In men with no sperm or very low counts, DNA or chromosomal damage should be suspected. In 10% to 15% of men with counts below 5 million, there may be a defect (DNA deletion) in their Y chromosome. In azoospermic men, there are certain regions of the Y chromosome (A2Fb region) where, if there is a deletion, sperm will not be found on testicular biopsy. If conception occurs in the men with low counts, there is a 100% transmission of this deletion to male offspring.

If adequate sperm are present on biopsy and hormone levels are normal, the problem is likely due to a congenital ductal abnormality or acquired obstruction of the duct system, and a scrotal surgical exploration may be necessary to find the location. Although this is done on an outpatient basis it is a longer procedure, depending upon what surgical procedures might be necessary to correct the obstruction, and more lengthy recuperation may be necessary. (RISK—MODERATE; PAIN—MODERATE; COST—MODERATE TO HIGH)

Obstruction can occur at any level beginning just within the testicle and progressing through the epididymis, vas deferens and ejaculatory duct. Some men have a congenital absence of the duct system or it can develop as the result of injury, infection or as the consequence of surgery. At times, the tubular system is present but functioning abnormally. This can occur

Problems with sperm usually have nothing to do with masculinity or virility.

with spinal cord or other neurological injuries or conditions that affect the ability of the bladder neck to close at the time of ejaculation. If the bladder neck fails to close, the ejaculate that enters the urethra flows back into the bladder (retrograde ejaculation) and leaves the bladder at the time of the next urination. This occurs most commonly in diabetes and following bladder-neck surgery. A class of drugs called alpha-adrenergic agonists can sometimes be effective in treating retrograde ejaculation by helping the bladder neck close at the time of ejaculation, but can cause severe side effects including high blood pressure, palpitations and abnormal heart rhythms. If drugs are not effective, we can only try to obtain sperm from the urine, buffer it to the proper pH and use it for IUI or IVF.

In a man with a history of infection or with a testicular trauma, tests designed to detect antisperm antibodies in the blood or seminal fluid may be useful. Tests designed to detect infection with common organisms (such as chlamydia or ureaplasma) also might be employed. (RISK—NONE; PAIN—NONE; COST—LOW)

In some selected cases, a sperm penetration assay (SPA) might be performed. This is more commonly known as the hamster test, because it records the percentage of hamster eggs penetrated by a man's sperm. The ability of sperm to penetrate the shell around the egg (zona pellucida) is usually specific to a particular species. In the hamster this shell can be removed by the use of enzymes, which allows the penetration of human sperm. In general, penetration below 10% is considered abnormal. However, the test results are not that specific, since pregnancies occur in couples with an abnormal hamster test (even those in which the SPA is zero) and some men who fertilize hamster eggs very well cannot achieve pregnancies. Today we rarely find a use for this test. In men with good counts and motility we now use other parameters such as a strict assessment of morphology to determine if ICSI will be required to assure a good fertilization rate. Others may use it to determine the best method of fertilization in IVF cycles. (RISK—NONE; PAIN—NONE; COST—MODERATE)

Finally, a relatively new test may be used which goes beyond the microscope and tests of sperm function. This test approaches the problem of male infertility from another angle, measuring and comparing the levels of sperm nuclear DNA damage. The Sperm Chromatin Structure Assay (SCSA) classifies men into one of three categories indicating their chance of fathering a viable normal pregnancy. In general those men with DNA Fragmentation Index (DFI) of less than 15% have an excellent prognosis, between 15% and 29.9% have a good prognosis, and over 30% have poor fertility potential. Increased DNA fragmentation in sperm may be the result of many factors including disease, diet, drug use, high fever, elevated testicular temperature, air pollution, cigarette smoking and advanced age. The role of this test in the infertility workup has not yet been established. But it might be most useful in the couple that have otherwise unexplained infertility, recurrent early pregnancy loss or multiple ART failures. (RISK—NONE; PAIN—NONE; COST—MODERATE)

Tubal problems

If obstruction of the tubes is found by hysterosalpingogram, laparoscopy would help confirm the location and cause of the obstruction. In addition, laparoscopy might uncover unsuspected adhesions around the tubes and/or ovaries or even pelvic endometriosis. In any of these instances, after completion of the other basic portions of the workup your doctor could proceed directly to treatment with no further testing. In fact, many times it is possible to correct these problems at the time of the diagnostic laparoscopy; surgery through the laparoscope (pelviscopy) is a technique many gynecologists have acquired and many reproductive endocrinologists have developed to advanced levels.

If a tubal problem is suspected, it is usually worth going through the laparoscopy to determine if it can be repaired and not require advanced techniques.

Even if the tubes are markedly dilated and obviously not repairable, laparoscopy is important before IVF to remove or interrupt the tubes to prevent the fluid in the tube from backing up through the uterus, where it can interfere with implantation. In one very specific case, obstruction of the tubes near the uterus, a radiologic technique may be used to directly catheterize the tubes.

In many cases, the tubes may be opened during a laparoscopy. (RISK—MODERATE; PAIN—LOW TO MODERATE; COST—HIGH)

Cervical factor

If the cervical mucus is full of inflammatory cells, antibiotic treatment may be prescribed. If the mucus is poor in quality or quantity, a small dose of preovulatory estrogen may be prescribed or, more commonly, the sperm can be washed and placed in the uterus (intrauterine insemination). If the PCT shows immobile or shaking sperm, further testing for antisperm antibodies may be performed. In most instances of an abnormal PCT, a trial of four to six intrauterine inseminations is recommended. Approximately one-third of these patients can expect to be successful. (RISK—LOW; PAIN—NONE; COST—LOW)

"ALL OF YOUR TESTS ARE NORMAL"

That's what about 5% to 10% of patients will hear at the conclusion of this set of tests. They will be categorized as having "unexplained infertility." This does not mean that there is no cause for their infertility problem, only that it has not yet been found. Other tests now need to be done, but there is little or no agreement among infertility specialists as to exactly where these fit into the workup.

"All your tests are normal" is very frustrating news.

Cultures and DNA probes

In couples who are unsuccessful in conceiving without an apparent reason, a variety of tests to determine both common and uncommon causes of infection of the genital tract may be performed at some time during the workup. These may include cultures or DNA probes for chlamydia and gonorrhea, common organisms implicated in infertility. A study from Italy correlated infertility with a subclinical chlamydial infection in the endometrium of patients who had normal-appearing tubes at laparoscopy. A culture of ureaplasma organisms may be done when there is a history of early pregnancy loss.

For example, Barbara and Tom, both 28, came in with a history of eight previous early pregnancy losses. They had been to several doctors; thorough workups had included chromosomal tests to insure that no genetic factor was present. This was some time ago, before the clinical availability of culture methods for ureaplasma. Specimens from Barbara's cervix were sent to one of the research labs testing for this organism. You guessed it! Her culture was positive for ureaplasma. Both she and Tom were treated with a long-acting tetracycline for 10 days and went on to have two healthy children in two successive pregnancies. (RISK—NONE; PAIN—NONE; COST—LOW)

Hormone levels

Certain hormone tests, specifically thyroid function tests and prolactin, may be ordered even if ovulation appears to be normal. Minimal elevations of prolactin can affect the luteal phase of the cycle and cause infertility despite the fact that all other tests are normal. An elevated prolactin can suddenly explain "unexplained infertility." Similarly, minimal alterations in thyroid function can also disturb ovulation.

In a small number of patients, correction of an underlying medical problem may lead to pregnancy. Several years ago Janet, 28, went through the entire workup with all tests normal except for a low normal sperm count on her husband, Michael, 32. When Janet came in complaining of fatigue, a complete medical workup showed slightly high blood sugar. A glucose tolerance test confirmed that she had early diabetes. She was placed on a proper diet and required insulin for adequate control of her blood sugar. When her sugar was controlled she conceived quickly and now has two girls. (RISK—NONE; PAIN—NONE; COST—LOW)

Even if all the initial tests are normal, the problem may still be fairly simple and treatable.

Ultrasound

An uncommon cause of unexplained infertility can be failure of the follicle to rupture at a normal diameter or to even rupture at all (luteinized unruptured follicle, or LUF). In order to detect this possibility, a series of vaginal ultrasound examinations can be done to trace the growth of the follicle to a proper peak diameter and its eventual rupture. The ultrasound probe is placed in the vagina and sends sound waves into the tissues. The waves send back an echo, creating a picture of the internal organs. When used vaginally, the probe is very close to the pelvic organs and the quality of the image is better than when the probe is placed on the abdomen. Another benefit to the vaginal probe is that there is no need to fill the bladder to capacity, which can be uncomfortable.

In order to evaluate follicle dynamics, scans will be done shortly before the anticipated day of ovulation and every one to three days until a normal follicle diameter is reached. The patient will also monitor her LH surge and will return two days following the surge to confirm collapse of the follicle. In one study, women with unexplained infertility and a confirmed abnormality of follicle growth and collapse had a very high cumulative pregnancy rate with ovulation induction compared to a rather low rate in women with normal follicle dynamics. (RISK—NONE; PAIN—NONE; COST—LOW TO MODERATE)

Antisperm antibodies

Infertile couples manifest antisperm antibodies in about 15% to 20% of females and 5% to 10% of males (contrasted to about 1% to 2% of the fertile population). In patients with abnormal mucus penetration the incidence of antisperm antibodies is much higher. Of the tests done for immunologic infertility, the immunobead test is believed to be the most specific. In this test, small beads with antibodies attached are mixed with sperm. If 10% of the sperm bind to the beads the test is considered positive. In couples with a normal postcoital test, these studies are not usually done until late in the workup. In fact, in the face of a normal PCT, many centers do these tests only in anticipation of going on to assisted reproductive procedures or if the sperm in the semen analysis show marked clumping or vibratory movement instead of forward motion. (RISK—NONE; PAIN—NONE; COST—LOW TO MODERATE)

We hear a lot of questions about antisperm antibodies. We don't do a lot of testing for them because the progression of treatments are designed to overcome them if they are present.

In the usual instance of unexplained infertility, intrauterine insemination (IUI) will be recommended, first with the patient's spontaneous cycle, then with the patient on fertility drugs (discussed in chapter 7). Since IUI is also the treatment for antibodies in either partner, we generally reserve antibody testing until after IUI and before ART. In preparation for the ART cycle, the presence of antibodies may indicate that IVF would maximize fertilization compared to GIFT. In some instances of antibodies in the male, a very large number of sperm must be added to the egg for fertilization to occur in vitro, or ICSI may be advised.

ON TO TREATMENT

Fifteen years ago, a much larger portion of patients would have fallen into the category of unexplained infertility. For those patients we would have had to say, "We do not have any specific treatment to offer you. Keep trying. Good-bye and good luck." Today we have a series of what are now considered conventional treatments for the couple with unexplained infertility as well as those in whom we have found an apparent problem. Since a basic principle is to do the safer, simpler and less expensive treatment first, we'll consider these conventional procedures in chapter 7 before going on to ART.

CHAPTER 7

Honey,
It Worked!

Although this is a book about IVF, GIFT and other types of assisted reproduction, we have spent a good deal of time outlining how the reproductive
system works, and when it sometimes doesn't work, how to find out why.
We are now about to embark on a discussion of some of the conventional
treatments for the various causes of infertility.

There are two reasons we are spending so much time on conventional infertility issues. The first is that it is impossible to understand the
complex issues regarding assisted reproduction without understanding the
basics of the human reproductive process along with why and how it can
malfunction. After all, in school you can't take Biology 102 until you have
completed the necessary prerequisite, Biology 101.

The second reason is to make an important point. We said it before
when we were discussing testing, and we say it again here because it is one of
the most important points to understand if you are considering ART procedures. You always do the safer, simpler and less expensive procedures first!
In order to make an informed decision regarding your need for the ART procedures you must be sure that all other reasonable avenues of treatment
have been exhausted. Remember that conventional treatment often works.

BASIC MATH

Before we go on to describe the pre-ART infertility treatments, you need to
know about the mathematics of reproduction.

Rule 1: Monthly conception rate

For the average "normal" young couple without any infertility problem, the chance of conceiving in one cycle—their monthly conception rate—will be between 20% and 25% if they have intercourse at the proper time of the cycle. This probably represents the maximum efficiency of the human reproductive system. It is important that you keep this in mind as you evaluate success rates of various treatments and your own response to treatment. For example, if a treatment is recommended and it does not work the first month, don't be discouraged. Even if it did totally correct your problem, according to this rule you still have only a maximum 20% to 25% chance of getting pregnant that first month. Many couples who do not understand this get discouraged and give up before they have given a specific treatment an adequate chance.

It is possible to learn how to calculate your chances of becoming pregnant each month.

Rule 2: Cumulative conception rate

The next logical step is that you must also look at the success of a treatment from the viewpoint of time. If in our "normal" couple we tried to calculate the chance of getting pregnant, it would naturally depend on how long they tried. If they tried for only one month, their conception rate would be, let's say, 20%. Yet you cannot say that this couple has only a 20% chance of getting pregnant. Let us go further out in time and look at a hundred "normal" couples. After one month 20 couples would have gotten pregnant, and 80 would not have conceived. In the second month, 16 would conceive (20% of 80 couples) and 64 would be left not pregnant:

Your age is an important factor in determining your conception rate.

Month	# Couples left	# Pregnant (Cumulative %)	# Not Pregnant
1	100	20 (20)	80
2	80	16 (36)	64
3	64	13 (49)	51
4	51	10 (59)	41
5	41	8 (67)	33
6	33	7 (74)	26
7	26	5 (79)	21
8	21	4 (83)	17
9	17	3 (86)	14

Month	# Couples left	# Pregnant (Cumulative %)	# Not Pregnant
10	14	3 (89)	11
11	11	2 (91)	9
12	9	2 (93)	7

So the cumulative conception rate in this group of "normal" patients should be 93% in 12 cycles. In fact, the true pattern does not strictly follow this rule, because all women are not the same. Included in these hundred women will be some who are highly fertile and some who have inherent low fertility or even a specific infertility problem. Actually, about 80% of couples attempting pregnancy will conceive within one year.

Using this cumulative rate, you can see how we can arrive at the time interval of one year as significant in defining infertility. If you have been trying for only six months, there is still a 26% chance you would not have conceived even if you were "normal." Since as many as 26% of normal couples would not conceive by six months, it does not pay to begin a workup at that time unless there are extenuating circumstances, such as age or a recognized infertility factor.

As with testing, safer, simpler and less expensive is the way to go with treatment.

The cumulative conception rate is also important to keep in mind if you are planning to go through an ART procedure because the implication of this rule is that in order to achieve the maximum chance of success, you will have to consider going through more than one cycle. If a program has, for instance, a 20% take-home baby rate in your age group and you go through one cycle, you have a 20% chance. Over four cycles the cumulative success rate would be 49%, based on these theoretical calculations. Actually a U.S. study through SART showed no change in success for a second cycle, a 15% to 20% reduction in the third, and a 25% reduction for a fourth cycle. As with natural fertility, as more cycles go by, the remaining patients tend to be on the whole somewhat less fertile. There is no single factor more important to a final successful outcome than having repeated cycles. Persistence is the key ingredient of success.

Rule 3: Your conception rate

You need to think of your infertility problem in terms of what it does to your monthly conception rate. You can then estimate how a particular treatment will modify your monthly rate and project it to a cumulative conception rate. This will give you an idea of how long you may wish to try a specific treatment.

Let's say your problem is azoospermia and you have decided to use donor sperm to overcome the problem. You can assume that the monthly conception rate with donor sperm is about 15%. You could calculate the cumulative rate as follows:

Month	# Couples left	# Pregnant (Cumulative %)	# Not Pregnant
1	100	15 (15)	85
2	85	13 (28)	72
3	72	11 (39)	61
4	61	9 (48)	52
5	52	8 (56)	44
6	44	7 (63)	37
7	37	6 (69)	31
8	31	5 (74)	26
9	26	4 (78)	22
10	22	3 (81)	19
11	19	3 (84)	16
12	16	2 (86)	14

Constructing your own table based on your monthly conception rate will help you determine how long to stick with a specific treatment.

After 12 cycles of artificial insemination all but 14% of otherwise normal women theoretically would be pregnant by donor insemination. Again, it is not actually this high because some of the women will have other fertility problems. So, if you are not pregnant by this time, it might be safe to assume that there may be an additional factor over and above the azoospermia, and further tests would be indicated. This would probably not be true after six months, when 37% of otherwise normal women would not have conceived. And it certainly does not make sense to stop after only three months of donor insemination because, at that point, we know there is a 61% chance that you would not be successful. It would be too soon to stop.

We can't say it too often: Perseverance pays off! Now you know how to figure out how long to persevere.

Rule 4: The exception to the rule

This is a modification of Rule 3. As you go further out in time, the pregnancy rate does not always approach 100% and the not-pregnant rate 0%, since our treatments are not perfect. There are often periods of time after which no pregnancies occur. For example, if we treat endometriosis with surgery, most of the pregnancies occur in the first year. From one to three years there is a decrease in the monthly conception rate, and after three years virtually no pregnancies occur. This can happen either because scarring from the endometriosis may have recurred following surgery or the couple may have, at this point, other factors for which they need further evaluation and treatment.

Monthly and cumulative pregnancy rates for most infertility factors and treatments have been worked out and published. Success rates of new developments are often reported in this fashion too, so this information can be obtained.

HOW SUCCESSFUL IS TREATMENT?

That pre-ART large 1980 study cited in chapter 5 not only discussed the causes of infertility in its patient population but also related the cause to actual results of treatment. One of the most interesting aspects of the study projected what the success rate should have been based on the cumulative conception rate for that particular condition if the patients had continued treatment indefinitely:

	Pregnancy rate	
	Actual *Percent*	*Expected* *Percent*
Endometriosis	31	52
Male factor	38	74
Lack of ovulation	44	79
Tubal factor	26	48
Luteal phase problems	46	58
Cervical factor	26	45
Uterine factor	33	38

Remember, at that time only conventional treatments were available so the rates for all of these are better today than they were before 1980, due largely to better conventional treatments and the advent of assisted reproduction.

The fact that the expected rates were much higher than the actual rates reinforces one of our most important points: Many people give up too early! This is not to say that you should try a particular treatment indefinitely. You should, along with your doctor, be able to rationally determine how long to pursue any and all treatment, using the concept of cumulative conception rates. It's like what they say about the stock market: many experts know when to buy a stock, but few know when to sell. Or, as Kenny Rogers advises in his song "The Gambler," you've got to "know when to hold 'em, know when to fold 'em." In infertility, there is usually good rationale for the selection of a particular treatment, but few guidelines on how long to persist. It takes a lot of experience to know when to move on to the next step.

Current actual pregnancy rates are better today because of more effective conventional treatments.

SPECIFIC TREATMENT
Lack of ovulation

Most treatment for anovulation falls into one of three regimens:

- clomiphene citrate (cc)
- human menopausal gonadotropins (hMG) or follicle stimulating hormone (FSH) with or without clomiphene
- gonadotropin-releasing hormone (GnRH)

Exceptions to use of these drugs would be in patients with documented hormone problems that can be overcome by the administration of a specific hormone to correct the problem. Patients falling into this category would include those with an elevated prolactin level with or without galactorrhea or evidence of a microadenoma of the pituitary gland. These people will be treated specifically with bromocriptine (Parlodel) or cabergoline (Dostinex), which will reduce the level of prolactin, eliminate the galactorrhea, shrink the microadenoma and allow ovulation to return to normal.

Bromocriptine is taken orally. It is relatively inexpensive and significant side effects are infrequent. The dose is usually increased gradually based on the reduction in prolactin. It takes from four to six weeks to relieve the galactorrhea, reduce serum prolactin and resume menses. The success rate is fairly high, with about 80% of patients responding with ovulation and over 60% becoming pregnant. The cost of bromocriptine averages about $2.20 U.S. a tablet as it is now available as a generic. Cabergoline was released in March 1997, and it is claimed to be more effective and better tolerated than bromocriptine. A tablet of cabergoline costs about $40 U.S., but it is taken only twice weekly. Both are similarly efficacious in reducing prolactin levels and the size of microadenomas.

Another example of the use of specific medication occurs in women who may have symptoms of excessive hair growth, acne and lack of a menstrual cycle due to excessive adrenal hormones. These women can be treated specifically with a cortisone-like drug such as dexamethasone, usually taken at bedtime. Again, this treatment is specific, effective, relatively inexpensive and free of side effects with short-term treatment. A third example involves women who are low in thyroid hormone and whose lack of ovulation can be corrected with simple and inexpensive thyroid hormone pills. Women with PCOS can specifically treat their insulin resistance (IR) with one of several drugs designed to treat IR, such as metformin which can lead to spontaneous ovulation in about 30% of cases.

Clomiphene can have some negative effects on fertility so you may want to limit your time on this drug.

But the vast majority of patients with ovulatory problems will be treated with the three major drugs.

CLOMIPHENE CITRATE
(CC—SEROPHENE, CLOMID)

The first drug available for ovulation induction was discovered by accident. It is an antiestrogen and was being studied as a contraceptive agent designed to block the implantation process in animals. When it was applied to humans it was noticed that it increased gonadotropins and caused ovulation. For well over 30 years it has been used as the first-line drug for the induction of ovulation.

Clomiphene is used in patients whose ovulatory problem is caused by a malfunction in the hypothalamus (due to the causes discussed in chapter 5) and in patients with polycystic ovaries/Stein-Leventhal syndrome. On a practical basis, clomiphene is often tried first in patients who are producing adequate amounts of estrogen because it is relatively inexpensive, easy to monitor and readily available to all physicians. It is taken orally, starting the third to fifth day of the cycle. A pelvic examination or ultrasound is usually done prior to starting treatment to make sure that no ovarian cysts are present. The drug is usually taken for five days and, if ovulation does not occur, the dose is increased in succeeding cycles.

As infertility treatments go, the cost of clomiphene is modest. Retail cost can vary but is around $5 U.S. a tablet for generic clomiphene, $10.50 for Clomid and $9 U.S. for Serophene. You may want to inquire from the pharmacist which brand he or she is giving you and compare the costs of each, since generic clomiphene, Clomid and Serophene are pharmaceutically equivalent. Side effects are not usually a problem but may consist of enlargement of the ovaries and/or abdominal discomfort. Risks include:

- multiple pregnancy in about 8% of patients (most often twins)
- development of ovarian cysts
- overstimulation of the ovaries (rare with clomiphene)

Overstimulation is a potentially serious problem causing an imbalance in the body's fluids and electrolytes (discussed in the section on hMG therapy, below). Minor side effects include hot flushes, breast tenderness, headache, mood changes, nervousness, dizziness, nausea and vomiting, and fatigue. In addition, it can also rarely cause potentially serious visual disturbances that should be reported to your doctor. In our experience, most patients on clomiphene feel perfectly fine. There is no evidence that clomiphene causes birth defects when used for induction of ovulation.

Success rates vary tremendously from study to study and range between 30% and 90%. In general, about 50% to 90% of women with abnormal menstrual cycles will achieve ovulation with clomiphene and about half of those will get pregnant if given an adequate trial. If all other factors are normal, the conception rate for clomiphene-induced ovulation should approach those of cycles in which ovulation occurred spontaneously. Failure to achieve pregnancy after successful ovulation with clomiphene may be due to any of the following factors:

HONEY, IT WORKED!

- an unwanted effect from the clomiphene, such as decreased cervical mucus or poor endometrial development
- poor-quality eggs because the hormonal environment of the ovary is not normal
- other causes of infertility that may be present
- lack of persistence. In one study of patients with no other fertility factors, the pregnancy rate approached 100% when corrected for the 44% of patients who dropped out before completing the recommended number of cycles.

Your cycle will likely be monitored with a basal body temperature chart, ultrasound and/or urinary LH testing. Some physicians will check a serum progesterone level during the luteal phase to check its adequacy. With some patients who do not ovulate, physicians may add a shot of hCG (a pregnancy hormone that simulates the LH surge) about eight days after the clomiphene is finished. Some choose to follow the follicle development via vaginal ultrasound and then administer hCG when the follicle reaches mature size. Ultrasound done two days later can assure that the follicle has actually ruptured.

The majority of pregnancies occur within the first four to six cycles of treatment. This is based on a monthly conception rate estimated by one group as 22% if no other fertility factors were present, which does not really differ from couples with normal fertility. This group of physicians felt that the rate declined after 10 months of therapy. You can construct your own table to determine how long you should stick with this treatment.

HUMAN MENOPAUSAL GONADOTROPIN
(HMG—PERGONAL, REPRONEX)
PURE FOLLICLE STIMULATING HORMONE
(FSH— BRAVELLE, FOLLISTIM, GONAL-F)

HMG, consisting of both FSH and LH, or pure FSH is generally used in patients who do not produce their own gonadotropins and secrete inadequate amounts of estrogen. It is also helpful in those patients who do not respond to clomiphene. In the late 1950s and early 1960s gonadotropins were first extracted from the urine of menopausal women in Italy, and it was not long before they were tried for ovulation induction. There were major problems from the start because the tools for monitoring its use were rudimentary and the multiple pregnancy rate was high. At first, doctors monitored their patients with pelvic examination, vaginal smears for estrogen level, observation of the cervical mucus and urinary estrogen determinations. Monitoring has vastly improved with the rapid serum estrogen tests and pelvic ultrasound. Recently, the use of vaginal ultrasound probes has made monitoring more comfortable and even more accurate.

More precise monitoring of hMG cycles has resulted in a reduction of the multiple-pregnancy rate from 28% to less than 10% and the almost complete absence of high-order multiple pregnancies (four or more babies). Patients considering hMG therapy should be aware, however, that although ultrasound monitoring reduces the risk, it is not absolute. Generally, follicles above 14 to 16 millimeters mean diameter are considered mature and capable of ovulation. However, follicles below this size can sometimes result in pregnancy. Just as with IVF, some surprisingly small follicles can yield mature eggs. Before you accept hMG therapy, be sure that you will be adequately monitored by a vaginal ultrasound and that estrogen measurements are available if needed. While some obstetricians and gynecologists have the facilities to do this, others don't.

Because of the high cost of hMG and its side effects, efforts should first be made to achieve pregnancy by simpler means. Currently the retail cost of one vial of intramuscular hMG (Pergonal, Repronex) is about $35–$45 U.S. with the subcutaneous FSH (Bravelle) costing slightly more per ampule. With 15 or more vials possibly necessary to complete the cycle the cost of medication often exceeds $700 U.S. for one cycle. Add to that three or four pelvic ultrasounds and a rapid serum estradiol and you are likely to spend over $1500 U.S. on one cycle of treatment. This has led some physicians to use a combination of clomiphene and hMG (cc/hMG) that requires less hMG, thus cutting costs somewhat.

The expense also leads patients to look for ways of cutting costs. We recently encountered a patient on hMG therapy for anovulation who was very concerned about the costs of treatment. She convinced her employer to offer a "drug card" with their health plan and all she paid was $5 for her entire supply of hMG. Others travel to other countries to get these drugs for less money.

There are many different ways of prescribing hMG or FSH, but most physicians start at a dose of one to two vials a day, starting on the second to fifth day of the cycle. The low dose, slow method of administration is superior, according to recent studies. One large study found that it results in fewer mature follicles, less medication used, lower cost, a smaller incidence of hyperstimulation and a multiple pregnancy rate of only 4%. In this protocol only one vial a day is given the first week, increasing by one-half vial as necessary. The patient is then seen again after four to seven days of injections, at which time the response may be assessed by ultrasound or checking estradiol levels, or both. The dose is adjusted, and the patient returns in one to three days, depending on the number and size of her follicles. When the follicles reach mature size in an acceptable number (one to three), the serum estradiol may be checked and hCG is given to simulate the LH surge, triggering ovulation. Ovulation should occur about 36 to 44 hours after the hCG. The patient is instructed to have intercourse accordingly, or in some cases she will have insemination, depending whether or not other problems such as a male factor are present.

The risks of hMG or FSH are similar to, but considerably more significant than, those of clomiphene. Side effects may include ovarian cysts, abdominal distention and pain, multiple pregnancy and ovarian hyperstimulation. Most of these do not progress and will usually resolve if the hMG or FSH is stopped, hCG is not given and the patient does not become pregnant. Overstimulation can be mild, with fluid retention, enlarged ovaries and abdominal discomfort. When severe, significant fluid imbalance may require hospitalization. Other side effects include allergy to hMG or FSH, pain, rash, swelling and irritation at the injection site. Mood swings may occur while on the medication. In addition, you may notice an increased amount of cervical mucus because of the increased amounts of estrogen. Overall, the incidence of birth defects in patients using hMG or FSH to induce ovulation is not any higher than that of the general population.

A form of pure urinary FSH (Bravelle) can be injected subcutaneously (under the skin) rather than deep in the muscle. The most recent development has been the availability of Follistim and Gonal-F, the first FDA-approved gonadotropins to be manufactured using recombinant DNA technology rather than being obtained from human sources. This gives it the advantage of not only subcutaneous injection but also no risk of transmission of human disease.

The benefit of a pure FSH product to certain patients is that pure FSH has practically no LH in it and therefore may be an advantage to patients who have an elevated level of LH. Patients with polycystic ovaries and an elevated LH fall into this category. If we give more LH, it can stimulate the production of certain hormones called androgens, and these can interfere with development or health of the follicle. Comparative studies of the circulating levels of LH and FSH after injection of the two drugs has shown higher levels of FSH and lower levels of LH with pure FSH. Bravelle, Follistim and Gonal-F have the additional advantage of being much easier to administer and much less painful, and can be administered by the patient herself. As with everything in life, with added benefit comes added cost. An ampule of Gonal-F or Follistim averages $55–$60 U.S.

The GnRH pump is a pain to deal with, but very effective for certain patients.

GONADOTROPIN-RELEASING HORMONE (GNRH)

GnRH has been studied in women with a wide variety of causes for their anovulation. It is highly effective in hypothalamic amenorrhea, and much less effective in PCO. The main requirement has been that the patient must have normal pituitary function, although recent studies show it is effective in higher-than-usual doses if the pituitary is impaired. Like hMG and pure FSH, it must be given by injection, but its action is completely different. Instead of being a gonadotropin, it stimulates the pituitary to secrete its own gonadotropins in normal sequence. It simulates a normal cycle. Therefore, as you would expect, you avoid the greater chance of multiple pregnancy and overstimulation associated with hMG.

The catch is that GnRH must be administered in pulses, usually every 90 minutes. Since it is impractical to take injections every 90 minutes around the clock, it is administered by an automatic pump worn around the waist with a needle inserted under the skin or into a vein. The cycle is monitored by vaginal ultrasound every few days to document the growth and collapse of the follicle. The pump is disconnected after ovulation is verified and then hCG is given to support the corpus luteum.

Except for some tissue reaction at the needle site, there are no serious side effects or complications. Data regarding effectiveness is optimistic, showing fairly high ovulation (over 90% with hypothalamic amenorrhea) and success rates (about 30% per ovulatory cycle). The cost for one cycle of treatment including monitoring would be in the neighborhood of about $1,000 U.S., slightly less than for gonadotropin ovulation induction. However, the commercial preparation of GnRH is not currently available in the U.S.

Unfortunately, there are causes of lack of ovulation and menses that are not treatable with these measures. But infertility due to premature ovarian failure or surgical removal of the ovaries is now treatable with the use of donor eggs through IVF techniques (discussed in chapter 12).

Clair, in her early twenties, is a good example of the type of expense and difficulty some patients with significant ovulatory problems must endure. She was diagnosed as having Kallman's syndrome, a combination of lack of ovulation because of low gonadotropins and loss of the sense of smell. This can be very difficult to treat, but it responds well to the GnRH pump. When she started treatment, the pump was not available. She went through six cycles of hMG-hCG without getting pregnant, using up to 60 ampules of hMG each cycle, costing over $2,000 per cycle for medication alone. When the GnRH pump became available, she conceived on her first try.

With azoospermia, after the workup it's almost, "Go directly to ICSI!"

Male factor

When you consider that a fairly large proportion of infertility is due to the male factor, it is surprising that treatment options for the male have been limited until recently. Nearly 20 years ago, all we could offer the couple with a significant male factor infertility was artificial insemination with semen from a donor, artificial insemination with the husband's semen into the cervical mucus or repair of a varicocele.

During the last decade, we've seen a great deal of interest in the workup and treatment of male factor infertility. This interest has paralleled advances in ART and the need to prepare the sperm for these advanced techniques. It bears repeating that changes in habits, when possible, should be recommended first to try to maximize the couple's chances of conceiving. For the male partner these would include changes in sexual frequency and timing; eliminating heated spa-type baths; changing from briefs to boxer shorts; and avoiding drugs, smoking and exposure to toxins.

Again, just as we categorized conditions causing male infertility according to the results of the semen analysis, we can break down treatment into the same categories.

NORMAL SEMEN ANALYSIS

If the female's evaluation and the initial semen analyses were normal, the man may be tested with more sophisticated tests of sperm function. These may include the sperm penetration assay (SPA, or hamster test), which evaluates the ability of his sperm to penetrate a hamster egg with the zona removed. Just as with other male factors, pregnancy may be possible with intrauterine insemination or IVF, sometimes by modifying the way in which sperm are prepared.

AZOOSPERMIA

In the complete absence of sperm, a hormone workup will help reveal the nature of the problem. If the man's gonadotropins (FSH and LH) are very high, it can be assumed that he has testicular failure. Recently, retrieval of sperm from a testicular biopsy for use in intracytoplasmic sperm injection (ICSI) has been possible in one-half of such cases. The only other treatment available is artificial insemination with the semen of a donor. If the couple is unwilling to have donor insemination, or unable to afford ICSI, they could consider adoption.

If his gonadotropins are normal or slightly elevated, he may have an obstruction of the ductal system and could have an operation called a scrotal exploration to determine the location of the obstruction and attempt to correct it. This is major surgery, with all of its risks, at a cost of about $3,000 to $6,000. It is an outpatient surgery procedure usually performed under general anesthesia. The variation in cost will generally reflect the complexity of the repair and the time required to perform the operation, from one and a half to five hours. Before the scrotal exploration, the urologist may recommend a biopsy of the testicle as a separate procedure to determine if enough sperm are present before proceeding on to the more serious scrotal exploration. The biopsy is also an outpatient procedure that can be performed under either local or general anesthesia at a cost of about $1,000.

In cases of congenital absence of portions of the tubular system, microsurgical procedures are now being used to retrieve sperm directly from the epididymis for use in conjunction with ART procedures involving the direct injection of sperm into an egg (intracytoplasmic sperm injection, or ICSI). In fact, now in any case of obstruction, whether congenital or acquired, microsurgical epididymal sperm aspiration (MESA), or a testicular biopsy usually yields sperm which can be used in ICSI. In percutaneous epididymal sperm aspiration (PESA) sperm can even be retrieved in the office by passing a tiny needle through the skin into the epididymis.

In the face of low gonadotropins with low testosterone levels and the presence of the sugar fructose in the semen, the man would need further evaluation of his pituitary hormones. Fructose is produced by the seminal vesicles, and its presence in the semen makes blockage of the tubular system unlikely. As in the woman, if his prolactin is significantly elevated with or without evidence of a pituitary microadenoma, he would be treated with bromocriptine. If his gonadotropins are low, he can be treated with hCG and hMG.

A special category of obstruction is the case of a man who has had a vasectomy and wants it reversed. This can be accomplished by microscopic surgery or laser-assisted microsurgery. In addition to the area of the vasectomy's intentional blockage, other areas of obstruction may develop in adjacent locations and must be searched for and bypassed. In general, the success of vasovasostomy will be related to the length of time that has elapsed between the vasectomy and its repair, and the skill and experience of the surgeon performing the procedure. Now MESA in conjunction with ICSI is yielding excellent results in couples in which the man has had a vasectomy, obviating the need for the major surgery required to reverse the vasectomy. If sperm cannot be found in the epididymis, testicular biopsy (TESE or Testicular Sperm Extraction) is often used successfully in obtaining sperm for use in ICSI. This can also sometimes be done with a needle rather than a surgical biopsy, but sperm are not as reliably obtained.

OTHER ABNORMALITIES

A more subtle abnormality that may be found is a varicocele. If detected, surgery may be considered after other nonsurgical problems, such as hormonal or environmental causes, have been looked for and corrected. A well-designed study from Israel published in 1995 showed distinct improvements in semen quality and fertility over the one to two years after surgery to repair varicoceles.

Of course, our basic premise applies here: that the simple, safe and less expensive treatments must be explored first. Therefore, in the face of

If you need MESA, PESA or TESE, seek out a urologist who has had a great deal of experience with these specific procedures and is confident he or she can retrieve sperm in most cases.

consistently abnormal semen analyses and normal tests of pituitary function, other causes of the abnormal semen must be considered: chronic use of drugs, infection, stress and exposure to toxic agents such as X-rays, pesticides, industrial chemicals or heat. Then if there are no other apparent causes for the abnormal semen analysis or there are other abnormal tests of sperm function, a varicocele should be searched for and surgery should be considered.

Special tests such as a venogram to help verify the presence of a varicocele are sometimes necessary and can be conducted on an outpatient basis. The varicocele is repaired through a 1.5-inch incision in the groin. Thus the veins are blocked above the testicle. This blockage of the flow of blood from the testicle does not cause damage because there are two other vein systems leaving the testicle. The discomfort after surgery is moderate and can be managed with oral pain medication. Most men can go back to work in three to four days and resume strenuous activity in three to four weeks.

Improvement in the semen analysis or fertility cannot be expected for at least three months. In properly selected men there will be a 60% to 70% chance for improvement in the semen, but possibly not until up to one year after surgery. The pregnancy rate after surgery reaches 40% to 45%, while men not treated have rates in the range of 15% to 20%. So, at best, varicocelectomy can improve pregnancy rates by two to three times. A recent review of seven randomized studies by researchers at the University of Maastricht in the Netherlands and McMaster University in Canada was more pessimistic, finding a 22% pregnancy rate after surgery, compared to a 19% rate when men had no treatment. An alternative to surgery would be ART procedures. But most urologists would recommend varicocelectomy in the case of an obvious varicocele with indications of abnormal semen and especially if the affected testicle is smaller than its mate. With all treatments of the female, including ART procedures, the chance of success will be better with the male factor improved as much as possible.

If the semen analysis reveals agglutination (clumping), a test for antisperm antibodies may be done. If antibodies are found, then high doses of steroids may be prescribed for short periods, although many practitioners are concerned about rare serious complications from steroids. Finally, the husband's sperm can be used for artificial insemination into the uterus after washing (AIH-IUI), as is commonly done for cervical mucus problems. If conventional treatments for sperm antibodies are not successful, then ART may be done and is highly successful. If the level of antibodies is high, ICSI may be advised.

Small volume or the complete absence of semen can occur as the result of retrograde ejaculation, or ejaculation backward into the bladder. If the retrograde ejaculation is due to a medical condition such as diabetes, semen can be obtained by use of drugs that close the bladder neck. If retrograde ejaculation is the result of a complication of trauma, spinal injury or previous surgery, sperm can be harvested from a urine specimen (after masturbation) and then prepared for artificial insemination. If the specimen is voided into culture medium and the acidity of the urine is adjusted by adding baking soda, the sperm will survive for a brief period of time in the urine. In some instances it is necessary to adjust the concentration of the urine.

UNEXPLAINED POOR SEMEN QUALITY

In many men with reduced count, motility and/or morphology, no apparent cause is found. Intrauterine insemination (IUI) following sperm washing can be successful, particularly with mild to moderate abnormal sperm. Most pregnancies will occur within four to six cycles of IUI. IUI in conjunction with hMG or pure FSH increases the chance of fertilization because there are more eggs available. Finally, IVF is highly effective, since 50,000 to 500,000 sperm are concentrated around the egg. If more than a mild male factor is present, ICSI is generally advised. ICSI may be particularly important with low strict morphology since the implantation rate is reduced with regular IVF, but is normal with ICSI. This may be because placing a large number of abnormal sperm around the egg may adversely affect embryo quality, causing a toxic effect on the embryo.

ENDOMETRIOSIS

The treatment of endometriosis has traditionally fallen into two general categories—medical and surgical. Now emerging is a third category—no treatment. This is because an accumulating body of evidence indicates that infertility patients with minimal to mild stages of endometriosis who undergo no treatment may have the same conception rate as those treated by

With all the advanced techniques available, it is our impression that we are seeing a reduced number of varicocelectomies being performed in our patients.

medications or surgery. That's probably because women with this degree of endometriosis are not truly infertile, but "subfertile," with a 1% to 3% lower than average possibility of pregnancy per cycle. Actually, endometriosis treatment is very complex and dependent on symptoms, location and degree of the disease. (A thorough consideration of endometriosis is beyond the scope of this book.)

At issue currently is whether it is necessary to treat endometriosis in an infertile woman when the degree of the disease is minimal. The pregnancy rate resulting from no treatment (31% to 75% over 18 months) is very similar to the rate when operative or medical treatment is used. The issue of "no treatment" is somewhat moot, however, because when laparoscopy is done to make the diagnosis, the implants can easily be cauterized or lasered through the laparoscope, thus preventing progression of the disease. If your endometriosis is minimal and it was treated at the time of laparoscopy, you may want to try to conceive without going through a course of medical therapy that may not be necessary.

Insurance considerations may determine which medical treatment is suggested for endometriosis. Make sure you are getting what is best for you, not for your insurance company's bottom line.

MEDICAL TREATMENT

The first hormonal treatment for endometriosis was based on the fact that pregnancy seemed to have the effect of improving endometriosis. Physicians thus tried to create a pseudopregnancy state with the use of hormones. This was accomplished by using either synthetic progesterone-like compounds (progestins) or birth control pills. Birth control pills are still used for this purpose, although more effective drugs are now available.

Birth control pills In the early days of hormonal treatment, continuous use of the birth control pill was popular because it was safe, effective, convenient and inexpensive. Since the subsequent pregnancy rate was fairly low (15% to 30%), other medications were developed and are now used more frequently.

The patient can be started on one birth control pill per day, but instead of stopping the pill after three weeks, it is continued for a total of nine months. If the patient develops bleeding while on this regimen, the dose of the pill may be gradually increased. It has been thought that patients should not have any menstrual periods while on this treatment to allow areas of endometriosis to subside. The use of the pill is relatively safe, although increasing to higher doses will increase the risk of blood clots and other complications of oral contraceptives.

Common but minor side effects include nausea, breast tenderness, headaches, irritability, fluid retention and spotting. One advantage of the pill is its low cost. A month of continuous therapy should cost less than $30 U.S.

Progestins If a woman is unwilling to take birth control pills or should not because of previous problems with blood clots, she may be put on a progestin, one of the synthetic compounds that has action similar to progesterone. Common ones used are medroxyprogesterone acetate (Provera) and norethindrone acetate (Aygestin). They can be given as daily pills or as a long-acting injection (Depo-Provera). It is a fairly innocuous medication as far as side effects are concerned and cost is low. We do not feel that the long-acting injection should be given to infertility patients because it can cause prolonged amenorrhea. It is best to fully suppress the disease and then try to conceive without delay.

There had been a great deal of concern about studies relating long-term progestin therapy to breast cancer, especially in postmenopausal women. These findings are highly controversial and should not be of concern since they have not been found with continuous use of progestins to treat endometriosis for short periods.

Danazol (Danocrine) This has been a popular method of hormonal suppression of endometriosis. Danazol acts to suppress the ovary and create a kind of pseudo-menopausal state. However, the fact that it is related in structure to the male hormone testosterone accounts for most of its side effects. These can include unwanted hair growth on the face and body, acne, deepening of the voice, weight gain and decreased breast size, as well as amenorrhea or abnormal bleeding. It also may have a detrimental effect by reducing "good" HDL cholesterol. In addition, the drug is costly, averaging about $200 U.S. for a month's treatment at the maximum dose. The pregnancy rate (30% to 60%) is higher than with the use of the birth control pill.

Gonadotropin-releasing hormone (GnRH) agonists Potent long-acting forms of GnRH agonists such as leuprolide (Lupron) are given by daily injection or every four weeks in a long-acting form (Lupron Depot). They initially stimulate gonadotropins, but as they are continued they suppress the pituitary. The resulting reduction of gonadotropins causes the ovary to almost cease its production of estrogen. Since endometrium is dependent on estrogen for continued growth, the endometriosis shrinks. Pregnancy rates are similar to results using danazol.

Its side effects are related to a lack of estrogen and include hot flushes, vaginal dryness, decreased libido and even some bone loss. Unlike danazol, it does not appear to have a detrimental effect on HDL cholesterol.

Another GnRH agonist commonly being used is nafarelin (Synarel). Synarel has the advantage of not requiring injections since it is administered as a nasal spray. Synarel was the first GnRH agonist approved for the management of endometriosis, pelvic pain caused by endometriosis and treatment of endometriosis lesions. Although Synarel is not specifically approved for treating infertility, treatment of the endometriosis could result in improved fertility, as with other medical and surgical treatments. A third alternative is goserelin acetate (Zoladex), which is administered monthly as an implant under the skin. All three GnRH agonists are limited to six months of use, largely because of concern over bone loss as a result of lowered estrogen levels.

Today the GnRH agonists are the drugs of choice for physicians specializing in infertility.

SURGICAL TREATMENT

Surgical options for endometriosis include either laparoscopy or open surgery through a conventional incision. The current trend is for more aggressive use of the laparoscope utilizing electrocautery, lasers and other surgical techniques (pelviscopy) through the laparoscope to destroy areas of endometriosis (implants), remove cysts, break up adhesions and even remove tubes and ovaries when necessary. The advantage of laparoscopy over conventional surgery is that it is done through very small incisions, is usually an outpatient procedure, requires less recuperation and can be less costly when you factor in hospitalization costs and recuperation time.

Many times very adequate treatment of even unsuspected endometriosis can be done at the time of an initial diagnostic laparoscopy. Before submitting to the initial diagnostic laparoscopy, it might be a good idea to ask if the surgeon is experienced and prepared to treat any conditions found at that time. In general, substantial amounts of endometriosis can be dealt with adequately through the laparoscope. More severe degrees of endometriosis may require an operation through a conventional incision. In addition, the combination of endometriosis with other abnormalities such as tubal problems or fibroids needing removal might require open surgery, although even some cases of tubal obstruction can now be treated through the laparoscope.

In the past the question of whether mild to moderate amounts of endometriosis interfered with fertility had not been resolved. However, a large multi-center Canadian study reported in the *New England Journal of Medicine* that laparoscopic treatment of mild to moderate endometriosis significantly enhances fertility.

The conception rates following laser treatment of endometrial implants are similar to those using electrocautery. Just be sure that your doctor feels comfortable handling mild to moderate degrees of endometriosis through the laparoscope so you won't be subjected to needless additional surgery or medical therapy.

Following surgery, hormonal treatment may be considered. With more extensive disease, some studies have suggested that combination therapy may enhance conception. A new wrinkle in the relationship between Lupron treatment improving conception rates was reported in *Fertility and Sterility* in October 2002. In that report, German researchers found an improvement in ART pregnancy rates when patients had a six month post-surgical course of Lupron immediately before the ART cycle. Two mechanisms were postulated for this observation. First, high fertilization rates can be expected when FSH is suppressed. Second, prolonged amenorrhea can have a positive effect on endometrial factors resulting in better implantation rates.

Tubal problems

The most important advance in tubal surgery has been the use of microsurgical techniques: the operating microscope, small sutures, microsurgical instruments and new tissue-handling techniques to reduce the risk of postoperative adhesions, such as peritoneal patches (Interceed, Gore-Tex). The most recent advance is the ability of many surgeons to perform these procedures using the laparoscope. The laser has been used in tubal infertility

A large multi-center Canadian study showed that laparoscopic treatment of mild to moderate endometriosis enhances fertility.

surgery, but its use is still controversial. Although many infertility surgeons advocate it and find that it saves time and facilitates certain aspects of tubal repair, there is no solid evidence that success rates are improved by the use of the laser.

Before we discuss success rates with surgery, you must realize that relatively few surgeons have enough personal experience to be able to quote meaningful success rates based on their own experience. Here is an opportunity for you to be a good consumer. Find someone in your community with a prominent reputation for this type of surgery. Generally, such an individual will have done at least a hundred microsurgical cases and does them on a fairly regular basis. The rates quoted below assume you have found a highly experienced surgeon.

The chance of success depends on the type of disease being treated:

- The best pregnancy rates occur when surgery is done purely to correct adhesions (lysis of adhesions) with essentially normal tubes. These adhesions can range from mild to severe. Surgery to remove adhesions will result in a 50% to 70% conception rate, with the better rate occurring when adhesions are mild.
- If the blockage in the tube is close to the uterus and the damaged area can be removed with the remaining ends put together (anastamosis), success rates will also be in the range of 50% to 70%. Newer methods are being used to catheterize and reopen this type of obstruction without surgery, and preliminary results are encouraging regarding pregnancy.
- When the damage involves the fimbriated end of the tube but the tube is open, plastic surgery to reconstruct the fimbria (fimbrioplasty) yields average conception rates of 40% to 60%.
- If the tube is closed at the fimbriated end and has to be opened (salpingostomy) and then repaired, the results are relatively poor. You can expect a success rate of 10% to 40%. If the tube, in addition to being closed, has also developed into a large hydrosalpinx, the pregnancy rates are worse still, averaging 5% to 10%.
- A totally separate category consists of women who have had their tubes "tied" and who later decide they want to become pregnant.

Depending on the method used to tie the tubes, the results of techniques to reverse sterilization can vary from poor to good. Some skilled physicians can now successfully reverse tubal ligations by using the laparoscope, sparing the patient a large scar and prolonged recovery.

The first step in the process is to determine how the tubes were tied. If it was performed by placing a clip or Falope ring through the laparoscope or by tying with a suture, the outlook for success would be good (80% to 90%). Electrocautery using a bipolar instrument would yield fair results, while cautery using the older unipolar technique destroys more of the tube, reducing results further (50% to 60%). Additionally, repair of an older tubal ligation in which the fimbria was removed (fimbriectomy) is even lower (40% to 50%).

If cautery was used, a laparoscopy should be done to see if there is enough tube left to anticipate good results. It is generally recognized that at least 1½ inches of the normally 4- to 5-inch tube is required to expect a reasonable chance of success. In summary, you can expect success rates for the following procedures:

	Percent
Clip or Falope ring	90
Ligation with suture	80
Bipolar cautery	70
Unipolar cautery	60
Fimbriectomy repair	40

This leads us to the logical conclusion that, with the advent of IVF and with the success rates of some centers above the 40% range, surgical procedures that do not yield pregnancy rates above 30% to 50% should be discouraged. Patients anticipating low success rates from tubal reversal should be counseled to consider IVF. The cost of a major tubal repair would usually be in the range of $12,000 U.S., including doctor, assistant, anesthesia and hospital. The woman would also run the risks of major surgery and require many weeks of recuperation.

If a couple is willing to commit to several cycles of IVF in a center with even a 20% take-home pregnancy rate, their cumulative success rate would be 20% after one cycle, 36% after two cycles and 51% after three cycles. Major surgery and recuperation are avoided and the cost may be similar. One of the factors in the cost is the availability of insurance, but at present most insurance plans cover neither the surgery nor IVF.

If a tubal repair is successful, you get a bargain in that if it works a second time, it is at no extra cost. Another factor which might make tubal repair more attractive is the new technique to perform reversal of tubal ligation through the laparoscope, reducing costs, need for hospitalization and recuperation time. In a 1996 study of 54 patients from CHA General Hospital in South Korea, the overall pregnancy rate following laparoscopic tubal reanastamosis was 77.5% with only one ectopic pregnancy among the 38 pregnancies.

There is still a place for tubal surgery: when anticipated results are better than ART procedures, or when surgery, but not ART, is covered by insurance.

The decision of whether to have surgery or IVF can be complex. The table opposite puts all of the variables into perspective. Faced with the same factors, different couples may reach different conclusions based on which factors are important to them. For example, if the nearest IVF center is four hours away, it may be better to travel once for tubal surgery, since the IVF cycle requires several visits.

Luteal phase defect (LPD)

This infrequent problem is the inadequate production of progesterone (too little or for too short a time) resulting in a poorly receptive endometrium, or one that starts to break down before implantation has become established. Diagnosis of LPD has been highly controversial because of the inaccuracy of diagnosis and variable result of treatment. Several types of treatment are possible.

Since there is a deficiency in the production of progesterone, the doctor can either prescribe progesterone by daily injections or vaginal gel (Crinone), or twice-daily vaginal suppositories. This would be continued from just after ovulation until obtaining the results of a pregnancy test two weeks later. If the pregnancy test is positive, the progesterone is continued, usually as suppositories. If it is negative, the progesterone is stopped and the menstrual period will occur. Both the injections and suppositories

Treatment Options for Tubal Problems

	SURGERY	IVF
Type of Procedure	major incision 4- to 6-week recovery	nonsurgical minimal recovery
Success Rate	5% to 90% depending on nature of disease, surgeon	up to 40+% depending on center and age
Another Pregnancy	possible	further cycle and expense
Tubal Pregnancy	5% to 25% of pregnancies [a]	1% to 10% of pregnancies depending on problem
Multiple Pregnancy	1%	up to 40% depending on center [b]
Time to Pregnancy	up to 5 years [c]	1 to several months
Insurance	?	?
Cost	$12,000 U.S.	$10,000 U.S.

Luteal phase defect can also be a cause of recurrent miscarriage.

(a) Rates for tubal pregnancy are often quoted per total number of patients, but only a percentage of patients become pregnant, so the proportion of pregnancies that are ectopic is actually much higher. With reversal of tubal ligation it is less than 5%, but with badly damaged tubes, it could be over 25%.

(b) The multiple pregnancy rate in a particular center rises in parallel with the success rate. Consequently the better centers usually transfer fewer embryos to try to reduce the percentage of multiple pregnancies.

(c) Pregnancies after surgery can occur as soon as the next month or as long as five or more years later. A couple should generally wait at least two years following surgery before going on to an ART procedure, although a shorter period of time could be reasonable if more than one pregnancy is desired or if the couple is older.

are fairly inexpensive and relatively free of side effects. Remember, the progesterone itself could cause a delay in your period, so the lack of a period while you are on the progesterone does not necessarily mean that you are pregnant. You should not stop the progesterone before taking a pregnancy test unless a menstrual period occurs.

Another approach is the use of clomiphene to improve an inadequate luteal phase. It is taken in the same manner as in patients who are not ovulating. Clomiphene increases progesterone secretion by stimulating better follicle maturity. In some women with LPD, ovulation may be abnormal. One paradoxical aspect is that the use of clomiphene itself can result in an inadequate luteal phase by having an anti-estrogen effect on the endometrium.

Small doses of hCG have also been employed on the third, sixth and ninth days following ovulation to treat this problem. This is generally only done when LPD occurs during ovulation induction. Again, this is inexpensive, effective and free from side effects.

To be effective, the progesterone or clomiphene must be continued for six to twelve cycles. It is common to try six months of progesterone and then to consider a change to clomiphene, since some patients with LPD may have inadequate ovulation. It is recommended that a biopsy be done to confirm that the defect has been corrected. If the endometrium remains abnormal after treatment, pregnancies occur infrequently and usually miscarry.

Vivian, 32, was a runner before she started trying to conceive. Although told that running could result in lower luteal phase progesterone levels, she did not want to stop. Two endometrial biopsies showed a consistent defect, but on ultrasound her follicles behaved normally. A repeat biopsy after treatment with progesterone suppositories confirmed correction of the defect. She became pregnant during the third cycle of treatment and delivered a healthy girl. She now runs while pushing a stroller!

Cervical problems

One of the more popular infertility treatments has become intrauterine insemination (IUI) with washed sperm. Previous treatments, including antibiotics to decrease inflammation, estrogen to improve mucus production, guaifenesin (Robitussin) to thin the mucus and insemination into the cervical mucus, were not very effective. Placing the sperm in the uterus bypasses the mucus and eliminates the cervical problem as a factor. It is known to be useful in the treatment of poor-quality mucus or mucus that has antibodies which clump and immobilize sperm. As mentioned, this technique is also successful for mild to moderate reductions of semen quality.

Although the chance of success varies with the individual problem, IUI yields about a 30% conception rate over three to six cycles, or 5% to 10% per cycle. In such couples the monthly conception rate without treatment might be 1% to 3%. It is entirely possible that this treatment "telescopes" successes into the treatment cycle which may have occurred spontaneously within another year or so of trying on their own. But we have not met many infertile couples willing to keep their lives perpetually on hold.

Treating cervical mucus problems with IUI is very easy and successful.

The procedure is usually scheduled based on the results of the urinary LH testing kit. Based on the woman's cycle, she is instructed when to begin testing and to schedule the insemination on the day following detection of the surge. The test is done in the afternoon or early evening so as not to miss the surge, which usually begins early in the day but may not be detectable in the urine until several hours later. On the day of insemination, the husband masturbates a specimen into a sterile, nontoxic plastic container. Preferably, the couple have avoided intercourse for two to three days before the anticipated day of insemination. After the specimen liquefies, it is washed in a nutrient medium. This can be done by a variety of techniques and in any one of several media. The washing procedure produces a concentrated pellet of motile sperm that is mixed with medium and placed into the uterus through the cervix by means of a thin plastic tube.

The wash and insemination are relatively inexpensive, currently costing around $250 U.S. per cycle. Side effects are rare but may include cramping. The risk of complications is low and related chiefly to the possibility of introducing infection. Many physicians administer a prophylactic antibiotic at the time of the procedure to prevent infection. One method of improving the success of the technique is to rest on the procedure table for 10 minutes after the IUI. At the 2000 ASRM Annual Meeting, researchers from McGill University randomized 116 patients into either an immediate mobilization group or a bed rest group. The pregnancy rate for the bed rest group was 29%, significantly higher than the 10% pregnancy rate for the patients who got off the table immediately.

Uterine problems

While uterine problems are relatively uncommon causes of inability to conceive, they can cause miscarriage. If fibroids are constricting the cavity and thought to be related to infertility or early pregnancy loss, they can be removed. Removal by hysteroscopy is often possible. This involves placing a telescope through the cervix under general anesthesia. Surgical instruments placed through channels in the scope can both cauterize and cut to remove certain types of fibroids. Hysteroscopy can also be used to cut adhesions bridging the uterine cavity (Asherman's syndrome) and to correct certain specific congenital abnormalities, such as a uterine septum. Even though hysteroscopy is usually done as a day surgery, the costs are significant.

The ultimate treatment for uterine problems is the use of a surrogate to carry the baby.

If fibroids need to be removed through an abdominal incision, the procedure (abdominal myomectomy) would carry all the risks, recuperation time and costs of any major abdominal surgery. Risks include bleeding, infection and anesthesia. In addition, there would be a significant risk of the development of adhesions at the sites where fibroids were removed. Some surgeons are using a laser to make the incisions in the uterus to try to reduce inflammation around the incision, with hope of diminishing the tendency to form adhesions. Estimated costs of an abdominal myomectomy today would probably be upwards of $10,000 U.S., depending on medical costs in your area.

Endometrial infection with ureaplasma is treatable with the long-acting form of the antibiotic tetracycline (doxycycline). Both partners are treated for 10 days with minimal cost and small chance of complications or side effects.

Tuberculosis should be treated medically, but treatment will not result in resolution of the infertility and IVF will be required.

The physical abnormalities caused by prenatal DES exposure currently cannot be treated directly, but other causes of infertility should be sought out. Treatments that increase the chance of a multiple pregnancy should be avoided as much as possible since DES-exposed individuals do not tolerate multiple pregnancy well.

Any serious uterine condition can ultimately be overcome by retrieving eggs from the infertile woman and using a surrogate to carry the pregnancy safely.

Unexplained infertility

If none of the tests has shown an abnormality, the cause of the infertility is said to be unexplained. In some such couples there may be sperm defects or egg abnormalities that have not been detected by standard tests. For example, examination of sperm for more minor defects of sperm morphology (strict morphology) has shown that many failures of fertilization with IVF are explained by a very low percentage of sperm that are truly normal. In some cases this can be remedied in vitro by adding a large number of sperm to each egg or utilizing ICSI. In other instances, the sperm may look normal but be unable to penetrate the egg. This possibility may be evaluated by testing the sperm with hamster eggs. Since the importance of this factor can't be fully known until the sperm are placed with the woman's eggs, the usefulness of the hamster test is limited. On the other side, we now know that some women have poor-quality eggs. However, most couples with unexplained failure to conceive have normal sperm and eggs; the problem is that sperm and eggs are not meeting in adequate numbers to achieve fertilization.

The number of sperm getting to the egg and staying there may be decreased by either fewer coming up the genital tract or more being removed from around the egg by scavenger cells in the pelvis. Actually, the sperm don't make their way up the genital tract under their own steam, but require contractions of the woman's reproductive organs. Problems can be caused by alterations in the muscular movements of the uterus or lower-than-normal levels of contraction-producing substances in the man's semen. Women with an infertility problem may also have increased numbers of scavenger cells (macrophages) in the pelvic cavity, which can reduce the numbers of sperm available. In other women the tubes may not have the normal capacity to pick up the egg.

In line with these basic problems of getting sperm and eggs together, such patients are often advised to have a short course of IUI. Then, to increase the numbers of eggs available to meet the sperm, the ovaries are stimulated with hMG-hCG or FSH-hCG, as in the anovulatory patient. The use of hMG or FSH/IUI makes sense before going on to IVF because it yields over 30% success over three cycles at about half the cost of GIFT or IVF. Finally, GIFT or IVF is the most direct solution, wherein the eggs and sperm are placed directly together either in the fallopian tube or the laboratory.

A study of the cost-benefit ratio of hMG with IUI compared to assisted reproductive techniques (ART) showed that the pregnancy rate for one cycle was inferior to average in vitro fertilization (IVF), gamete intrafallopian transfer (GIFT) and zygote intrafallopian transfer (ZIFT) rates. However, two cycles were comparable to IVF or ZIFT and inferior to GIFT. Three cycles were superior to IVF and ZIFT and comparable to GIFT, and four cycles were superior to the average success rates of all three ART procedures, at a lower cost. It is important to remember that this comparison was based on *average* ART success rates and thus groups achieving much better than average success might alter the conclusions reached in this study. In addition this study was done when ART success rates were not as good as they are today.

The use of hMG or FSH/IUI should be considered in all patients before going on to ART, except in those who have a documented tubal or severe sperm problem.

It is clear that one should not persist with unending cycles of gonadotropins with IUI before moving on to ART. In a 1991 study in *Fertility and Sterility*, all pregnancies occurred in the first four cycles of treatment. A January 1999 report in the *New England Journal of Medicine* concluded that superovulation with intrauterine insemination is three times more likely to result in pregnancy as intracervical insemination and twice as likely to result in pregnancy as either superovulation and intracervical insemination or intrauterine insemination alone. Age is a potent factor in the outcome of this as well as all treatments. In a 1991 review of 306 cycles from the University of Toronto published in the journal *Human Reproduction*, the pregnancy rate was 15.5% per cycle in women less than 36 years of age and 7.2% in women older than 36.

Many well-meaning friends, family members and even health professionals will give these couples advice to relax, forget it or adopt a baby. Denise, 38, who recently had a baby girl after eight years of infertility, tubal surgery and three IVF cycles, said, "If one more doctor told me to go on a vacation, I was going to scream." Interestingly, alternative methods of treatment using relaxation and stress reduction techniques may be helping to improve the chance of success. More about that in chapter 14.

Most of the time one of these conventional treatments will end up with the wife calling her husband with her positive pregnancy test in hand and exclaiming, "Honey, it worked!" But when it doesn't, you get introduced to the alphabet soup of assisted reproduction.

CHAPTER 8

Alphabet Soup

By the time you are ready to consider the techniques we call assisted reproduction, you may already have been through many years of evaluation and treatment. Now you are faced with a veritable alphabet soup of choices. IVF? GIFT? ZIFT? ICSI? AH? PGD? Which procedure should you choose?

In many cases, the selection of a procedure will be based on what type of problem is causing your infertility. But in some cases, especially when the cause of the infertility is unexplained or there is a male problem, several options may be available. The clinical procedures that are currently available include:

- IVF (In Vitro Fertilization). This is the cornerstone in the ART repertoire, where the egg and sperm are combined in the laboratory, incubated, and the resulting embryos are transferred into the woman's uterus. The acronym sometimes used for this procedure is IVF/ET or IVF/ER, indicating embryo transfer or replacement. In 2001 99% of all ART was IVF.
- GIFT (Gamete IntraFallopian Transfer). In this procedure the physician transfers a mixture of eggs and sperm into the fallopian tube during a laparoscopy, allowing fertilization to take place in the normal location. GIFT represented less than 1% of all ART in 2001.
- ZIFT (Zygote IntraFallopian Transfer). With this method, which is a mixture of IVF and GIFT, fertilization takes place in vitro, but the resulting fertilized eggs (zygotes) are placed into the fallopian tube. In the 2001 SART/CDC report ZIFT accounted for 1% of all ART.
- ICSI (IntraCytoplasmic Sperm Injection). This is a variation of IVF in which fertilization is achieved by direct injection of a single sperm

into the egg. It is utilized when the male partner has a significant problem with his sperm or when IVF is planned and there is a significant concern regarding fertilization. ICSI was performed in 50% of ART cases in 2001.

- AH (Assisted Hatching). This is an additional variation in IVF in which a small hole is made in the shell surrounding the embryo to facilitate implantation.

- FET (Frozen Embryo Transfer). The cryopreservation (freezing) of extra embryos (and later transfer) allows the chance of pregnancy when the "fresh" cycle is unsuccessful. It allows for an additional pregnancy at a later time. Embryos can be frozen at different stages from the "2PN" (the egg is fertilized and shows the male and female pronucleus (PN) through the blastocyst stage). The 2PN stage is used primarily when all conceptuses (one-day-old embryos) are frozen, for example when the woman has a high risk of ovarian hyperstimulation. The cleavage stage (embryos have divided into two to eight more cells) is used when transfer is done on Day 2 or 3 and blastocysts are frozen when a Day 5 transfer is done. There is no known limitation on the duration of storage. The longest storage with a successful pregnancy at Reproductive Partners is eight years, only because couples rarely wait a long time before returning for another pregnancy. The risk of an abnormal offspring has not been reported to be any different from regular IVF. In fact, in one report it was significantly lower.

- PGD (Preimplantation Genetic Diagnosis). This technique is also a variation of IVF. It involves removing a polar body (genetic material next to the maturing egg), or a cell from the dividing embryo for genetic analysis to avoid the transfer of genetically abnormal embryos or embryos carrying a genetic abnormality linked to the sex of the offspring (generally the male).

As you can see, many of these procedures are very similar and some, as defined by certain groups, may overlap. Others may be done in conjunction with IVF. In a few centers both GIFT and IVF may be done on the same patient at the same time, with transfer of eggs and sperm into the tube, and embryos into the uterus. Alphabet soup indeed!

A GOOD DOSE OF REALITY

Before we embark on a thorough discussion of each of these techniques, a closer look at the chances of success and failure is in order. Remember, although the success rates of these procedures continues to improve, the average chance of delivery from the transfer of fresh non-donor embryos in 2001 was only 35% under age 35, 28% between 35 and 37, 20% from 38 to 40, 10% at ages 41 and 42, and 4% over age 42.

These statistics may not sound terribly encouraging on the surface. But, as indicated previously, a reproductively normal couple has only about a 20% chance of delivering a baby as a result of a single month's attempt, and IVF patients are not reproductively normal. When you consider that many of these couples were hopelessly infertile before this technology, 40,687 babies in a single year (2001) of ART represents enormous progress.

TECHNIQUES

IVF

The procedure of in vitro fertilization/embryo transfer consists of four basic steps:

1. Ripening of the eggs
2. Retrieval of the eggs
3. Fertilization of the eggs and growth of the resulting embryo(s)
4. Transfer of the embryo(s) into the uterus

Before a patient is placed into the program, certain tests are advisable if they have not been done recently. We recommend a semen analysis, semen culture, possibly a test for antisperm antibodies in both partners, evaluation or treatment for chlamydia and a "trial transfer." The transfer is the most critical part of the process and a rehearsal of this process with a mapping of the cervical canal is most useful. In addition, most programs test for certain serious sexually transmitted diseases (testing for HIV, hepatitis B and C, HTLV-I and syphilis are required by California law).

Aspirin in IVF

A recent addition to most routine ART protocols is one of the oldest treatments in medicine. A 1999 article in *Fertility and Sterility* showed a "baby" aspirin a day to be useful in improving the results of IVF. In a randomized,

When you look at the success rates of various ART procedures you have to keep in mind that the natural rate of conception is only 20%.

controlled and double-blind placebo-controlled study, 149 patients went through IVF cycles with the only difference being the use of a single, 100 mg aspirin (available in the U.S. as 81 mg) a day in one group and a placebo in the other. Patients in the aspirin group had statistically better numbers of eggs, higher estrogen levels, more uterine and ovarian blood flow and almost double the implantation and pregnancy rates of the placebo group.

EGG DEVELOPMENT

In the initial attempts at IVF, the natural cycle of the woman was used. After the first successes it became apparent that the efficiency of the process could be improved by the development of multiple eggs. Currently, there are a variety of stimulation regimens incorporating human menopausal gonadotropins (hMG) or pure follicle stimulating hormone (FSH), with or without clomiphene citrate (cc):

- clomiphene with hMG/hCG or FSH/hCG (cc/hMG/hCG)
- hMG/hCG or FSH/hCG
- hMG/hCG or FSH/hCG combined with a GnRH analog (agonist or antagonist)

In any of these regimens hMG (Pergonal or Repronex) or pure FSH (Bravelle, Follistim or Gonal-F) can be used interchangeably, although Bravelle is somewhat less potent than Follistim or Gonal-F. In some protocols both hMG and FSH are used. A major advantage of pure FSH is the subcutaneous route of injection, which most patients can accomplish themselves with minimal instruction. Although some hMG preparations can be given subcutaneously, some individuals can have a marked local reaction.

Until the introduction of GnRH agonists, cc/hMG/hCG was the most common regimen. In most cases cc would be started on Day 2 or 3 of the cycle and continued for five days. The hMG was started before the cc was stopped (overlapping) or sometimes given simultaneously with the cc. A number of studies utilizing endometrial biopsy in women not going on to transfer have reported that the use of cc in some women interferes with the development of secretory changes that prepare the endometrium for implantation of the embryo.

Somewhat less common had been the use of hMG/hCG without cc. Again, stimulation is usually started on Day 2 or 3 of the cycle. The dose of hMG is higher, thus the number of daily injections and cost are also higher. Although no comparative study has been reported to prove greater success with avoiding the use of cc, we know that the retarded secretory development of the endometrium is prevented, and it had been empirically observed that some of the highest reported success rates had been by programs, including our own, using hMG without cc. Pure FSH has the theoretical advantage of lower LH levels during egg maturation and a recent compilation of reports confirmed that in IVF cycles not using a GnRH agonist, success rates with pure FSH were superior to hMG.

With both of these regimens the main problem has been the response of the pituitary gland to the development of multiple follicles. Estrogen levels rise to concentrations higher than in a normal cycle, triggering the premature release of luteinizing hormone (LH). LH, in turn, may cause early aging of the eggs or even release of the eggs from the ovary. In those cycles with a full surge of LH, either the cycle must be canceled or egg retrieval must be timed by frequent blood or urine LH measurements. In some cases there is a higher baseline level of LH without the surge, which has been associated with a lower rate of pregnancy.

The use of a GnRH agonist has reduced the cancellation rate from 30% to less than 10%.

Now the most common approach is to suppress the pituitary with a GnRH agonist (GnRH-a) to prevent premature release of LH. This reduces the rate of cancellation because of an LH surge, and the inconvenient frequent monitoring of LH is not necessary. A number of programs, including our own, have reported markedly decreased cancellation rates along with increased pregnancy rates. An analysis combining various studies comparing success rates with and without GnRH-a showed a twofold increase in the pregnancy rate with GnRH-a.

We have used pretreatment with a GnRH agonist, leuprolide acetate (Lupron), for most of our ovarian stimulations for well over 15 years. We feel that the use of Lupron provides more control over the stimulated cycle, an increased number of eggs and embryos, and better egg quality. Our rate of cancellation has decreased from about 30% to less than 10% and now is usually because of a poor ovarian response. We feel that this improved rate is most important since the inconvenience and psychological impact of cycle cancellation are considerable. These factors, together with the cost of the canceled cycle, more than offset the increased drug costs with the combined treatment.

Over the last few years the majority of programs, including our own, have used pretreatment with a cycle of birth control pills (OC), overlapping with Lupron. This allows us to "program" the cycle by varying the duration of OC therapy rather than by extending the ovarian suppression with GnRH-a, which can cause menopausal symptoms. It also markedly reduces the incidence of ovarian cysts resulting from the stimulatory phase of the GnRH agonist. Sometimes for scheduling purposes we still use the mid-luteal start. The mid-luteal start cycle begins about a week following an ovulation that has been documented by a urinary ovulation-detector kit. The patient comes in for an initial vaginal ultrasound scan to evaluate the baseline appearance of the pelvic organs and a blood test to prove that ovulation has occurred. If the scan is normal and the test shows evidence of ovulation, she is started on daily injections of Lupron subcutaneously. These injections can be given by her partner or self-administered. After 10 days of Lupron, or later if her menstrual period has not started, she returns for another scan and a blood test to see if her estrogen level is suppressed. A normal scan and suppressed estrogen level allow us to start her on hMG injections. The dose given is based on her weight, a count of her early (antral) follicles and a measurement of her FSH level on Day 3 of her menses, or according to her previous individual response to hMG. Again Bravelle, Follistim or Gonal-F may be given instead of, or in combination with, hMG. Since the hMG injections are intramuscular and therefore more difficult to give (the patient's partner or a friend is generally taught to do this), another option for providing some LH effect is to use a very small dose of hCG, which can be given subcutaneously. Pure FSH has become the predominant method of stimulation, although with many protocols a small dose of hMG or hCG is advised to prevent adverse effects of very low LH levels in some women who become oversuppressed with OC, GnRH-a or GnRH-antagonist (GnRH-ant).

Most recently, it has been possible to block excessive LH secretion and LH surges using a GnRH antagonist (Antagon, Cetrotide). Since it works immediately, the GnRH antagonist can be started when the lead follicle is 12 to 14 mm, resulting in many fewer injections. In order to retain flexibility for scheduling, the cycle is commonly preceded by OC. Stimulation is then begun after 4 to 5 days off the OC, using pure FSH with or without a small dose of hMG or hCG. When the GnRH-ant is started, the dose of stimulation is maintained at the same level or increased, because of the marked suppression of the patient's own circulating gonadotropins. Most programs add a small dose of hMG or hCG during GnRH-ant therapy because of the marked suppression of LH by the antagonist. There has been some concern whether the pregnancy rate is equal to agonist cycles, although it is generally felt that lack of experience with these new agents may have been the main reason for the slightly lower outcomes reported.

On the sixth day of stimulation (Day 5 with antagonist) the patient returns for a scan, which may result in a modification of her dosage. Repeat scans are done every one to three days. When the follicles reach close to mature size, blood tests for estrogen are done. When the size and number of the follicles and resulting estrogen level indicate that the eggs are mature, hCG is given and preparations are made for retrieval of the eggs.

EGG RETRIEVAL

If the eggs are not retrieved within 36 to 38 hours of the hCG injection, spontaneous ovulation may occur. Therefore, the timing of the trigger injection of hCG is crucial. If we schedule the egg retrieval for 9:30 a.m. two days hence, instructions are given to take the hCG precisely at 10:30 p.m. The precise timing of this injection has led to a number of interesting situations.

One of our patients was a movie producer who had a preview of a major motion picture scheduled for the night his wife needed her hCG precisely at 9:00 p.m. They silently tiptoed out of the theater and looked for a place to give the injection. You may never have thought about this, but there are not many good places in a packed movie theater to give an injection. They ended up in the ladies' room and unpacked their syringe, needle and vial of hCG. They mixed the hCG and she received her injection right on time. Both of them were hysterical when they realized that if anyone had happened to come into the room she probably would have thought, "Look at those Hollywood types. They can't even sit through a movie without shooting up!" Another similar situation occurred when a couple was required to attend a business meeting in a restaurant the night the hCG was required. Again, promptly at the assigned hour, the couple excused themselves, headed for a corner of the kitchen, and proceeded to "shoot up" in front of an amazed audience of waiters and busboys.

Today, eggs are usually picked up by vaginal ultrasound–guided egg retrieval. The earliest attempts were by laparoscopy, but it is rarely necessary now to do it that way. In 1985, laparoscopy was reported to account for 94.2% of egg retrievals. By 1988 only 13% were by laparoscopy. Now it is only occasionally necessary to retrieve the eggs by laparoscopy if the ovary cannot be safely aspirated vaginally.

If the retrieval is by laparoscopy, an anesthesiologist will administer either a general or epidural anesthetic. The anesthesiologist must be careful not to use agents that may be toxic to the eggs. The epidural is an injection of local anesthetic into a space near the spinal column. Little medication gets into the bloodstream, and toxicity is not a problem. The patient feels numb from the ribcage down and tolerates the laparoscopy well. The surgeon makes a small incision under the navel and inserts a telescope. Additional incisions are made to accommodate instruments to manipulate the ovaries and puncture the follicles to remove the eggs. Each follicle is punctured, the follicular fluid is removed and then culture medium may be flushed into the follicle and aspirated until the egg is found. The fluid is handed to an assistant, who passes it to the embryologist. This is continued until all the follicles have been emptied. When the procedure is finished, the incisions are closed with small stitches or paper strips.

Laparoscopy is considered an operative procedure. It requires an anesthetic and carries the risks of complications that can occur with any operation. That is not to say it is an unsafe operation. But there is the chance of bleeding, infection, injury to the bowel or other organs and reactions to the anesthetic. It also requires several days of recuperation. In order to make IVF a less expensive and more widespread technique, a search was begun for a more economical, safe and acceptable procedure to retrieve the eggs.

The first attempts at egg retrieval were made by using abdominal ultrasound to guide a needle into the follicles of the ovary through the bladder, but this technique was technically difficult and painful. It was through the development of vaginal ultrasound probes that an alternative technique blossomed. The placement of the ultrasound probe into the vagina brought it very close to the ovary, thus giving a sharp image. The addition of a needle guide to the probe allowed direct access to the ovaries. However, there are still some rare patients in whom the ovaries are inaccessible who need to have the retrieval done by laparoscopy. The advantages of ultrasound-guided follicle aspiration are that it is done with sedation rather than anesthesia and it is not a full surgical procedure—with consequently less risk, expense and recuperation time. Any of the complications mentioned with laparoscopy could occur with ultrasound retrieval, but they would be less likely. Almost all patients who have experienced both methods of retrieval prefer the ultrasound route.

The two most common techniques for pain relief are conscious sedation, using a narcotic and a sedative, or deep sedation, most often using propofol. Although the latter requires an anesthesiologist or nurse anesthetist, we prefer this method because it is difficult to pick out the few individuals who will have significant pain in spite of conscious sedation. Also patients are less anxious knowing that they will not experience pain during aspiration.

An intravenous line is started and after a mild sedative is injected through the IV, the patient is positioned as she would be for a pelvic examination. The vagina and surrounding area are washed with an antiseptic solution. Paper drapes are then put around the area and the antiseptic is washed out of the vagina with culture fluid. The ultrasound probe is then covered with a sterile sheath, the needle guide is attached and the probe is placed into the vagina. The follicles are visualized on the screen. Once all of the preparations are complete, deep sedation can be started. The needle is placed through the vaginal wall into the ovary and into the first follicle. The follicle is aspirated, may be flushed with medium, and reaspirated. Often all the follicles are aspirated by a single entry into the ovary.

In most patients, the preparation may cause the only significant discomfort during this procedure. A study of conscious sedation showed that listening to music by earphones also reduced discomfort by drawing attention away from the procedure. Of course with deep sedation, the patient will not hear, feel or remember any of the procedure. After the procedure is completed, the patient is watched for a period of time before going home.

The number of eggs retrieved can vary tremendously, up to 30 or even more. You must remember, however, that this is not a numbers game and, in general, the more eggs produced, the lower the average quality. Also, because of the risks of hyperstimulation, your physician must be somewhat conservative in advising how much medication to take. As the eggs are identified by the embryologist, they will be categorized according to apparent maturity and quality. He or she is looking for mature, good-quality eggs that will fertilize and form a good embryo. If a lot of eggs are retrieved, many may be immature and those will likely result in a lower fertilization rate. It sounds great to say, "I produced 24 eggs!" But remember that you are after a baby, not eggs. Don't be disappointed if there are only four to fertilize. It's more important that those four are of good quality. We have had many pregnancies with only one embryo to transfer.

If assisted hatching is planned for a three-day transfer the patient is started on oral doxycycline, an antibiotic, and Medrol, a steroid, the evening of the retrieval day. The night of the day following the retrieval the patient is started on progesterone injections to prime the endometrium for implantation. Most patients who have been stimulated to form many eggs have estrogen levels far in excess of normal. The elevated level of estrogen needs to be balanced by higher amounts of progesterone to form an appropriate endometrium. It has also been found recently that supplemental estrogen is helpful for implantation, since the patient's estrogen level starts to plummet about eight days after the initial injection of hCG. Follow-up doses of hCG or estrogen by mouth or skin patch will prevent the levels from falling too low. The progesterone injections and the estrogen will be continued until 16 days after egg pickup, when the pregnancy test is done, and continued if the pregnancy test is positive. Progesterone by vaginal suppository, gel or capsule may be equally effective, although the data is not entirely consistent on this issue. We do not hesitate to use this approach if the injections become problematic.

It is amazing how well most patients tolerate the vaginal egg retrieval procedure.

FERTILIZATION

While the patient is being observed following the pickup, the eggs are taken to the laboratory, where they are incubated until insemination. The incubation period allows the eggs to further mature (remember that the eggs are retrieved early so ovulation will not occur). The husband will produce a semen sample in a sterile container by masturbation. An additional sample may be requested on the day before retrieval and placed in a special medium (test yolk buffer) to enhance the ability of the sperm to penetrate the egg. The specimen is washed, incubated, and then an appropriate number (usually 50,000 to 100,000) are placed in the medium with the egg. In some cases the man will be asked to give an additional specimen if insufficient sperm were produced in the first ejaculate.

Obtaining the semen specimen is a crucial part of the process. It would seem fairly straightforward for a man who probably has provided a number of previous specimens for testing and insemination. But, as Murphy's Law states, "Whatever can go wrong probably will." We know of a number of incidents in which an adequate specimen was not forthcoming. Rarely, a man simply may not be able to perform under the tremendous stress of the importance of this particular specimen. We have, on occasion, had the wife quickly recover from her retrieval to help her husband obtain the specimen. And there have been times when in the excitement of the moment the specimen missed the cup and landed on the floor.

Perhaps the most unusual incident involved a couple who were Orthodox Jews. According to their beliefs, masturbation is not permitted and all previous specimens had been collected by intercourse, using a nontoxic condom. That's not a problem. But it was also their belief that the husband could not have intercourse with his wife until a certain period of time after her menses and only after she participated in a ritual bath. At that time, we were not using Lupron, and since her follicles developed very quickly, the cycle had to be canceled. Now many rabbis feel that exceptions can be made to these rules if a greater good is to be achieved through the procedure. Some of our patients of various religions have searched until they have found a sufficiently flexible cleric to advise them.

It would be possible to fill a book with interesting "obtaining the semen specimen" stories.

Assuming that sperm can be obtained and the eggs inseminated, the next morning the eggs will be examined for evidence of fertilization. We hope to see two structures in each egg, the male and female pronuclei, indicating that fertilization has taken place. At this time abnormal eggs, those that may have fertilized with more than one sperm, will be discarded. Those that did not fertilize may be inseminated again and fertilization will be checked the next day. In some cases, embryos are frozen at this stage.

Two, but more commonly three days after the retrieval, the eggs are checked again. This time we are looking for evidence that the fertilized eggs, now embryos, have divided. They will be scored according to their number of cells and other characteristics. The previously unfertilized eggs will be checked again for evidence of fertilization. Selection will be made on the basis of embryo morphology (appearance) as to which will be:

- discarded because they did not fertilize, divide, or are abnormal
- frozen
- transferred into the uterus

EMBRYO TRANSFER (REPLACEMENT)

The selection of how many embryos to transfer and which ones to use takes a great deal of experience and is probably the second most important decision couples have to make in connection with ART procedures. (The most important decision is which center to select to do the ART procedure, and this will be considered later.) In some places a limit to the number of embryos to be transferred is written into law, such as in England where no more than two embryos may be transferred. In England the government pays for ART procedures as part of the national health plan, so limiting costs for multiple pregnancies is a higher priority than maximizing the chance of becoming pregnant. The English Human Fertilisation and Embryology Authority has complete control over all reproductive medical procedures, including strict limitations on the number of embryos to be transferred. In the United States and Canada there is no legislation limiting the number of embryos in IVF or the number of eggs in GIFT that can be placed back into the woman's body. SART and ASRM developed guidelines in November 1999 for U.S. fertility clinics to follow, which has achieved a better balance between a successful outcome and the risks and expense of multiple pregnancy. The guidelines include:

When thinking about how many embryos to transfer, remember the "more is better" misconception.

* Most favorable prognosis (e.g., female partner under age 35 with embryos of sufficient quality and quantity for freezing and improved embryo quality as judged by morphologic features): usually no more than two good-quality embryos should be transferred.
* Above-average prognosis patient (e.g., female partner under 35 without sufficient embryo quality or quantity for freezing): usually no more than three embryos should be transferred.
* Average prognosis patient (e.g., female partner age 35 to 40): usually no more than four good-quality embryos should be transferred.
* Below-average prognosis patient (e.g., female partner age greater than 40 or multiple failed cycles): usually no more than five good embryos should be transferred.
* Donor egg cycles: the age of the donor should be used in determining the number of embryos to be transferred.

Most couples are willing to take our strong advice to follow the SART/ASRM guidelines when it is made clear that multiple pregnancy, even twins, is associated with many potential complications for both mother and infants. Even with careful selection of the best embryos their success rate will not be enhanced enough by transferring more embryos to warrant the increased risks. Curiously, the rate of multiple pregnancy has been higher than one would calculate it should be. This observation suggests that additional embryos actually help each other develop and implant, and thereby increase the chance of success. The chance of multiple pregnancy also increases in proportion to the success rate of a program, as it is an index of embryo quality and therefore the quality of the laboratory. In specific instances, such as with an abnormal uterine cavity or when twins would complicate a medical condition of the woman, a single embryo may be transferred.

The embryo transfer, done in the dark and quiet, is almost a mystical experience.

The selection of the particular embryos to be transferred is based on experience. The physical characteristics considered favorable are:

- greater number of cells
- uniform size and shape of the cells
- absence of fragmentation of the cells
- areas of thinning of the zona (shell)

But, in the final analysis, these factors only lead to tendencies toward a better implantation. We know that sometimes very irregular embryos can develop into healthy pregnancies. So, although we can try to limit the risk of multiple pregnancy, currently we simply do not have the means to tell with certainty which embryos will implant. Additional embryos that are of adequate quality are then frozen for later use.

Over the past several years, investigations into the differing environment of the fallopian tube and uterus and the corresponding requirements of the embryos during development—over the first two days after fertilization when they normally reside in the fallopian tube and the following two days when they are in the uterus—have resulted in the development of "sequential" media which support in vitro development of healthy blastocysts that can then be transferred on Day 5 after retrieval. This allows better selection of the best-quality embryos, allowing transfer of only one or two high-quality blastocysts. The risk of triplets is minimized (there is a low incidence of identical twinning associated with the procedure) and the uterus is more quiescent for the embryo transfer. More success is shifted to the fresh cycle, whereas the results with embryo freezing of blastocysts have not been not as high as with cleaved embryos. This technique is most applicable to couples with many good-quality follicles, eggs and embryos, for whom the risk of high order multiple pregnancy is the greatest. One of the most difficult situations we encounter is when no embryos reach the blastocyst stage. There is no transfer and then the couple feels they could have been successful with Day 3 transfer. Some programs that have made blastocyst culture routine feel that an embryo that failed to develop in vitro also would have failed in vivo. Most programs, including our own, take a middle-of-the-road position in offering this option for women with a good number of follicles. It is particularly applicable to women between age 35 and 40 for whom transfer of more than two embryos is often considered.

The woman is given Valium orally about an hour before the transfer. She is placed in the pelvic examination position in a darkened, quiet room. Her mate can sit by her side, holding her hand. The incubator holding the embryos to be transferred is quietly wheeled into the room. As a speculum is placed in the vagina, the partner has an opportunity to come over to the incubator to look through the microscope and view the potential offspring. This is a special moment and a very emotional one. After all those years, tests, treatments and disappointments, there they are—embryos, any or all of which have the potential to develop into their children. After rejoining his partener, the embryos are drawn up into a small plastic catheter which will be threaded into the uterus through the cervix. The cervix is washed by the doctor and the catheter is placed according to a map drawn during a trial transfer done prior to this cycle. Many centers, including our own, are now performing ultrasound-guided embryo transfers in order to assure placement of the embryos in the proper position in the uterus. When ultrasound is employed, the transfer is performed with the patient's bladder full. The full bladder assures a better ultrasound picture and has the additional benefit of straightening the cervical canal in many cases, making the transfer easier to perform. The embryos are expelled from the catheter. The catheter is withdrawn and the patient rests in the transfer bed for 30 minutes. She is instructed to rest at home for the next two days and then avoid strenuous activity, exercise and intercourse for the next two weeks until the pregnancy test.

SUCCESS AND FAILURE

Not every patient who enters the program completes the cycle. Cancellation of the cycle can occur during any of the four stages. We have cited several instances above. However, most cancellations will occur during the stimulation. These may be the result of:

- development of only one or two follicles;
- failure of any follicles to develop; or
- development of too many small follicles, which could lead to hyperstimulation and result in a very high estrogen level that could inhibit implantation.

Failure is the most difficult aspect to deal with for both the patient and IVF team.

At times, poor fertilization may result in not having any embryos to transfer. With ICSI now advised for instances where a significant problem with fertilization is anticipated, this is rarely due to the male. We recently had a patient who had gone through several unsuccessful cycles before we saw her. Six eggs were retrieved but only three fertilized. On the second day it was noted that none of the fertilized eggs had divided, which is extremely unusual. One of the previously unfertilized eggs had fertilized. The transfer was postponed until the next day, when only the egg that had fertilized on the second try had divided. From six promising eggs, only one embryo was available for transfer. It was transferred on the third day following retrieval, but with only a very small chance of success. She did not get pregnant. In her case it was now obvious that her multiple failed cycles involved poor-quality eggs, whereas their previous poor performance had been attributed only to a sperm problem. The appearance of her eggs to the experienced eye was very unusual. She was matched with an egg donor. As you will see in chapter 12, she will now have an excellent chance of success.

Assuming a couple completes the cycle, what are their chances of having a baby? According to the 2001 SART/CDC report with 384 centers reporting, the clinical pregnancy rate was 32.8% of fresh, non-donor ART cycles begun in all age categories. Almost 83% of those pregnancies resulted in live births: 53.1% singletons and 29.1% multiple-infant births. In fresh cycles when a donor was used the live birth rate was 47% per transfer; 27.4% live birth rate per transfer in frozen donor cycles. (For the detailed success rates of individual programs for the latest survey as reported to the SART/CDC Registry, go to the cdc.gov website. For the detailed 2001 National Summary see Appendix I.)

"Natural cycle" IVF

The first attempts and success with IVF were performed within the woman's natural cycle. In an attempt to make the process more efficient various stimulation protocols were developed. Some reproductive specialists believe that there is still occasionally a legitimate place in today's practice of assisted reproduction for "natural cycle" IVF. In 2001 less than 1% of ART cycles were unstimulated. Unstimulated IVF's benefits include lower costs, fewer injections, better acceptability for women who may have ethical or religious problems with embryo freezing and the disposition of extra embryos, and virtually no risk of multiple pregnancy. With the lower cost a couple can afford to go through more cycles.

Natural cycle IVF is now rarely done probably because of the low success rates.

EGG DEVELOPMENT

With availability of GnRH antagonists, it is now possible to allow full maturity of the follicle without fearing an LH surge. By giving the antagonist and supporting the follicle with hMG, the oocyte is allowed to fully mature. An injection of hCG is then given and the retrieval will be scheduled for 35 hours later.

RETRIEVAL

The retrieval will be performed using a vaginal ultrasound probe just as in stimulated cycles. One of the major limitations of natural cycle IVF is the difficulty in achieving a high retrieval rate from these large follicles that tend to fold in as they collapse. Use of a double-lumen needle allowing repeated flushing with less concern about losing the egg may improve the efficiency of this option. The fact that only one follicle is being retrieved means that less sedation is necessary and the observation period after the procedure is shorter.

FERTILIZATION

Fertilization technique is identical to that in stimulated cycles but, of course, only one egg is available for insemination.

TRANSFER

Transfer technique is identical to stimulated cycles, but with the advantage that the endometrium is more favorable for implantation since it is not disturbed by the pattern and level of hormones accompanying ovarian stimulation.

Use of a GnRH antagonist for the natural cycle has recently been reported to result in a 17% delivery rate per egg retrieval. Unstimulated cycles, which comprised less than 1% of all ART cycles, were not reported separately in the 2001 SART/CDC report. Further refinements and simplification of monitoring and egg retrieval could make this a cost-effective option in the future.

GIFT

In GIFT (gamete intrafallopian transfer) the sperm and eggs (gametes) are placed together and transferred into the fallopian tube by means of a catheter during a laparoscopy. The apparent differences between IVF and GIFT are that GIFT requires that the tubes must be open and normal, and the partner needs to have an adequate semen specimen. Obstructed fallopian tubes are one of the primary reasons for performing IVF. In GIFT, fertilization takes place in its normal location, the fallopian tube. It also eliminates the most critical part of IVF, the embryo transfer. Although for many years the average success for GIFT exceeded IVF, as the quality of IVF laboratories has continued to improve, the success rates of IVF and GIFT are now equal. There are few properly controlled studies comparing IVF and GIFT in the same patients, although those that have been done have shown no difference.

If the woman needs an ART procedure because of endometriosis, pelvic adhesions with normal tubes, or mild male factor or unexplained infertility, the couple may choose IVF or GIFT. In general, men with significant sperm problems or women with abnormal tubes should not have GIFT. Some specific indications for GIFT are failed donor insemination, since the fertilizing capacity of the sperm is particularly high; difficult transcervical embryo transfer; and perhaps women over age 40 or with multiple failed cycles of IVF. Dr. Bill Yee, medical director of Reproductive Partners Medical Group, Inc., has had extensive experience with the GIFT procedure. He feels that the success rate may be higher in some women with GIFT because fertilization and embryo development take place in the normal environment. He says, "What Mother Nature did for millions of years in developing the fallopian tube makes it the best site for the egg and early embryo." But he does not feel locked into the GIFT decision. The tubes should be perfectly normal with no previous surgery performed on them. He takes a careful look at the tube and makes sure he can pass a catheter at least four centimeters into the tube before transferring the eggs and sperm. If the tube appears abnormal or he cannot pass the catheter, he will convert the cycle to IVF.

In cases where the cause of infertility is mild male factor, Dr. Yee would proceed with GIFT if a good number of eggs develop because more eggs than the number to be transferred will be fertilized in vitro, allowing direct observation of the fertilization process and detection of fertilization problems. In such cases, if the woman developed only a few eggs, he would suggest converting the cycle to IVF. Other factors to be considered are insurance coverage for one procedure and not the other, and the age of the patient. The eggs of women of advanced age may do better in the natural environment.

As of July 1988 the ASRM developed the following standards for consideration of the GIFT procedure:

Dr. Bill Yee feels that the fallopian tube is the best environment for fertilization to take place.

Our experience is that more insurance companies cover GIFT than IVF. Add this to the list of criteria for GIFT.

- The patient and her partner have been investigated using ASRM minimum standards.
- The patient has at least one normal fallopian tube and a cause of infertility not amenable to less invasive techniques.
- The facility performing the procedure has a laboratory and personnel that meet the ASRM's minimum standards for IVF.
- GIFT is performed in a facility that is prepared to carry out IVF as an alternative if GIFT does not prove a feasible option.

These are good rules to remember and to apply to a program if you are considering GIFT.

Basically, a GIFT cycle consists of three steps:

1. Development and ripening of the eggs
2. Retrieval of the eggs
3. Transfer of the eggs and washed sperm into the fallopian tube

Before a patient enters a GIFT program, the same basic tests may be done as those carried out prior to an IVF cycle. The only exception is that there is no absolute need to perform a trial transfer, since an embryo transfer would not be anticipated unless the fallopian tubes were found to be abnormal. Documentation that the tubes are open is prudent if it has not been confirmed recently. The main reasons for performing GIFT are prolonged infertility as the result of:

- unexplained infertility
- endometriosis
- a mild male factor

Don't let anyone talk you into an ART procedure prematurely. Here are the standards for consideration of the GIFT procedure.

EGG DEVELOPMENT

In order to achieve maximum efficiency of the GIFT process, stimulation of the ovaries similar to that for IVF will usually be carried out in order that an average of four eggs can be transferred to the fallopian tube. As with IVF, stimulation protocols can vary considerably among programs. But, in general, the administration of the drugs and monitoring of the cycles with ultrasound and estrogen levels are similar to what we described with IVF.

EGG RETRIEVAL

Once the hCG is given, the retrieval is scheduled 34 to 35 hours later. It is done by transvaginal ultrasound or laparoscopy, as described in the section on IVF, since this is the means by which the eggs will be replaced in the tube.

TRANSFER

The difference between GIFT transfer and the laparoscopy for IVF is that after the eggs are retrieved, the embryologist will categorize them as to quality and maturity, select the best for transfer and load them together with sperm into a special catheter for placement into the tube. The catheter will then be passed through one of the instruments and carefully placed into the fallopian tube. The ASRM/SART guidelines allow one more egg to be transferred than embryos in each prognostic category outlined above in the IVF transfer. At present usually three to four eggs and an appropriate number of sperm are then injected through the catheter at least four centimeters into the fallopian tube, allowing fertilization to occur in its normal place in the body. The embryos then make their own way down the tube and into the uterus for implantation.

When the procedure was first developed, half the eggs and sperm were placed in each fallopian tube. That is, if four eggs were transferred, two with appropriate numbers of sperm would be placed in each tube. Recently, pregnancy rates have been reported to be as high and even higher by transferring all the eggs and sperm into one of the tubes.

We now put all the eggs with sperm into one tube.

SUCCESS AND FAILURE

The average chance of a GIFT procedure resulting in a live birth is the same as for IVF, although not all patients treatable by IVF are candidates for GIFT. The most significant problem that cannot be treated with GIFT is, of course, tubal obstruction. In 2001 the SART/CDC Registry included the delivery rates for GIFT procedures along with IVF in the total ART success rates. Less than 1% of the cases of ART were GIFT in 2001.

There is, according to this report, a great variation in success in clinics doing ART. The implications for the consumer are obvious. For programs with a good IVF laboratory and physicians experienced with operative laparoscopy, achieving good success with GIFT is not difficult, but neither of these prerequisites can be assumed. Comparing outcomes for IVF and GIFT is difficult since the success rates of each are not reported individually for centers that do both in the SART/CDC report. It is further complicated by differences in patient populations undergoing each procedure. Since GIFT is done earlier in the infertility evaluation and IVF is sometimes done after failed GIFT procedures, the GIFT success rate should be slightly higher than IVF to consider it clearly more successful.

A definite limitation of GIFT is less ability to minimize high order multiple pregnancy compared to IVF. With increasing emphasis on transferring only one or two embryos, it is likely that GIFT may be done only for specific indications in the future. One of those indications may be in the woman aged 40 to 42 in which the couple does not have an absolute cause for their infertility, leaving age as a major factor. In a 1998 study published in the *Journal of Reproductive Medicine* the authors found a delivery rate of 25% per stimulation cycle in 24 consecutive stimulation cycles in women aged 40 to 42 between 1988 and 1997. This is a far better rate than the average success rates for IVF reported in the SART survey for those years in that age group. But before you get too excited, remember that more favorable patients are generally selected for GIFT, which can partially explain the disparity.

ZIFT

ZIFT requires both an ultrasound egg retrieval and laparoscopy to place the zygotes into the fallopian tube.

This procedure is similar to basic GIFT, except that instead of sperm and eggs, fertilized eggs (zygotes) are placed into the fallopian tube. The advantage over a transfer into the uterus is to allow the embryos to spend time in the natural environment of the fallopian tube and then enter the uterus in the normal manner, without the potential adverse effects of an embryo transfer. The benefit of placing embryos rather than sperm and eggs is that you then know that fertilization has occurred, avoiding one drawback of the GIFT procedure. Also, fertilization occurs more reliably in the laboratory, where a high concentration of sperm can be placed close to the egg. This is especially useful if the problem is a male factor or if you have unexplained infertility, both of which result in a reduced chance of fertilization.

ZIFT will consist of four parts:

1. Development and ripening of the eggs
2. Retrieval of the eggs
3. Fertilization of the egg and growth of the embryo
4. Placement of the embryo into the fallopian tube

EGG DEVELOPMENT

The stimulation protocol for these procedures will vary, depending upon the preferences of a particular program. Basically, the same drugs and monitoring will be employed as for IVF or GIFT.

EGG RETRIEVAL

Vaginal ultrasound–directed retrieval would be performed as if in an IVF cycle.

FERTILIZATION

Again, the eggs and sperm would be brought together in the laboratory and fertilization would be "in vitro" as in IVF.

PLACEMENT IN THE TUBE

This is the aspect in which ZIFT procedures differ from IVF. Depending upon which stage of embryo is going to be selected for placement in the fallopian tube, a laparoscopy would be scheduled at the proper interval after the retrieval. Strictly speaking, the embryos would be transferred into the woman's fallopian tube 18 to 24 hours after fertilization. At this point the embryo has not yet divided and is still a single cell, hence the name zygote. However, the term ZIFT is also loosely applied to all transfers of embryos into the fallopian tube, including cleaved embryos which are typically transferred two days after the retrieval at about the four-cell stage.

The success rate of ZIFT is not much better than for GIFT.

SUCCESS AND FAILURE

The 2001 SART/CDC Registry results showed that less than 1% of ART cycles were ZIFT. Success rates were included in the total ART for each center, so it is difficult to compare ZIFT with IVF or GIFT success rates of an individual center. Again, any advantage over IVF depends on the specific rates for IVF and ZIFT in the individual center.

ICSI

ICSI (intracytoplasmic sperm injection) has revolutionized IVF because it has allowed us to offer treatment to men for whom no treatment was available. Not only will it help couples in whom the male has just a few, barely swimming sperm in the ejaculate, but thanks to advanced techniques for aspirating sperm from the ductal system and techniques for harvesting sperm from testicular biopsies, it can also aid men who ejaculate no sperm. These sperm-harvesting techniques include MESA (microsurgical epididymal sperm aspiration) and PESA (percutaneous epididymal sperm aspiration), an office procedure where sperm can be obtained by passing a tiny needle through the skin into the epididymis. Testicular sperm extraction (TESE) can be used to obtain sperm in many men. This is also an office procedure, sometimes done with a needle rather than as a full surgical biopsy, but sperm are obtained less reliably this way. It is usually done with a large biopsy needle under local anesthesia.

This new micromanipulation treatment, which was developed in Belgium and introduced into the United States in 1993, evolved from previous attempts at micromanipulation such as PZD (partial zona dissection) and SUZI (subzonal insertion), which did not enjoy the success that ICSI has attained.

ICSI has revolutionized the treatment of severe male infertility.

The IVF cycle is conducted exactly in the manner described above, with a very few exceptions. After the eggs are retrieved, instead of mixing the sperm with the egg, the embryologist utilizes a thin glass pipette to immobilize the sperm, sucks it up into the pipette and then injects it directly into the egg's cytoplasm. Since the egg is the size of a pinpoint, it is a sophisticated technique requiring a high-powered microscope, tiny glass pipettes and instruments that translate hand movements into extremely fine movements of the pipettes.

SUCCESS AND FAILURE

In the 2001 SART/CDC report, 50% of ART cases involved ICSI. The success rates for ICSI are the same as for IVF, indicating that the manipulation has very little effect on the egg. However, since the female partners of these men are reproductively normal, there may be some small adverse effect, also reflected in reports of slightly reduced embryo quality with ICSI. Most data indicates similar rates of abnormalities with ICSI and IVF, although some reports suggest a minor increase of chromosomal anomalies, many of which are related to the man's genetics or his sperm, rather than the procedure itself. Because of these concerns, prenatal genetic testing with a fetal karyotype is suggested for ICSI pregnancies. Recently concerns about a higher rate of some very rare abnormalities may be associated with IVF and ICSI, specifically Beckwith-Wiedemann syndrome which includes kidney problems, low blood sugar and an increased risk of childhood tumors.

In a proportion of men (10% to 20%) with very low or absent sperm in the ejaculate, the man may have a chromosome defect or a genetic defect not visible on routine chromosome analysis (Y chromosome microdeletion) that could pass on a similar problem with infertility to male offspring. Rarely, such a chromosomal defect could cause a serious abnormality in the offspring. We therefore suggest a karyotype for men with fewer than 5 to 10 million sperm per ml in the ejaculate. In men with congenital absence of the vas deferens, one can assume the male is a carrier for cystic fibrosis (CF). Since such men can have a mutation not screened for in the standard CF panel, it is recommended to test the female partner. If she is a carrier, the couple could elect to have their embryos tested for CF.

AH (Assisted Hatching)

One of the most frustrating aspects of assisted reproductive technology for patients and fertility professionals alike is having to deal with failure. This is especially true in couples who have attempted assisted reproductive procedures many times, and also in those whose time is running out because of their age. Assisted hatching is offering hope to couples who fall into these categories.

Assisted hatching was developed from the observation that embryos with a thin zona pellucida (shell) had a higher rate of implantation during in vitro fertilization. It was postulated that creating a minor defect in the zona might result in a greater chance of the embryo "hatching," or shedding its shell, allowing for a better chance of implantation in the endometrium.

Initial controlled trials at New York-Cornell Medical College showed an increase in implantation in all women studied and particularly in those over age 38 or with an elevated FSH level on Day 3 of the menstrual cycle. Couples with multiple failed IVF cycles also appear to benefit from assisted hatching. AH may be helpful for these infertile couples because their embryos lack sufficient energy to complete the "hatching" process. It is thought that some women may fail multiple cycles of IVF because their eggs have a thicker shell; therefore they have a better prognosis with assisted hatching. In addition, hatched embryos implant one day early, which may allow a greater opportunity for implantation to occur, particularly if the endometrium is advanced by the ovarian stimulation.

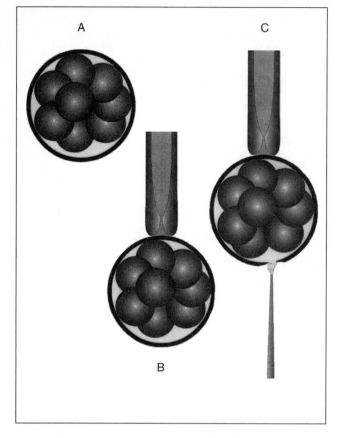

Figure 5   Micromanipulation of Embryos

The addition of assisted hatching to the standard IVF protocol does add extra laboratory manipulation and therefore added costs. There is a small risk of damage to the embryo during the micromanipulation process or at the time of transfer, and there may be a slight increase in identical twinning compared with regular IVF. In our practice we have not observed such an increase. This may relate to whether a large enough opening is made in the zona to prevent pinching of the embryo during the hatching process.

The IVF cycle is conducted in the routine manner until the evening of the day of retrieval, when the patient is started on four days of a steroid, methylprednisolone, and an antibiotic, tetracycline, to protect the embryo from inflammatory cells. The fertilized embryos are allowed to develop until the third day following the retrieval, since the more advanced embryo is more resistant to the effects of inflammatory cells.

The assisted hatching procedure, like ICSI, is carried out by a technique known as micromanipulation. In small dishes the embryos (Figure 5), which now contain an average of six to eight cells (A), are stabilized by a holding pipette (B), while on the opposite side a small pipette containing acidified Tyrode's solution creates a small defect in the zona (C). The size of the defect is critical; if it is too small it may pinch off the embryo during hatching and either reduce the chance of implantation or cause identical twinning. The embryos are then rinsed to remove any excess acid solution and returned to the incubator for a few hours before transfer into the uterus.

SUCCESS AND FAILURE

This relatively small variation in the IVF procedure has yielded dramatic results. First, we discovered that there is a learning curve for this procedure that requires a certain amount of experience with the technique before patients can reap maximum benefits. Our second conclusion was that assisted hatching improved the success rate in women between 35 and 40 so much that it began exceeding the results of our women under 35. Since the initial results with AH reported at Cornell showed an improved outcome at all ages, we have therefore also done this procedure in the younger women.

The bottom line for couples who fall into the poor-prognosis category because of age, previously failed cycles or elevated FSH levels on the third day of their menstrual cycle is that they should consider adding assisted hatching to the regular regimen of in vitro fertilization. It is important to be sure that the center they choose has enough experience with the technique to assure it has passed the early part of the learning curve and is achieving an enhanced success rate.

FET (Frozen Embryo Transfer)

One of the developments in assisted reproduction that has increased the efficiency of IVF procedures is embryo freezing (cryopreservation). Sperm freezing has been routine for some time and techniques to freeze embryos are currently being employed in most programs. Most recently, techniques have been developed to successfully freeze oocytes. Since we now have the technology to stimulate the production of many eggs and have efficient techniques to retrieve those eggs and fertilize them, the ability to freeze the embryos and utilize them in multiple cycles improves efficiency. One stimulation and retrieval can provide embryos not only for a transfer during that IVF cycle but also for additional frozen embryo transfer cycles.

One example of this ability is the story of Jane and Terry Mohr. The story of the birth of their "triplets" 21 months apart was reported nationwide and described in detail in *Redbook* magazine. Jane's first pregnancy at age 33 was an ectopic pregnancy in the left fallopian tube. Her second pregnancy was also discovered to be ectopic, this time in the right tube. The tube was surgically opened, the pregnancy removed and the tube repaired. Her third pregnancy, stimulated by clomiphene, was also ectopic, in the

Assisted hatching has had the greatest impact in achieving success rates in women up to age 43 similar to those in women under 40.

right tube. By this time, after three ectopic pregnancies, her doctor referred her for in vitro fertilization, fearing that her tubes were too severely damaged to try again.

She entered the UCLA IVF program (when Dr. Meldrum was there) and on June 26, 1986, 10 eggs were retrieved. Nine of those eggs fertilized and four were implanted into her uterus two days following the retrieval. The remaining five were frozen. On February 15, 1987, their son Cooper, weighing 3 pounds 14 ounces, was born by caesarean section in Jane's eighth month of pregnancy when she developed toxemia. When Dr. Meldrum moved his program to Redondo Beach, the Mohrs asked that their frozen embryos also be moved, since they lived close to the new center. In March 1988, Jane returned to have her frozen embryos transferred. Three of the five had survived the freeze and thaw and were transferred into the uterus. On November 29, 1988, twin daughters Hannah Christina and Mollie McKenna were born, each weighing more than five pounds. Cooper and the twin girls are technically triplets, conceived during the same cycle but, through assisted reproductive technology, born almost two years apart. Since then we have had many couples who have had up to three deliveries eight years apart from the same egg retrieval.

The use of frozen embryos makes the whole IVF process more cost-effective by increasing total success at little added cost.

Freezing embryos is an option all couples going through IVF should consider. However, even for those who have no ethical problems with embryo freezing, many decisions have to be made regarding disposition of the frozen embryos in the event of divorce or death—or even a cross-country move. In divorce, the couple may choose to assign the embryos to one or another of them, donate them to another couple or discard them. In case of the death of one member of the couple, the other could take possession. If both die, the frozen embryos could be donated or discarded. Difficult as this is to think about, these decisions must be made prior to the actual procedure.

A most unusual situation regarding frozen embryos was the widely publicized case of Risa and Steven York. In 1986, the Yorks went through an IVF program at the Jones Institute for Reproductive Medicine in Norfolk, Virginia. After failed attempts at IVF and frozen embryo transfers, the Yorks moved from New Jersey to California and requested that their one remaining frozen embryo be transferred to a comparable facility in Los Angeles. The Jones Institute refused and offered them four choices. They could have the embryo transferred into her uterus at the Jones Institute, or have it donated to another couple, destroyed or used for experimentation.

The Yorks sued, but a federal judge refused to grant a preliminary injunction and ordered a trial to begin some time later. This was a problem for Mrs. York, 39, because her increasing age might reduce her chance of becoming pregnant. This case raises the question, "Just whose embryo is it?" The mother's, the father's, or the doctor's? We believe that a couple's embryos are the property of the couple and decisions as to the disposition must remain their sole right. But happily for the Yorks, this matter did not go to court. A settlement was reached in September 1989 whereby the clinic released the embryo and the Yorks released the clinic from any liability and agreed to drop their $200,000 lawsuit for emotional stress.

The nation's population of frozen embryos is growing. A survey in 2003 concluded that there were close to 400,000 embryos frozen in fertility clinics throughout the U.S. There are bound to be other conflicts like that between Mary Sue and Junior Davis. In this divorce case, Mary Sue wanted to keep the embryos in storage in case she wanted to use them or donate them to another couple. Junior Davis wanted them destroyed because he felt that their use after the divorce would force him into unwanted fatherhood. If that happened, would he have to pay child support? Logically, the embryos would be treated as property in a divorce settlement, to be awarded to the partner with the predominating cause of infertility. However, at the trial court level the case was decided in favor of Mary Sue, based on the judge's ruling that the embryos were children and custody was awarded based on child custody law. Finally, the Tennessee Supreme Court ruled that Junior Davis's constitutional rights would have been violated if he was forced to become a father against his will. The U.S. Supreme Court refused to review the ruling and the embryos were destroyed.

Most of the time there is no conflict. The couple usually have a single purpose—to have a baby—and frozen embryos can increase their chances. The frozen embryo transfer consists of four steps:

1. Freezing of the embryos not being transferred during the IVF cycle
2. Storage of the embryos
3. Monitoring of the frozen embryo cycle
4. Thawing of the embryos and transfer to the uterus

FREEZING

Most IVF programs now freeze embryos at the time of embryo transfer, rather than at the 2PN stage, thus allowing the best embryos to be chosen from all that are available. This in turn has allowed programs to reduce the number of embryos transferred to minimize multiple implantations. Since the best embryos are transferred fresh, and there is some adverse effect of freezing, the success rates are somewhat lower with FET. On the other hand, the endometrium is likely to be more receptive than it is following ovarian stimulation. There may be some specific instances when the stimulated endometrium or the quality of the luteal phase prevents implantation in the IVF cycle itself. A couple in our program who experienced two very early (biochemical pregnancy) losses is an example. Her embryo quality was good and we speculated that difficulty with implantation might be the issue. She delivered twins from frozen embryos transferred in a natural cycle. In her specific case, she produced very high-quality embryos, but her stimulated endometrium may have been the problem.

The frozen embryo cycle is a very easy process for the patient compared to the complete IVF or GIFT cycle.

Occasionally, all the embryos are frozen because the risk of hyperstimulation is lower if pregnancy does not occur. This has become less common since the use of "coasting," which involves keeping the patient on Lupron while stopping the gonadotropin to allow the estrogen level to fall into a range where hyperstimulation generally does not occur.

STORAGE

The embryos are maintained in a frozen state in liquid nitrogen with an alarm to prevent inadvertent thawing due to, for example, rare failure of the insulation of the storage tank. The embryos theoretically can be maintained in a frozen state indefinitely. Provided they are kept immersed, they will probably remain unchanged for the reproductive life of the woman, which is the current ethical guideline in the United States for the duration of storage.

MONITORING THE FROZEN EMBRYO CYCLE

As you would expect, we do not want to place these valuable embryos into the uterus unless the endometrium is perfectly primed for implantation with the correct hormonal sequence of a normal ovulatory cycle. At the onset of a menstrual period the woman is started on estrogen, usually in the form of either a pill or a skin patch. An estrogen level may be obtained on the fifth day of the cycle to adjust the dose to achieve optimal levels. The dose is gradually increased to mimic a normal cycle or kept constant at a moderate dose. On the 14th day of the cycle an ultrasound is performed to measure endometrial thickness. We generally want an endometrium to be nine millimeters thick. If the thickness is not sufficient, the estrogen is continued and sometimes increased. If a follicle is seen on ultrasound, a progesterone level is obtained to insure that spontaneous ovulation has not occurred. Premature ovulation would mature the endometrium too quickly and make it out of phase with the embryos. Progesterone is then started and the thawing and transfer are scheduled. In some programs, a GnRH agonist is given to suppress the ovary before estrogen is given. We have found this not to be necessary except in those rare patients whose ovarian function is not suppressed by the estrogen replacement therapy.

THAWING AND TRANSFER

The timing of the thaw and transfer is based on the age of the embryos. Currently, about 70% of the embryos survive the freeze and thaw. The transfer procedure is carried out in the same manner as in the IVF cycle we previously described.

SUCCESS AND FAILURE

Frozen embryos were used in approximately 14% of all ART cycles in 2001 with a live birth rate of 23.4% per transfer using non-donor eggs. In cycles when donor eggs were used the live birth rate was 27.3% of transfers performed in 2001. Remember that these patients did not have to go through stimulation or retrieval. Instead of looking at this rate only, we should actually add 23.4% and 27.3% to the success rates of the IVF non-donor and donor cycles from which they resulted. (Keep in mind that only about half of couples using their own eggs have extra embryos to freeze.)

PGD (Preimplantation Genetic Diagnosis)

PGD is a relatively new procedure which can be used to screen embryos in couples who have a family history of certain genetic diseases, or to determine if abnormal chromosomes may be present in embryos of couples in which there are no known genetic concerns. The primary indication for

PGD is for the couple known to be at risk for a genetic disorder. For example, if a couple have had a child with cystic fibrosis, or they have been found to both be carriers through routine screening, their chance of having an affected child is 25%. Rather than becoming pregnant, having prenatal testing and aborting an affected fetus, the couple may choose to undergo PGD. In other instances, only one parent may be affected, but 50% of the offspring will be abnormal (dominant disorders). The third most common indication for PGD is for sex-linked disorders, in which only male embryos are affected, as in hemophilia, where there is an abnormality on the X chromosome which becomes dominant when there is not a second X as there is in a female (XX). Thus only males (XY) are affected. In this instance, only female embryos would be transferred. Finally, a couple may choose PGD because of repeated miscarriage and because one partner has a chromosomal translocation (when part of a chromosome is attached to another chromosome, resulting in some embryos having less or more genetic material than normal).

A more controversial indication for PGD is the screening of embryos in women of advanced age for aneuploidy (errors in the number of chromosomes). This concept has not yet been accepted because of additional costs of several thousand dollars, an error rate estimated at 10% and potential damage to embryos in the process without good evidence of its efficacy. It sounds like it makes sense. The main reason for the lower rate of success and increased miscarriage in older women is that a high proportion of their embryos are genetically abnormal. If one can identify the normal and abnormal embryos accurately and without affecting the viability of the biopsied embryos, the pregnancy rate could increase and the rate of miscarriage could be lower. One team that has been performing this procedure for several years on selected patients with a good ovarian response has reported improved results, but the final verdict is not yet in on this application of PGD.

OBTAINING AND EVALUATING
THE GENETIC MATERIAL

Micromanipulation techniques are used either to remove the polar body next to the egg, which contains a set of the egg's chromosomes discarded during egg maturation, or to remove a cell from the Day 3 embryo, usually at the six- to eight-cell stage. Various genetic analyses can be done to determine whether a normal set of chromosomes is present, or whether the embryo carries an abnormal gene. The current technique of fluorescent in situ hybridization (FISH), which uses specific probes for errors in five to nine particular chromosomes may be eventually replaced, once it's fully developed, by comparative genomic hybridization (CGH), which enables enumeration of every chromosome in a cell. When there is a known metabolic disease in the family, biochemical analyses can be applied to determine the carrier or disease state of the embryo. Abnormal embryos are then discarded and only normal, chromosomally "balanced" embryos are transferred.

SUCCESS AND FAILURE

There are no nationwide general statistics available on the impact of PGD on success since neither the 2001 SART/CDC report nor the CFAS survey looked specifically at PGD cases. But we do know that there are potential pitfalls. One drawback is that up to 10% of embryos may be designated as abnormal when they are in fact normal, because of errors in the chromosomes of individual cells, which may be simply relegated to the placenta. The converse is also possible. An embryo could be deemed normal chromosomally and yet be abnormal, because many techniques evaluate only nine pairs of chromosomes. Secondly, the biopsy procedure itself could have an impact on the viability of an embryo. As techniques become refined both for the biopsy and preparation of the cells at the individual IVF center as well as for the analysis of several key chromosomes, this technique may prove helpful to improve outcomes especially in older women. A third concern is the added cost of the procedure, approximately $5000 U.S., to the already expensive IVF process. As these concerns are resolved, at some point in the future PGD may become part of the IVF routine to assure that all embryos transferred are chromosomally normal.

Although the technique holds great promise for eliminating the chance of a genetic or chromosomal disease, the ethical issues created by the process have prompted some countries to limit or completely ban the technique. It is banned in Austria, Germany, Ireland, Switzerland and portions of Australia, and limited by legislation in France, Spain, Sweden and the U.K. Other countries such as Belgium, Israel, the Netherlands, Italy, Greece and the U.K. have a national oversight agency that controls the procedure, while in the U.S. and Canada it is subject only to state or provincial laws without specific reference to PGD.

IVF, GIFT OR ZIFT: WHICH TO CHOOSE?

GIFT and the other procedures that utilize the fallopian tube for supporting gametes and embryos initially arose out of the frustration with low rates of success with IVF. Unless the IVF laboratory is functioning at a very good level, the fallopian tube is a better environment for the nourishment and growth of these cells. Today in the average ART program, IVF success is equal to GIFT. The comparison is further complicated by the fact that different groups of patients are appropriate for the two procedures. In one study in Australia in the 1980s the same group of patients was allocated to either IVF or GIFT and the success rates in the study were identical, even at a time when average IVF rates were much lower than GIFT.

At first glance, the GIFT procedure seems inherently more logical. First, it would seem that fertilization and embryo development must occur more normally in the location where these events usually take place. Second, the embryos do not reach the uterine cavity prematurely in GIFT. (In IVF embryos have been routinely transferred to the uterus after about 48 to 72 hours to avoid prolonged exposure to potentially suboptimal culture conditions.) Third, with GIFT the embryos enter the uterus in a normal manner, without irritation and potential displacement of the embryos from the upper part of the uterus where implantation normally occurs.

However, these benefits can be counterbalanced by inherent advantages of IVF. First, from animal studies, it appears that a lower percentage of eggs become normally fertilized with GIFT than with IVF. Since the eggs are aspirated from the ovary several hours before they would normally ovulate, these less-than-fully-mature eggs may not fertilize or may fertilize abnormally. You would not know this with GIFT since you can't observe fertilization. Also, a much lower concentration of sperm is achieved in direct contact with the egg than in IVF, due to very large areas within the folds of the tube. Second, if pregnancy does not occur and extra eggs do not fertilize, there is no way to know whether the failure was due to lack of fertilization or of implantation. The other major difference between IVF and GIFT is the need for laparoscopy for the latter as well as a major form of anesthesia. For most women who have had prior surgeries and anesthesia, the prospect of a procedure without incisions and done under deep sedation is enough to sway the decision toward IVF. On the other hand, laparoscopy can add significant diagnostic aspects and the possibility of treatment for some women. Endometriosis may be evaluated and cauterized or vaporized and the status of the tubes and adhesions can be assessed. In the recent case of one GIFT procedure we cauterized endometriosis and washed the pelvic cavity to remove the sperm-engulfing scavenger cells (macrophages) that are thought to reduce fertility in this disease. Although pregnancy did not occur with GIFT, she conceived on her own the following month, after seven years of infertility and multiple cycles of hMG/IUI.

One further difference between IVF and GIFT is the risk of tubal pregnancy. Although surveys have shown virtually equal rates (3.9% of pregnancies for IVF and 3.2% for GIFT in the 1994 SART survey), tubal pregnancies with IVF occur almost exclusively in women with abnormal tubes, whereas most women undergoing GIFT have normal tubes. Therefore, in the women for whom either GIFT or IVF is appropriate, there is probably a small increase in the risk of ectopic pregnancy with GIFT. In women with tubal disease, the risk of ectopic pregnancy with GIFT varies from 5% to 17%, depending upon the extent of the tubal damage. That's why Dr. Yee emphasizes careful observation and cannulation of the tube prior to proceeding with the tubal transfer.

You can see that the choice of GIFT versus IVF is not easy and depends on the success rate achieved with GIFT or IVF in a particular program, the potential for diagnostic information and the patient's outlook toward surgery, anesthesia and tubal pregnancy. Unfortunately, the current SART/CDC format does not show the individual success rates of IVF and GIFT in the clinic-specific reports, so objective information is not available.

Then what about ZIFT? It is not yet clear whether ZIFT carries a significantly higher rate of pregnancy than GIFT. In the 1994 survey it did not; 29.1% for ZIFT versus 28.4% take-home baby rate per retrieval for GIFT. It may be considered an option when a difficult transfer is anticipated in a patient who otherwise would require IVF. However, it does require both vaginal egg retrieval and laparoscopy, with accompanying increased discomfort and expense. Again, in programs that have good IVF success rates there appears to be no advantage of ZIFT, as shown in two well-controlled studies.

If your tubes are blocked, the choice is easy: IVF is the only appropriate method for you. If your problem is unrelated to a tubal factor, you have a choice. Now, you also have the facts. To summarize:

	IVF	GIFT	ZIFT
Laparoscopy mandatory	−	+	+
Anesthesia mandatory	−	+	+
Ultrasound retrieval	+	+/−	+
Fertilization known	+	−	+
Fertilization in normal location	−	+	−
Requires normal fallopian tube	−	+	+
Provides diagnostic information	−	+	+
Severe male factor requiring ICSI	+	−	+

COSTS

Costs will vary depending on geographic location and may vary considerably within a geographical area.

The estimated cost of an IVF or GIFT cycle, exclusive of medication at this writing, is $7,000 to $10,000 U.S. depending on many factors, including which additional procedures, such as ICSI, PGD and AH, may be required. There is also great geographic variation in the costs, as well as some differences among programs in different parts of the same city. ZIFT will be more expensive because it requires independent costly procedures for both egg retrieval and transfer. The cost of freezing and maintaining embryos is relatively small as opposed to going through another complete cycle to obtain more embryos. It is usually several hundred dollars for the freezing and $1500 to $2000 U.S. for the frozen embryo transfer cycle.

What hurts most is that, unlike many other high-tech medical procedures, insurance usually does not pay for IVF. Some insurance companies specifically exclude IVF or may argue that IVF is elective or not medically necessary or not treating the underlying problem. See chapter 2 for more information on insurance coverage.

Our take-home message regarding costs is to ask for a full accounting of what your charges will be and when you will be expected to pay them. Most programs will have you pay up front because of the high costs of running an ART program and the uncertainty and delay of insurance payments.

Now that you are knowledgeable about the procedures and their costs, on what basis should you choose a physician, group or ART program that most closely meets your needs? The next chapter will tell you.

CHAPTER 9

Dr. Perfect, I Presume?

You need a full arsenal of information to be a clear-headed, informed consumer when setting out on your quest for the practitioner and program best equipped to help you win the battle of infertility. Basic armament includes your knowledge that not all doctors are equally competent and that you need the services and understanding of one who is professionally excellent. You also know that cooperation and patience are going to be required on your part and you should realize that once in a while the wrong chemistry between medical expert and client couple may sabotage an otherwise promising therapeutic plan. And you admit, however sadly, that Dr. Perfect practices only on Fantasy Island.

Your first determination has to be the type of doctor or program you need. This will depend to a great extent on where you are in the process of investigating your infertility problem. If you have never consulted a physician for your problem or have not had many tests, your own gynecologist is probably the best place to begin. He or she will probably be board-certified or a candidate for certification by the American Board of Obstetrics and Gynecology (U.S.) or the Royal College of Physicians and Surgeons (Canada) and may be a member of a national fertility society such as the American Society for Reproductive Medicine (ASRM) or the Canadian Fertility and Andrology Society (CFAS). Membership in ASRM or CFAS does not in itself mean that he or she is a great doctor but it does signify a certain level of interest in treating problems like yours. You can check the specialty board status of physicians by going to your public library and looking in the Directory of Medical Specialists or seek this information on the Internet. If you do not have your own gynecologist, read on. Most of the selection criteria and investigation we suggest will pertain to physicians with any level of specialization.

If you have already been through the basic testing and have tried various treatments, it may be time to move on. Now you may want to seek a more specialized level of care from a physician who has had training in reproductive medicine. He or she will have had specialized training and/or be certified or a candidate for certification by the American board in the area of reproductive endocrinology (for which there is no Canadian equivalent). This means that he or she has spent at least three extra years in a fellowship devoted exclusively to study in this field and usually limits his or her practice to this specialty. These specialists can be found in individual practice, medical groups, fertility centers and as directors of IVF programs.

How do you pick a doctor or center in which to place all your life's hopes and dreams?

SOURCES OF REFERRAL

You may or may not be under the care of a physician when you initiate your search for your own fertility specialist. You may be locked into a provider network through an HMO or PPO-type insurance, which will significantly limit or eliminate the possibility of making your own choice. You may be in a geographic area that has half a dozen IVF centers, or you may live in a rural area where a great deal of travel is required to reach any center. The following are referral sources generally available, some less effective than others:

Yellow Pages: In general, we do not suggest that you let your fingers do the walking to find any type of sophisticated medical service, especially ART. In fact, it's probably not a good idea to use the Yellow Pages to select any sort of health provider since you cannot obtain objective information from an advertisement. Certainly, the size of the ad is not in any way proportional to the quality of service or medical care you will receive. The Yellow Pages or ads in newspapers and magazines are probably okay to use in finding names and addresses of potential providers available. But remember that this may be an incomplete list; some of the best providers may choose not to advertise.

Internet: The Internet is great! Just punch in www.drperfect.com to find the doctor of your dreams. 'Fraid not. Although there is a great deal of "information" on the Internet, it is not any more objective than the Yellow Pages. If success rates are claimed, they should be in the form in which they are reported to SART/CDC. The size and sophistication of the web page is not in any way proportional to the quality of service or medical care you will receive, and information on the web is no better than any other advertising.

Medical associations: One method of selection often used is the physician referral service of the area medical association. We don't think this one is very good either. It is true that you will obtain the names of providers who are licensed and in "good standing" in the medical association. This means that they have paid their dues to the association and have not done a deed dastardly enough to get them thrown out, but it is no guarantee of quality. In addition, someone who comes very close to being your Dr. Perfect may choose not to be a member of this organization. The local medical association may be helpful to check whether any complaints have been filed against a particular physician, but it is not a good basis for making a quality selection.

Physician referral service: The same caveat is probably valid for physician referral services run by hospitals. These are purely mechanisms for bringing patients into that particular hospital's orbit. The referral service of a reputable hospital is a step up from the medical association because the hospital, at least, has certain requirements for staff membership in the areas of education and training and requires references and monitoring for new physicians, so a minimum level of quality is assured. But you're not looking for minimum standards. You're looking for excellence. Also, the referral service usually gives you the next three names on the list rather than one who meets your individual needs. Lately, some hospitals have been trying to meet more individual needs by using computer programs to match doctor and patient. The criteria used range from age of physician to schools attended and geographic location. This is somewhat helpful, but don't stop here.

Friend: Asking a friend for a recommendation is actually a pretty good way to start the selection process and is light years better than a referral from the county medical association. This is because at least some objective criteria can be used. But you have to dig deeper to establish the reasons for the referral. The friend's referral is based more on his or her needs than yours. Start making your list of what you want in a doctor or program and make sure that your friend is making the referral based on what you think is important. Chances are you'll find a competent physician, as well as one who is personable.

Support groups: Since the development of Alcoholics Anonymous, support groups have helped individuals and families with diverse medical problems. Infertility is no exception. The most prominent American support group for couples with infertility is Resolve, Inc., with headquarters in Massachusetts. They provide education, support groups, a bi-monthly newsletter, library and referral service, and have a nationwide network of chapters in most major cities. They will be some of the best-informed people about the infertility situation in your area. In Canada you can contact the Infertility Awareness Association of Canada centered in Ottawa with provincial branches.

Your physician: If you are currently under the care of a physician and he or she has offered you all the skill and expertise available to him or her, the next step would be to refer you to a higher level expert to continue your care. This is a reasonably good way to find a physician, but it does not mean that you can close your eyes and blindly charge off to the new Dr. Right. Your doctor could have referred you to Dr. Right because they have a friendly golf game every week.

Physicians also have a natural tendency to refer patients to their own hospital rather than to a nearby competitor, to get a new program going, or even to help one that is faltering at their hospital, despite the fact that the competitor may have a much higher pregnancy rate. Remember: your goal is to have the best chance of success, not necessarily to support the local hospital. You are looking for a service that does vary markedly in quality.

Or, perhaps your doctor knows personally that Dr. Right is an excellent physician and is also very personable and caring. Even so, your doctor's Dr. Right could be your Dr. Wrong—so ask some questions. A simple, "Why are you referring me to Dr. Right?" may provide important information. And even if the answer sounds good, you are not finished with your investigation, as you will see in a moment.

Physician-Friend: The best possible referral source you can have, if it's available, is a friend who is either a physician with firsthand knowledge of the medical community or another health professional who knows professionally and personally the reputations of the physicians you may wish to consider. This health professional–friend has your best interests at heart and also has objective information. In addition, by knowing you he or she can match you to a physician based on both your medical and your emotional needs.

Here's a breakdown of the major referral sources ranked from best to worst, according to objectivity and to the extent that each is mindful of your needs.

1. Physician or health professional–friend
2. Your physician
3. Support groups
4. Friend who has had good results
5. Prestigious hospital referral service
6. County medical society
7. Classified telephone directory, Internet or any advertising

Inside information from someone who is knowledgeable about the medical community is the way to go.

INVESTIGATION OF RESOURCES

Armed with your list of potential providers, you are now ready to embark on the second part of the process, your investigation of these resources. We suggest you set up a chart with criteria to be determined along the vertical axis and the providers you are considering on the horizontal axis. You will find similar graphs in consumer magazines such as *Consumer Reports.* You can conduct this investigation either by telephone or in person. To save time, you may be able to eliminate some potential providers by telephone answers to your most important questions. Each person's list of questions and concerns will be slightly different, since we all have different needs. But there are some that will be universal.

Before we outline the most common areas of concern, a word of advice: It may be just as important to you how the questions are answered as what the actual answers are.

- When you call, is the person you speak to friendly and helpful?
  Then, when you arrive at the office, are you treated as cheerfully as

you were on the phone? Or do you find yourself suddenly in the domain of a coldly efficient office staff who insist that you sign in, fill out the form and take a seat? Remember, your experience with the office staff may be a clue to the attitude of the physician in charge.

- Will this be a sit-down visit with your clothes on to obtain your history and discuss this huge investment in time, money and your future that you are about to make? In other words, does the first meeting occur in a relaxed atmosphere, or will you meet the physician or nurse-coordinator for the first time only when you are bereft of the "protection" of your clothing, literally exposed in stirrups, already positioned in the role of dutiful, submissive patient? "Hey, wait a minute. Why are my feet in stirrups? I just came to ask questions!"

- What about the doctor's attitude? Regardless of where the consultation takes place, it's important that the doctor show genuine interest in your questions and concern about your problem. Do you have the doctor's undivided attention, or must you share it with frequent phone calls and interruptions from the front office? You should be mindful, of course, that the best physicians are often in high demand. So, more importantly, pay attention to how your questions are answered. Are there hints of resentment in the answers? ("You don't need to concern yourself with that. That's my concern; I'm the doctor....") Are the answers honest, straightforward and clear, with facts to back them up? If the waiting room is packed, the doctor may be in a rush. You'll know this in advance of your meeting if you witness the doctor walking a patient down the hall and asking if she has any questions. So, be alert to indications of insincerity. ("Don't worry, sweetheart. Everything will be just fine....") Your Dr. Perfect will be the person who is concerned about you, interested in your problem, is honest, straightforward, one you can trust with your future and someone who has the technical skills to treat your problem.

- One more point about attitude—this time yours. Greet the doctor with a positive outlook. Many patients initially can be angry and hostile because they are frustrated with their infertility problem and give the impression that they may have been ripped off elsewhere. We suggest you begin your relationship with this potential Dr. Perfect with a clean slate. Tell him or her about yourself as succinctly as possible, leaving out extraneous material not related to the present problem. Tell him or her who referred you. Don't become argumentative. Try not to put the doctor on the defensive. You're there to make an assessment, not to score points in a debate. If you're nervous, that's okay. Remember, you're not the one who's auditioning, right?

TEN QUESTIONS

There are certain questions and concerns that we all would have regarding our entry into an ART program. There are also questions and concerns that may be unique to you as a couple. The following are just suggestions for you to include in your list of criteria on the graph you've already constructed.

Please don't confront the new doctor with your anger. He or she does not deserve it and it may start off your relationship on the wrong foot.

1. Success rate

The first consideration has got to be the success rate of the program. Over 420 ART programs were established in the United States by 2001 with only 384 of them reporting to the SART/CDC registry. As of 2001, there were 22 IVF programs in Canada, with 21 participating in the 2001 Canadian Assisted Reproductive Technology Success Rate report.

The pregnancy rates among these programs have been highly variable, with a small number of teams having little or no success. Therefore, obtain a definite figure for success of the program you are investigating based on their report to the SART/CDC. Ask to see their latest actual report, or you can check out the cdc.gov website. Do not accept "average" success rates for other programs; they have no relationship to the success rate of the particular program you are investigating.

It is important for you to understand how success rates are calculated because there can be a wide variation in rates, based on a program's experience, just by juggling the figures. The success rate is calculated by creating a fraction and then converting it to a percentage. The top number of the fraction (the numerator) represents pregnancies, the bottom number (the denominator) represents procedures.

The fraction would look like this:

$$\frac{\text{pregnancies}}{\text{procedures}} = \text{success rate}$$

But pregnancies could be any and all pregnancies, including:

- biochemical pregnancies (a positive pregnancy test without ultrasound confirmation of a pregnancy)
- clinical pregnancies that end as miscarriages or ectopic pregnancies
- clinical pregnancies that go past 12 weeks
- live births

Procedures could include any of the following:

- patients undergoing stimulation
- patients going on to egg retrieval
- patients reaching embryo transfer

Using this fraction, you can see that if we use the greatest number of pregnancies possible, including biochemical, in the numerator and the smallest number of procedures, only patients reaching transfer, in the denominator, the success rate will be very high. We do not feel that this gives an accurate indication of the success of a program.

Let's look at an example. Here are the raw data representing one year's experience of a hypothetical IVF program:

Procedures	Results
Stimulations—100	All pregnancies—20
Egg retrievals—90	Clinical pregnancies—13
Transfers—80	Live births—9

Here are the results, depending upon how these data are reported:

	All Pregnancies	Clinical	Live births
Stimulations	20%	13%	9%
Retrievals	22%	14%	10%
Transfers	25%	16%	11%

So you see that this IVF program, based on these raw data, could legitimately report success rates varying from 9% to 25%, depending upon what criteria were used. *We feel that the best reflection of the success of an IVF program is the rate of delivery (live birth) per egg retrieval.* By this method, our hypothetical IVF program should report a 10% success rate.

The delivery rate of living babies is the most important numerator. This is because the definition of clinical pregnancy may vary among IVF programs, the level of miscarriage may be higher with poorer technique and a live baby is what you are striving for. Using the "live-baby" rate can be somewhat impractical since there is an inherent nine-month delay from embryo transfer to delivery. Only well-established IVF programs can give a reasonably accurate take-home baby rate. In addition, by the time you obtain a rate based on take-home babies, it is based on techniques used and personnel involved over a year ago, a lengthy interval of time when considering ART procedures. If there have been such personnel changes, ask for the clinical pregnancy rate per transfer for the most recent year.

In the denominator we suggest egg retrievals rather than embryo transfer rate as the best reflection of IVF program quality, because cases not reaching transfer could reflect deficiencies in egg retrieval or laboratory techniques and may give a falsely high success rate. The percentage of canceled stimulations should also be examined because the success rate can be substantially influenced by allowing egg retrievals only when the results of stimulation are ideal.

We strongly suggest comparing only figures from a calendar year's experience. This follows recent guidelines from the Society for Assisted Reproductive Technology and prevents the possibility of a program quoting a rate from a selected period. Therefore, for practical purposes to get the most up-to-date information we suggest:

- For the year in which follow-up is available through the end of October, when the final data on deliveries are compiled:

$$\frac{\text{live births}}{\text{egg retrievals}}$$

- For the most recent full calendar year:

$$\frac{\text{clinical pregnancies}}{\text{egg retrievals}}$$

Using this formula, you can use the figure of 30% clinical pregnancy rate per egg retrieval in the under-35 age category as the minimum level of performance to warrant confidence in an ART program. Maximum rates have varied in a number of programs as greater than 50% or even more in the under-35 age category.

2. *Level of activity*

You need to know how many cycles of IVF and GIFT are done by the program in a year in order to gauge the significance of the quoted success rate. (A program is defined as a group of physicians who use the same protocols and laboratory, not by the total volume in a particular laboratory.) This does not mean that you should shy away from very small programs. On the contrary, many are excellent and afford you the individualization you may need. But, because of substantial variation based on chance alone, at least 100 cases are required to be able to quote a success rate that is a reasonably accurate reflection of the quality of the program. For example, in our program we have had streaks of up to seven successful IVF cycles in a row, but we also experience occasional "dry" spells. These variations can be easily demonstrated statistically to be based on pure chance. This is one of the reasons SART advises quoting experience based on at least one year. We also give patients our rates through the last several years since the larger the denominator, the more reliance can be placed on the calculated rate. When evaluating a small program you can compile results from several years to see if they are consistent.

3. *Stability*

A companion question will revolve around how long the program has been established. If they have not been doing ART for at least several years, inquire how they learned these procedures. In order to learn the fine details that have proven successful through years of experience, these individuals must have prolonged and extensive experience with an established, successful program. How long has the team been together? Are the current members of the team the same people whose success rate they are quoting?

There is some tendency for personnel in this sophisticated field to move from program to program. This is a complex process requiring a team composed of individuals with training and experience in pelvic surgery, reproductive endocrinology, andrology and embryology. The absence of one of these key people could have a devastating effect on an otherwise excellent program. In some cases there actually may not be anyone who was there when the quoted results were obtained.

4. SART membership

All qualified programs should belong to the Society for Assisted Reproductive Technology (SART), a specialty group of the American Society for Reproductive Medicine (ASRM). Membership in SART assures you a minimum level of expertise and activity. There is, however, no assurance of a reasonable success rate, since achieving a certain rate is not a requirement for membership. In addition they should be included in the SART/CDC report.

5. Cost

Although it is more difficult to assess the success of a small program, the individual attention suits many couples.

One of the most important considerations is the cost of whatever ART treatment you may need, and costs vary quite a bit. The cost of an IVF cycle runs $7,000 to $10,000 U.S. for each attempt, excluding medications. The largest variable will probably be geography, although centers in the same city may vary significantly. We certainly do not suggest that you "shop around" for the lowest price, but we do recommend that you fit cost into the equation relative to its importance to you. Do not compromise quality for cost, but if you are considering two similar programs, cost may become the deciding factor. Refer to chapter 2's discussion of payment schemes.

6. Qualifications of the director

The director of the center or head physician of the team must be highly qualified. In addition to being board-certified in obstetrics and gynecology, he or she may also be boarded or have at least finished a special fellowship in reproductive endocrinology. This is an area of medicine, as we have stressed before, where intensive teamwork is required. But the responsibility for the success of the team lies with its director, and there is no substitute for a qualified and competent physician in this role. That is not to say that every couple must see that person or be treated by him or her; that's not always possible in a program large enough to offer the quality we're talking about. A good director will assure that all physicians on the team are using the same techniques.

7. Psychological support

An experienced program should have readily available psychological support to optimize the couple's ability to cope with the stresses inherent in the process. Psychological issues can have a major impact on the success of an individual couple, since perseverance is a key to the ultimate chance of a pregnancy. Emotional stability and mutual support help a couple persist in their quest.

8. Flexibility

The director does not have to personally do all the work in a fertility program, but is responsible, more than any other individual, for its success or failure.

The flexibility of a physician's ideas and the program's protocols are very important. Is this the type of program that is going to fit you into a procedure because it is best for them, or will they individualize treatment? Do they try to push you into GIFT because they are having difficulty with their embryo transfer technique? Will they individualize the stimulation protocol to vary the dose and timing of drugs based on your needs, or is everyone treated the same?

9. Laboratory accreditation

At this time, all of the provisions of the Wyden Act have not been implemented, including a mandatory program of laboratory accreditation. However, there is a voluntary program through ASRM and the College of American Pathologists (CAP). Accreditation is not an assurance of quality, but it does guarantee that minimum standards are being used.

10. All treatment methods available

A quality operation should have all current methods of treatment available. An example might be embryo freezing. By limiting the number of transferred fresh embryos to two or three in younger women, the risk of multiple pregnancy can be better controlled. Freezing additional embryos can reduce costs considerably by allowing multiple embryo transfer procedures from one stimulation and retrieval. In some women, the uterus may not be receptive in the stimulated cycle. For example, Patty, whom you met in chapter 1, became pregnant only after a frozen embryo transfer.

ADDITIONAL QUESTIONS

You may have some questions that address your particular concerns, such as age, distance or prior surgery. Here are some examples:

- Doctor, I'm 41 years old. I know that you generally have very good results, but what are your results with women my age?
- We live about 400 miles up the coast. Since it would be so expensive for me to travel or stay here, can my doctor there start my medications?
- I had my tubes tied by Band-aid surgery. The other doctor told me that surgery to repair my tubes would be better than IVF. Is that true?
- My friend had some bleeding after her eggs were picked up. Do you ever have complications?

When you get on the emotional roller-coaster of fertility treatment don't under-estimate the importance of support from your friends, family, support groups and, if necessary, psychological counseling.

Now you have the tools you'll need for finding Dr. Perfect. Don't be afraid to use them and keep reminding yourself that having your baby is well worth whatever effort it takes. While you may not find Dr. Perfect, we believe that you'll come a lot closer to him or her than other couples who rely mainly on factors that have little to do with the quality of care they will receive.

CHAPTER 10

A Lifetime of Hope in About Thirty Days

It's amazing how much of what we do is timed according to the number of days it takes the moon to revolve around the earth. That interval of time is 29.25 days, approximately one month. It is usually how often we pay our bills, the period of time on one page of a calendar and the basic unit we use to rent an apartment or pay our mortgage. People see the time frame of 30 days as significant, often choosing it to reach a particular goal. For example, in advertisements on the back of comic books and magazines in the late 1950s bodybuilder Charles Atlas boasted, "In just 30 days I can make you a man." A book promised "Thirty Days to a More Powerful Vocabulary."

We could have titled this chapter "In Just 30 Days We Can Make You a Baby," but this concept does not agree with our outlook that it is the couple who makes the baby; we just help. It is true, though, that all of the ART procedures encompass an approximate 30-day interval. This is simply because these procedures are coordinated to the menstrual cycle, which averages 28 to 30 days. Having taken thousands of couples through these procedures, we know that they are investing not only their money and time, but also their hopes and dreams, in the events that will take place in the next 30 days.

THE PATIENT'S PERSPECTIVE

If you are planning to go through an IVF, GIFT or related procedure, you want to know what actually happens on a day-to-day basis. Although we can outline from the IVF team's point of view what each day involves, we enlisted the help of Cheryl Scruggs, one of our IVF patients, to provide you with a look at each day's activities through the eyes of a typical patient.

Before we start, we want you to understand how Cheryl and Jeff Scruggs came to need IVF. Cheryl, then 27, was a sales representative for Konica Business Machines. Jeff, 28, was a sales representative for the children's clothing company Osh Kosh B'Gosh. (They both felt that there was a certain irony that Jeff was in the children's clothing business while they were unable to have a child.) Their struggle with infertility was slightly unusual in that they had tried to conceive for only nine months before discovering their problem. Because of the severity of the problem, they immediately opted for IVF. Most other couples struggle for many years before reaching IVF or GIFT.

"In just 30 days we can make you a baby."

Cheryl had come in for a routine annual examination and had expressed her concern that she had been trying to get pregnant for nine months and nothing was happening. She remembers that "in my heart, I knew something was wrong." Because of her concern, she was started on a basal body temperature chart and a semen analysis (which was normal) was obtained for Jeff. Her BBT showed that she was ovulating. But a hysterosalpingogram showed that both tubes were closed and, in fact, looked as if she had a hydrosalpinx on each side.

In order to determine the exact nature of her tubal problem and what it would take to repair it, she underwent a laparoscopy. Her worst fears were confirmed. After the laparoscopy, Jeff was told Cheryl's tubes were indeed closed. In addition, the fimbriae at the end of both tubes were destroyed and each tube ended in a blind dilated sac. The extent of tubal damage and surrounding scar tissue indicated a poor prognosis for surgical repair. He was told that tubal microsurgery would yield only a 10% chance of pregnancy in her case. (Actually, Cheryl was lucky that the dilated tubes did not interfere with her subsequent IVF. We now advise removing or tying off a hydrosalpinx since in at least half of women, the fluid tracks back through the uterus and prevents implantation.) After the laparoscopy, Cheryl was too groggy to really discuss the findings, and an appointment was made for several days later to discuss the situation thoroughly.

> I remember driving home from surgery and no one had told me what they had found. Jeff said that we would talk about it after I got some rest. "No," I said, "tell me the results now!" Jeff, with tears in his eyes, said that my tubes looked really bad. They were blocked and scarred and basically nothing could be done to fix the problem. He said we could try surgery to fix the tubes or attempt in vitro fertilization. He said that the doctor felt that surgery was not my best option since there was only a 10% chance it would work. I was devastated to think I could never have my own child. My mom was so fertile and popped babies out right and left. How could I have problems?

Several days later, the options were discussed with Cheryl and Jeff: tubal repair, IVF or adoption. The best option appeared to them to be IVF. They were young, Jeff had a good semen analysis and their only problem was the tubal obstruction. Statistically, IVF had a higher success rate than tubal repair. Adoption was not an option they would select at this time.

Cheryl was in a hurry to get started, but there were obstacles. At that time, there was an 18- to 24-month waiting list before a patient could enter the program. Now there is no waiting period.

> I was very impatient because we wanted to get started. I felt deep in my heart that once we started we would reach our dream of having a baby. We kept a positive attitude and feel that this can make the odds better for success. We waited approximately nine months. I called the center almost every day. The nurse-coordinator thought I was neurotic and totally obsessed.

Cheryl's persistence paid off. The program was just at the point of changing its method of retrieval to a simpler technique that could become routine for most patients. Cheryl immediately volunteered for the transvaginal ultrasound method and was started in the program.

THIRTY DAYS HATH SEPTEMBER, APRIL, JUNE AND IVF…

In taking you through a "typical" cycle, we will be using the stimulation protocol, retrieval and transfer procedures along with instructions used at Reproductive Partners facilities in Southern California. Obviously, if you go through IVF at another center or choose another procedure altogether, you may have a slightly different experience. That does not mean that our way is right and theirs is wrong, or vice versa. As we've said before, there are many different ways of doing these procedures. So, if your experience differs, don't be alarmed.

With that caveat, let us begin. Most centers use Leuprolide (Lupron) to suppress the ovary. The preparation for the cycle begins when the patient first comes in to start Lupron. This will be either about three weeks after the start of a menstrual period or after two weeks of taking a low-dose birth control pill. Newer medications, Antagon or Cetrotide, might be used instead of Lupron, to suppress the LH surge. Antagon or Cetrotide would be started around the 5th or 6th day of stimulation.

When you start an IVF cycle, Day 1 is usually not the first day of your cycle.

Typically, after two weeks on the pill, the patient comes into the center for a vaginal ultrasound to ensure that the pelvic structures are normal. If the ultrasound is normal, the patient is instructed in the technique of injecting the Lupron. The injection is given subcutaneously through a tiny needle. During the next 10 days of preparation an injection of Lupron is required each morning. The patient remains on the birth control pill, creating an "overlap" for the first seven days of Lupron.

When Cheryl went through IVF, Lupron typically was begun one week after ovulation as determined by detection of the LH surge by a urine test or by a temperature chart. Seven days after the LH surge was detected, the patient came into the center for a progesterone level check to determine that ovulation had occurred and a vaginal ultrasound was done to ensure that the pelvic structures were normal. Now most cycles are begun on the second day of menses with tests for FSH and estradiol, and the patient is started on birth control pills. The Lupron test is then begun after two weeks of the birth control pills, overlapped for a week and taken for a total of 10 days.

By this time I was totally obsessed and overly anxious. Although I was about to start at a time when they were getting close to their summer break, I decided to go ahead anyway. I pushed them into letting me start. I felt as if I was up against a deadline to completely finish the process before they closed down.

After 10 days of Lupron, the patient will return to the center for an ultrasound scan and estrogen level test. The ultrasound detects cysts stimulated by the initial phase of Lupron, which may interfere with ovarian stimulation. The Lupron should suppress the estrogen level. If the scan is normal and the estrogen low, the patient is ready to begin stimulation. If her estrogen is not suppressed or if cysts are seen on the ultrasound, she will return every four days until everything is right. However, most patients are suppressed after 10 days.

Lupron injections are fairly easy to tolerate.

Because my cycle is normally so long, I was on Lupron longer than usual. I got very impatient and anxious, which I feel slowed my body's natural cycle and therefore made the process longer. I did not make it this time to the Pergonal. I was dropped because my period was so delayed and they could not have possibly finished my cycle before they were scheduled to close for two weeks for lab maintenance. Actually, Jeff felt it was better that we stopped then because I was really not in the right frame of mind.

I was very upset, almost mad at them. They told me I would have to wait until September to try again. Another three months; I couldn't believe it! I knew it would be the longest three months of my entire life. That night I cried and cried. We went to the support group sponsored by the center, but we didn't feel that it was to our benefit. Believe it or not, many of the people in the group were more emotional than I was. We actually felt that our emotions were in control. That summer went fast. We took a trip back east to see our families. We also spent a lot of time at the beach. All I wanted to do was get started. I knew it would work.

Day 1

Once suppression of the ovary is confirmed, the patient begins the gonadotropin stimulation regimen specifically prescribed for her using Follistim, Gonal-F, Bravelle (pure FSH) and/or Pergonal or Repronex (hMG). Lupron injections are continued and she can carry on normal daily activity.

When higher doses of Lupron are used, one of the hMG (Pergonal, Repronex) medications may be given as well to provide supplemental LH. Another option would be to inject a very dilute solution of hCG along with the pure FSH to provide LH activity.

Alternately, if the Antagon or Cetrotide regimen is used, stimulation begins four to five days after a one-month cycle of low-dose birth control pills.

The daily injections of gonadotropin are usually given between 7:00 p.m. and 9:00 p.m. The intramuscular form (Pergonal, Repronex) is generally too difficult for the woman to give to herself, so her partner will usually give it or make alternate arrangements. The subcutaneous form (Bravelle, Follistim, Gonal-F) can be given by the woman herself, like the Lupron. The routine dosage is two or three ampules daily, but may be up to six or more ampules a day. If the total daily dose is more than three ampules, we prefer to divide it into two injections: one in the morning, the other in the evening. In addition, the Lupron is continued each morning, but sometimes at a modified dose. So there may be up to three injections a day until the patient is ready for the hCG.

Before starting my second attempt, I had to start my period. As I expected, it was six days late. I couldn't wait to call the center even though I was scared to start the process. It was starting to bother me that all of our friends and family were having babies. It was now hard for me to be around babies. I really never felt jealous of these people. It just made me want one even more. I had not accepted the fact that we may never have children of our own, or that our only option might be to adopt. I felt guilty because I blamed myself for not being able to conceive. Jeff is a very supportive person and always told me it was "our" problem, not mine.

When I called the center, they told me to come in to start the Lupron. They taught me how to inject the Lupron into my thigh or abdomen. I really didn't look forward to the shots, but I knew that every injection was getting us closer and closer to possibly having our own baby. I would have done anything to have a baby, no matter what I had to sacrifice.

It was a strange sensation feeling the needle just below the skin and actually seeing the medication make a little bubble. With the Lupron, it was very important to place the needle just below the skin, not into the muscle. The spot

*where I placed the needle would swell up, get very hot and would itch for about
30 minutes. I also had hot flashes and would perspire. While taking the Lupron,
I felt somewhat tired, but not depressed. I was a little moody, so Jeff would rub
my back, hug me or do whatever would make me comfortable.*

Day 2 through Day 5 (starting ovarian stimulation)

After the visit on Day 10 or so to confirm suppression of the ovary, no visits
to the center are necessary for five days. The patient continues to take her
regimen of gonadotropins and Lupron injections and can carry on normal
daily activity.

*The Pergonal scared me a little mainly because of the size of the needle,
which was about one inch long. Jeff had to administer the Pergonal once a day
at 7 p.m. into my hip. I dreaded the shot because it did hurt some. But I was
willing to do anything to achieve a pregnancy.*

*Jeff tried to make it a comical situation. He'd say, "Okay, honey. Pull your
pants down and bend over. It's time for your shot." Jeff was a pro. He put the
needle in fast and I barely felt it go in. The first couple of times he didn't place
it in the right spot in my hip, which would cause my leg to ache for a couple of
hours. We called the center and they made us come in and take another lesson on
where to place the needle. After that, we had no problems.*

Day 6 to the Day of hCG

By this time, five days of stimulation have been given and it should be possible to evaluate the response. Most patients will receive hCG any time
within the next one to seven days. This is the point at which a determination may be made to continue the cycle or to "drop" it if there are not
enough follicles developing, or if one follicle is far more developed than the
others. If Antagon is used instead of Lupron, the patient would begin the
nightly Antagon injections around Day 5 or Day 6 of stimulation, or later if
the lead follicle is not large enough.

A vaginal ultrasound will be done and the dose will be adjusted, depending on the response of the follicles. If there is little activity, it may be
increased. If the ultrasound shows many follicles developing and the estrogen level rising rapidly, it may be lowered. The doctor will get the first indication of the adequacy of the stimulation at this point. The Lupron is

usually continued at the same dose unless there is a poor response in which case it may be lowered to half the dose. An appointment will be made to return in from one to three days, depending on the response.

Antagon or Cetrotide will usually be started when the lead follicle has a longest diameter of 14 millimeters. At this time one of the hMG (Pergonal, Repronex) medications will be added to the pure FSH to provide supplemental LH. Another option would be to inject a very dilute solution of hCG along with the pure FSH to provide LH activity.

> *The Pergonal made me even more tired. At this point I was seeing the doctor every day for an ultrasound. I responded very well to the Pergonal. Every ultrasound showed more and more eggs. I was very excited, yet felt nervous. I just prayed that all would go well.*

Day 7 to the Day of hCG

After seven days of stimulation have been given, a few patients will get their hCG injection on this day to trigger ovulation. Most will receive the hCG any time within the next three to four or more days. An estradiol level obtained as the follicles approach maturity could indicate that there are too many small follicles, producing an excess of estrogen. Rarely, this could make continuing the cycle too dangerous and force the process to be stopped. More recently, these uncommon instances of overstimulation can be handled by "coasting," which means stopping the gonadotropins and continuing the Lupron, allowing the estrogen level to fall into the acceptable range. With the use of Lupron to suppress the ovary prior to the use of the gonadotropins, we have experienced a dropout rate of less than 10%, compared to about 30% prior to the use of Lupron. The decision on which day to give the hCG is based on follicle size and, to a lesser extent, the estradiol level. Generally, it would be given anywhere from Day 7 to Day 12, with the average patient receiving her hCG on Day 10.

The most important features of the hCG injection are that it be given precisely at the time instructed and that it be given correctly. The hCG causes realignment of the chromosomes of the egg to ready it for fertilization. Since ovulation becomes increasingly common after 36 hours following the hCG injection, the retrieval will be timed to occur 35 hours after the hCG. If the hCG is given too early, the follicles might ovulate spontaneously. If it is given too late, the follicles might not be optimally ready for retrieval. If the injection is not given in its entirety, the lower blood levels achieved might compromise the cycle. If hCG is not given at all, the eggs will not mature and may remain stuck to the follicle wall.

Cheryl received her hCG after only seven doses of gonadotropins. (The average patient receives the hCG after 10 days of stimulation.) On that day she had 18 follicles measured, with several small ones noted. Her estradiol level was 2168. Because of the large number of follicles present and the estradiol over 2000, it was felt that the stimulation should go no further because a very high estrogen level may have a detrimental effect on implantation. She was scheduled to receive her hCG at precisely 9:00 p.m. and the ultrasound retrieval was scheduled for 7:30 a.m. two days hence.

We had plans to go to dinner with some friends at 7 p.m. We were only going five minutes away from home, but did not want to chance not being home by nine. We took the hCG shot with us. Our friends whom we were meeting had also been through IVF. They were successful with quadruplets (in Dr. Meldrum's program—the first in the country through IVF) and fully understood what we were going through.

When we arrived at the restaurant, we explained to the hostess that it was vital to us that I have this shot at exactly 9 p.m. and asked if they had a place we could use for a few minutes. We sat down for dinner and at 9 p.m. they ushered us into their food storage room. When we entered, we burst out with laughter. Around us were shelves with box after box of ketchup, salt, bacon bits, etc. I told Jeff that we needed to lock the door, but there was no lock. So, I took off my high heels and pulled my pants down. Jeff was laughing so hard that he didn't think he would be able to give me the shot. I was afraid that someone would open the door and see me with my pants down. Sure enough, just as Jeff was about to hit me with the needle, the door flew open. It shut immediately and all we could hear was laughter and apologies. Jeff finally gave me the shot and we returned to our table in hysterics.

Day 11 (the Day after hCG)

The patients return to the center for:

- ultrasound to check on the status of the follicles
- brief history and physical examination in anticipation of the retrieval procedure the next day

In cases when ICSI is not planned, a semen specimen is collected for 24-hour incubation. It is suggested that the last prior ejaculation be about two to four days before the first specimen of the cycle. Perhaps the most important feature of this visit is the thorough explanation of the retrieval procedure along with its expectations and potential complications. We go through the entire technical procedure, along with information about sedation or anesthesia and expectations of results, then discuss what will be done with the eggs after the retrieval. This is a good time for the couple to ask questions to relieve any fears or concerns they may have. Important decisions regarding embryo freezing and any required consents should be signed by this time. Even if general anesthesia is not given, we advise no food or drink after midnight.

Day 12 (the retrieval)

The patient is admitted to the center about an hour and a half before the scheduled time of the retrieval. An IV is started in her arm and some fluids and an antibiotic are given. An injection of a sedative is given through the IV. She is then wheeled on a stretcher to the procedure room.

She is placed in a position similar to that of a pelvic examination, with her legs supported by stirrups. Additional sedation may be given slowly through the IV for the prep. In some cases a general or epidural anesthetic is administered by an anesthesiologist. The nurse washes the area outside the vagina with an antiseptic solution and then inserts a catheter into the bladder to keep the bladder empty during the procedure. She then washes the inside of the vagina with the antiseptic. The washing of the vagina can be uncomfortable, but by this time most patients are fairly well sedated and tolerate it without too much discomfort.

The doctor washes out the antiseptic from the vagina with a special sterile solution. The area around the vagina is surrounded by sterile drapes. A sterile plastic cover is placed over the ultrasound instrument; a tube to guide the needle is attached and it is placed into the vagina exactly as it had been when the follicles were being monitored. The collection system is tested and the procedure is ready to begin. Most patients now receive an intravenous injection of propofol which results in a state of deep sedation in which she is rendered unconscious, but not at a general anesthetic level. During the entire procedure the patient's vital signs, blood gases and EKG are constantly monitored by the anesthetist. In the rare patient who does not want deep sedation, conscious sedation is administered. If the patient is not fully sedated we also find it helpful to have the patient listen to her favorite music through a set of headphones. Most non-anesthetized patients talk to the staff during the procedure and many follow the count of eggs retrieved and can find out the quality of the eggs from the person screening them.

Two things to bring with you to the retrieval: a pair of warm socks because your feet will get cold, and a tape or disc player to pass the time.

With the ultrasound visualizing the follicles, the needle is placed by means of the guide through the vaginal wall and into the nearest follicle in the ovary. Once the needle is in the ovary it is moved from one follicle to another. Each follicle is aspirated and may or may not be flushed until the egg is found. The fluid returns through the needle and tubing into a test tube. This tube is passed to a team member who labels the tube and quickly places it into the incubator, which is maintained at body temperature with a special 5% carbon dioxide atmosphere. The screener pours the fluid into a small dish and examines the contents under a microscope until the egg is found. Mature eggs are usually visible with the naked eye because of a halo of translucent tissue around them. Any comments regarding the quality of the egg will be noted and it is transferred to a test tube containing a nutrient medium for incubation.

The procedure is repeated until all the follicles on each side have been aspirated. The pelvis is then scanned to be sure that there are no additional follicles present and that there is no evidence of bleeding. The propofol is stopped and the patient awakens quickly. The drapes are removed, the patient's legs are taken out of the stirrups and she will be observed in the center for an hour or so until she is stable. During this time, her blood pressure and pulse will be monitored and she will be given some fluids and medication for pain or nausea, if needed.

We arrived at the center about 7 a.m. to prepare for the egg retrieval. They gave me a shot of Demerol, which I had an immediate reaction to. I broke out in a cold sweat, felt nauseous, and my blood pressure went down. I was getting sleepy and light-headed. Jeff was by my side during the preparation. He held my hand, kissed me, and was very comforting. I was scared, yet excited. During the procedure I really couldn't feel much except when the medication started to wear off. Then I could feel a tug in my ovaries as if they were extracting something. They got 23 eggs! Everyone was so excited. They took me to the recovery room and said I'd go home at 2 p.m. But I was extremely sick to my stomach and couldn't stop vomiting. I ended up staying until 6:30 p.m.

After the egg retrieval is completed, it is time for collection of the semen specimen. In non-ICSI cases we now routinely obtain an additional specimen on the day before egg retrieval, which is incubated in a special buffer (test yolk buffer) to enhance its ability to penetrate. It is suggested that the last prior ejaculation be two to four days before that specimen. The man masturbates into a sterile nontoxic container. The semen is then washed with nutrient medium in the laboratory. Approximately 50,000 sperm are added to each egg which, by now, has incubated for several hours. In the event of a male factor problem, a larger number of sperm may be added to each egg or ICSI may be performed.

The fertilization check is always a stressful time because you know it could all end here. But it rarely does.

> *As they wheeled me to recovery, they asked Jeff to collect his specimen. He was somewhat embarrassed, but was actually used to giving specimens as he had previously had sperm counts, antibody tests and the hamster test.*

Following the retrieval, medications are limited to acetaminophen (Tylenol) or codeine if there is any discomfort. If the couple is planning a three-day transfer with assisted hatching, doxycycline, an antibiotic, and methylprednisolone, a steroid, are started that evening. A light diet and rest are recommended. The couple goes to sleep at home as their eggs and sperm are uniting in the laboratory.

Day 13

Early in the morning the eggs are checked for the first time for indications that fertilization has taken place. Each egg is examined under the microscope for two pronuclei, indicating that genetic material from only one sperm and one egg is present. The occasional egg that may have been fertilized with more than one sperm (polyspermic) will have three pronuclei and will be discarded. Eggs that did not fertilize will be reinseminated. If there are more embryos than can be transferred during this cycle, extra embryos may be frozen at the pronuclear stage. A call will be made to the couple giving them the information regarding the status of their embryos and final arrangements will be made for the time of the embryo transfer two to four days later. The only other task remaining is to begin progesterone injections, which are given deep in the muscle each evening starting one day after the retrieval.

> *On Saturday we called to find out how many eggs had fertilized. We were delighted to learn that 15 had fertilized. One had been fertilized by more than one sperm, so we had 14 embryos to work with.*

Day 15 or 17 (embryo transfer)

This is the day of the embryo transfer. The patient may have a light breakfast and will take an antibiotic tablet. In general we recommend limiting fluids as we prefer she not have to get up to urinate during the hour or so of rest after the transfer. If the transfer will be guided by ultrasound we want her to have a full bladder. The transfer procedure is actually quite easy for the patient. She is given a dose of Valium so that she is relaxed. She is placed in the position for a pelvic examination with her legs supported by stirrups. Meanwhile, the embryos are being examined in the laboratory under the microscope and evaluated for the number of cells, consistency of size of each cell and the presence of fragments. The best embryos have the following characteristics:

- greatest number of cells
- uniformity of size of cells
- absence of fragmentation

When the best embryos have been selected for transfer, they are placed in a dish. The transfer catheter is rinsed with medium. The incubator is rolled into the transfer room, which is quiet and has had the lights dimmed. A speculum is inserted into the vagina and the cervix is washed with medium. If ultrasound guidance is used a nurse or technician positions the ultrasound probe on the abdomen.

The partner is then asked if he wishes to look at the embryos. He usually agrees. This is a very emotional moment as he looks at the two to four embryos, consisting of only a few to a cluster of cells, which may become his offspring. The embryos are drawn up into the catheter attached to a very accurate syringe and passed to the physician. It is up to the physician to carefully thread this catheter containing the embryos up through the cervix and into the uterus just a fraction of an inch away from the top of the cavity. The whole process depends on these embryos being deposited gently in the right place, allowing them the best chance of implanting.

About one minute after the embryos have been expelled the catheter is withdrawn and checked for retained embryos. If the catheter is empty, the speculum is removed and the bed is positioned so the patient is lying on either her stomach or back, depending on the position of the uterus, with her head angled down. She is allowed to rest for 30 minutes and then go home and continue bedrest for the next 48 hours. She will continue receiving progesterone each day.

> *We arrived at the center at 9:30 a.m. They put me in a hospital gown and gave me Valium. I was nervous and felt cold. The best part was that Jeff could come in the room during the transfer. I started to cry. I'm not sure why. Maybe it was just to relieve the pressure because I knew that this was "it." Would it work? We went into the quiet, dark room. Jeff was holding my hand and in my other hand was my rosary. Although I am not a practicing Catholic anymore, I have had that rosary since I was a kid and I felt I wanted it with me. I was praying and smiling.*
>
> *They brought the incubator in with the embryos in it. Jeff looked in the microscope and saw the four embryos. He said that it was an unbelievable feeling. He was possibly looking at his future child or even children. All the embryos were healthy and strong. They placed them into my uterus very carefully. There was no pain. After the transfer they took me to a room where I had to lie on my stomach with the head of the bed lower than my feet. I was unable to sleep and had no entertainment or radio. My head kept sliding into the headboard and my neck was killing me. Jeff went home for a while and came back to get me. I went home and was instructed to stay in bed for two days.*

Days 16 and 17

These two days are spent at home on complete bedrest. The only injection required is the dose of progesterone which will be given at about 7:00 p.m.

I couldn't do anything except go to the bathroom. No showers, no walking around, no cooking—nothing! Jeff brought all my meals upstairs and basically waited on me hand and foot. I read magazines, watched television and slept.

Day 18 through Day 27 to 29

Following the two days of bedrest, normal activity is allowed. We recommend against any strenuous physical activity, exercise or sports. We also advise against intercourse or even other stimulation to orgasm. We really don't know what effect activity has after the transfer, but after going through so much, it is better to be cautious. The progesterone injections are continued daily.

I was able to get up, but was supposed to take it easy. I went back to work the following Monday, but for only half-days. But, more than anything else, I worried. We had been through so much that if it failed, I now knew that I would be very upset.

Day 28 to 30 (the pregnancy test)

This is it! Years of trying, testing and treatment all culminate in one test this day. About two weeks following the transfer, the woman returns to the center for the pregnancy test. Actually, the pregnancy test can be done at any reliable medical laboratory. But if the patients live close to the center, we request that they do this test at the center, where we can share the news—good or bad—with them. Some couples come together; some women come and face the news alone.

If the test is positive, there are usually tears of joy. These tears are not always limited to the couple. The members of the IVF team, even those not directly involved in medical activities, share the intense joy of the successful patients. The couple will be told that the positive pregnancy test is a first step toward their goal and that there are still some hurdles to encounter. We offer our congratulations and discuss early pregnancy instructions. (We discuss those instructions and the special concerns in an IVF pregnancy in the next chapter.)

If the test is negative, there may also be tears shed, but these are the tears of bitter disappointment. Some patients want to discuss the technical aspects of their cycle at this time. Some express their disappointment.

Most, however, express surprisingly little outward emotion at this time. Perhaps they expected bad news, or perhaps they prefer to express their grief in private. In any event, we recommend to them that they return in a couple of weeks to air their feelings, review their cycle to see if any aspects of the process can be improved, and discuss their plans for the future.

On the day my pregnancy test was scheduled, I was already feeling a little sick, my breasts were tender, but I really believed that it was all in my head.

The night before the pregnancy test we went to dinner with our neighbors. When we went home they hugged us and by then we were all crying. We could feel their hope and concern. They wished us well. Earlier that week I had gone to lunch with my friend Jill, and she kept saying that she knew I was pregnant. I didn't want to get my hopes up because I was scared to death that it may not have worked. The two weeks after the transfer seemed like an eternity. Jeff and I talked a lot about the procedure and what would happen if it failed.

When we got to the center, they called me in to take my blood. They asked me how I felt, if my breasts hurt and if I was nauseous. When I said yes, they said those were good signs. They told us that it would take about 45 minutes. By this time I was really keyed up. My heart was beating fast and I didn't know if I could last another 45 minutes. We decided to go for a walk to kill some time. Jeff was nervous, too, but he tried not to show it. We made small talk while holding hands tightly. Secretly, I think we were both praying. After the walk, we went back into the center and sat down impatiently. My legs were shaking. We saw Minda, who had screened and cared for our eggs, come out of the lab to talk to us. I could see that she had tears in her eyes. My immediate thought was that it didn't work. She nodded her head, "Yes, you are pregnant." Jeff and I immediately burst into tears and held each other tight. I was, for once, speechless. Our dream had come true.

They then told us that my pregnancy hormone level was so high they were sure it was more than one. We were ecstatic because we actually wanted twins. We immediately went home and told all of our neighbors and called all of our family and closest friends. There were many tears of joy.

Day 31 and beyond

In 30 days, more or less, we have couples who must bear the disappointment of failure and figure out where to go from there. Will another IVF cycle be worthwhile? Will there soon be some scientific breakthrough that will make their chances better? Will their marriage even survive this disappointment?

On the other hand, we have couples who are about to embark on the journey through the next nine months that will, if all goes well, give them the child they have so longed for.

Two weeks later I was scheduled for my first ultrasound to see how many babies I had. During those two weeks, we pondered the thought of twins or triplets. Twins sounded wonderful; triplets maybe more than we could handle. The ultrasound showed twins.

We think their positive attitude and sense of humor were helpful in getting them through the cycle.

Cheryl's pregnancy went quite smoothly. She delivered twin girls by caesarean section because both babies were coming feet first. Brittany Marie weighed 6 pounds 11 ounces and Lauren Nicole tipped the scales at 6 pounds 7 ounces. From the start, Cheryl and Jeff considered their IVF cycle their "science project." They kept their sense of humor throughout this difficult period. They were fortunate enough to have the support of their family, friends and, most important, each other. They both feel that it was this mutual support that sustained them.

...GIFT AND ZIFT

These procedures differ from IVF in that an operation is required both to retrieve eggs and to transfer eggs and sperm into the fallopian tube in GIFT, and to transfer embryos in ZIFT. The stimulation phase will be similar to what we described in IVF. In ZIFT the egg retrieval will be identical to IVF. With GIFT, the laparoscopy is performed on Day 12, the day of retrieval. In the case of ZIFT, it is done on Day 13, 15 or 17 depending on the stage of embryos to be transferred.

The patient is admitted to the hospital in the day surgery area. An IV is started and the anesthesiologist explains the anesthetic options. These would include:

- Epidural, in which local anesthetic is injected near the spinal column. It numbs the tissues below the waist while the patient remains awake, but can be sedated.

- General anesthesia, in which the patient is given an intravenous medication to induce sleep, and then gas is administered through a tube placed into the trachea to reach a deep level of anesthesia.

If general anesthesia is chosen, the patient's abdomen is washed and drapes are placed around the lower abdomen before the anesthetic is given in order to reduce the period of time the eggs are exposed to the anesthetic. With the epidural, the anesthetic is administered first, since very little of the medication gets into the bloodstream.

A small incision is made in the lower margin of the navel. A thin needle is introduced into the abdominal cavity and a gas is put in to allow the surrounding tissues to fall away from the pelvic organs. The sheath for the telescope is then placed through the same incision and the pelvis is observed. Smaller incisions are made in the lower part of the abdomen for the other instruments to hold and move structures, to aspirate the follicles or to place gametes into the fallopian tube.

If GIFT is being done, the ovary is brought into view and each follicle is punctured, aspirated and flushed with medium until the egg is found. The eggs are identified, the quality is assessed and those suitable for transfer are chosen. With GIFT, usually three to four eggs with 100,000 sperm are placed into the better-looking fallopian tube. While the eggs and sperm are being prepared, the pelvis is inspected for any abnormalities such as endometriosis. If any endometriosis is found, it can be cauterized. The sperm and eggs are then drawn up into a catheter placed through one of the incisions and guided more than four centimeters into the tube. The eggs and sperm are expelled, the catheter is removed, all instruments are withdrawn and the incisions are closed. After several hours of recovery, the patient may go home and, after recuperation, may engage in light activity for the next two weeks or so, until the pregnancy test. She will also be taking daily progesterone injections.

In very rare cases combined IVF/GIFT may be done. If some of the eggs are less mature, they can be allowed to develop further before the sperm are added. Then if embryos form, a transcervical transfer can be done three days later, as with IVF.

In the case of ZIFT, the eggs will be retrieved as described for IVF and then transferred one day later. One disadvantage is the need for two separate procedures for retrieval and transfer. This increases cost, discomfort and risk. On the other side of the balance, studies have indicated a slightly higher success rate for ZIFT.

One of the most poignant accounts of a patient going through a ZIFT procedure was provided by Anne Taylor Fleming, the noted writer and media commentator, in a March 15, 1989, article in the *New York Times,* "Points West: When a Loving Nest Remains Empty." She described her second attempt at ZIFT.

Anne Taylor Fleming's article is reprinted here with the permission of the New York Times.

So I am—or was—a pioneer of sorts, pregnant with optimism throughout the two weeks of fertility drugs before the procedure and the two weeks after as you hold your breath for fear of dislodging any embryos that might have nestled within. It is suspended time; you live backward, taking inventory of the decisions that brought you to this point, and forward, imagining your barren years ahead. Your womb seems to be calling you to account, making you heed its emptiness. "At last I've got your attention," it seems to be saying. "Where have you been all these years?" But along with the deliberations and discomforts there are incredible highs. The process is akin to being in a demonic love affair, when the pull and punishment of the flesh are irresistible. When I found they had retrieved 11 eggs from my ovaries, I was elated. How could I miss? But, by nightfall, I was in despair: What if none of the eggs fertilized; what if on the most basic level my husband and I were hopelessly incompatible, our sperm and eggs unwilling to conduct their extra-corporeal courtship; what if by morning we had no zygotes?

The nurse called early to say we indeed had zygotes. Four eggs had fertilized. "Come get them," she said, and my heart leaped at the invitation. I dressed carefully and washed my hair, as if I were about to meet somebody special. Would I be able to hold onto one or any of them; would they continue to divide and grow inside me? Knowing the ZIFT odds, I was hopeful. No, that's not strong enough: I was crazed with hope as they put me to sleep, made a tiny slit in my navel and through a catheter dropped three of my embryos (the fourth was frozen for a future attempt) into my one good fallopian tube. All those embryos had to do is migrate down to my waiting womb. What could stop them now?

Something did, some something. My embryos didn't take hold; they vanished. When that was confirmed, two weeks to the day after the procedure had been performed, I myself vanished for a while into a fetal curl of grief. This was hardly a death, not even a miscarriage, just a noncarriage.

> *So what's next? For me, my remaining frozen embryo. It (he, she?) will be thawed and inseminated [sic] into my uterus in another month or so, after my body recovers from this last assault... Out beyond that I can try another ZIFT. The woman who went through it the same day I did is pregnant. With clenched teeth, I rejoice for her.*
>
> *How many rounds do I have left and how far am I willing to go before I give up or consider another course like adoption? I don't know.*

Apparently her attempts at biological parenthood were never achieved. In a February 11, 1998 commentary called "Baby Boom," on the "NewsHour with Jim Lehrer" on PBS, it was clear that her feelings remained unresolved.

> *I too went through a long and ultimately unsuccessful baby quest, stopping just short of using donor this or that because the questions for me were simply too intense. I figured menopause was the end. But now doctors tell me that I can get back in the baby chase; that it's never too late to give birth, a thought that feels both weird and hopeful and right and wrong all at the same time. Fertility clinics are now full of women like me, and every year there are more of us. In just seven years — from 1988 to 1995 — the number of American women in their child-bearing years who suffered from infertility went from 4.9 to 6.1 million, a 25% jump, in no small part because women are waiting longer to have their children. So more money and more effort will be thrown at the problem. The latest breakthrough is the freezing of eggs on their own so that the young and unready full of dreams and career goals can simply have a batch of their young, healthy eggs frozen in their early 20s and stored for future use. How weird it all seems.*

SUCCESS AND FAILURE

The most intense 30 or so days in the lives of these couples is now over. There can be only two possible results: success in the form of a baby in the next nine months; or failure by means of a negative pregnancy test, miscarriage, ectopic pregnancy or other obstetrical problem.

The couples who do not conceive have to deal with the bitterness of not having the opportunity of achieving their goal this time. They face an uncertain future and a decision of whether to try again, give up the fight or go in a different direction such as adoption.

Fortunately, for most, a second, third or fourth attempt will have almost the same chance as the first. In a multicenter study by SART, the results of a second cycle were identical to the first. The chance was 80% to 85% as high in the third cycle, 75% to 80% in the fourth and almost 60% as high for cycles in excess of four. This study and another from Britain refute the findings of one atypical study which showed a marked fall-off in success with subsequent cycles. There is no single factor more important to ultimate success than having repeated attempts. Does this sound familiar? Yes, persistence is the key to success.

There does come a time, however, to end the quest for a biologic child. For some, the knowledge that we all did our best to try to achieve their goal brings the mission to a conclusion, as expressed in this December 1994 letter from Mike and Carol Wallensack:

> *We each wish these days had ended differently. But be clear about this; you gave us the gift of hope. And the final outcome does not diminish your precious gift. For those days of hope we are deeply grateful to you.*
>
> *Truly, the greatest pain at the end of the road is parting with you.*
>
> *But it isn't really the end of the road, is it? It is more like a fork in the road. Because of your help, we are comforted knowing we did everything possible. Now we can leave our infertility behind and turn onto the road of adoption.*

In June 1995, Carol and Mike adopted Mark Wallensack.

For some couples, special problems may have been recognized during the first attempt. In chapter 12 we will discuss the role egg and sperm donors can play in overcoming problems with the production of normal healthy eggs or with fertilization. For others, new experimental procedures may be possible (chapter 13).

Those who are pregnant will enjoy the sweetness of their success. The positive pregnancy test, of course, is not the end point, but merely the beginning of the pregnancy that hopefully will lead them to their ultimate goal, a healthy baby. Yet there may be some potential hazards along the way; these we discuss in chapter 11.

CHAPTER 11

And Baby Makes Three...or Four

The key question to be answered for those who are pregnant as the result of an ART procedure is whether these pregnancies are at greater risk than those conceived in the usual manner. Of course, multiple pregnancies—of which there is a stronger likelihood when ovulatory drugs and ART procedures are used—are more risky in general. But, aside from the increased risks from multiple pregnancy, are there additional perils for the ART pregnancy or the baby? We will explore this issue after we give you some basic advice.

"CONGRATULATIONS, YOUR PREGNANCY TEST IS POSITIVE"

Those are the words you want to hear, but they do not necessarily reflect the ultimate goal you want to achieve. The positive pregnancy test is just one step, albeit a very important one, along the way. Yet many couples misinterpret the positive pregnancy test as a sign that they have achieved their final goal. Actually, one of four outcomes can occur following the positive pregnancy test.

Biochemical pregnancy

This is a situation in which fertilization has taken place, the embryo implants and starts to produce one of the pregnancy hormones (hCG), but something goes wrong with the implantation or the pregnancy fails to develop. A weakly positive pregnancy test indicates the presence of a pregnancy, although no evidence of a pregnancy can be detected by ultrasound. The hCG level gradually declines to zero without any clinical evidence of a pregnancy. This is not a rare phenomenon, and as noted in previous chapters, we do not feel that centers should include these biochemical pregnancies (usually about 5% to 10% of positive pregnancy tests) in their statistics indicating success.

Clinical pregnancy

In this case not only is there a positive pregnancy test, but we can also find other evidence of a pregnancy. The earliest evidence of a clinical pregnancy would consist of finding a pregnancy sac with or without fetal parts or a fetal heartbeat on an ultrasound examination. This is a very exciting moment for the couple, and we encourage the father to be present for this first ultrasound.

However, the pregnancy is still subject to all the risks encountered by any pregnancy, including miscarriage and other conditions that can lead to a poor outcome. In addition, there has been a minor increase in premature labor in IVF pregnancies besides that resulting from multiple births.

Ectopic pregnancy

Rarely the embryos can float into the fallopian tube, become trapped there and implant, creating a tubal ectopic pregnancy. It is more common in women with preexisting tubal disease but can occur in women with apparently normal tubes. The rate of ectopic pregnancies was reported in the 2001 CDC/SART survey as 0.7%.

Live birth

This is the outcome we are all working toward. But even with the birth of a live baby, there can be a chance of birth defects just as there is in the general population. So the goal we are hoping for is the birth of a healthy, normal baby.

You cannot assume that we will achieve this goal based only on a positive pregnancy test. Our joy at hearing that the pregnancy test is positive must be tempered with a small dose of caution. Placing too much emphasis on the positive pregnancy test can lead to great disappointment if it turns out to signify only a biochemical, ectopic or clinical pregnancy that is later lost through miscarriage or other accident of pregnancy.

Theresa's reaction following a biochemical pregnancy is a good illustration of how deep the disappointment can be. Happily, she had a positive pregnancy test following her IVF cycle. Now, you must understand that positive pregnancy tests evoke very strong emotions not only in the couple, but also among the staff as well. Theresa was a very outgoing person and had become friendly with almost everyone on the staff. Thus, when her pregnancy test was positive, there was much crying and hugging and congratulations from the staff. Theresa interpreted this activity to mean that the baby was practically in her arms. When her positive test turned out to indicate only a biochemical pregnancy, her distress was especially intense. She felt that the positive response from the center's staff made her disappointment more painful. Fortunately, several months following this experience she became pregnant as the result of a frozen embryo transfer and delivered a healthy, full-term baby. But because of this incident, we have instructed our staff, including physicians, to be mindful of the fact that the positive pregnancy test is news to be tempered with cautious optimism.

Consequently, these are the instructions we usually discuss with patients who have a positive pregnancy test:

We often have to remind successful patients and our staff that a positive pregnancy test is not the goal, but merely an important step in achieving the goal—the birth of a healthy baby.

1. We offer our congratulations, but moderate our joy with an admonition that although the positive test is good news, there is still a long way to go until they get to hold their baby. It's really too bad that we have to be somewhat pessimistic at this very happy news, but we feel it is our role to present all the facts to the couple in the proper perspective.
2. The woman should not engage in very heavy activity. This includes lifting, heavy housework and exercise. Other than these precautions, she may engage in normal activity.
3. A daily prenatal vitamin is recommended. Studies have indicated a significantly lower incidence of heart and spinal cord defects when prenatal vitamins containing 0.4 mg of folic acid are taken early in pregnancy, preferably even before conception.
4. Intercourse with or without orgasm and other means of achieving orgasm can lead to uterine contractions that may interfere with the

implanting embryo and therefore is not recommended until after at least the first 6 weeks. This extra-cautious approach was started early in our own program and, as a result or coincidentally, we have experienced a very low rate of miscarriage. Understandably, we have continued to advise this precaution, and our rate of pregnancy loss has continued to be lower than the national average. Bleeding is common in ART pregnancies, probably due to multiple implantations. This may be the reason that the uterus is not quite as stable as it is in other pregnancies.

5. Progesterone will be continued, but may be changed to vaginal suppositories rather than injections if progesterone levels are adequate and there is no bleeding. If there is any problem using the suppositories, or significant bleeding occurs, the injections are resumed. Some vaginal bleeding occurs in a large number of pregnancies, including both naturally-conceived and ART pregnancies, and does not necessarily mean that a miscarriage is occurring.

6. We recommend that the mother-to-be avoid caffeine, alcohol, smoking and all drugs—including over-the-counter preparations and, of course, any recreational drugs. The only exception is acetaminophen (Tylenol, Datril, Anacin-3), which may be taken for aches and pains and should be taken to reduce fever.

7. She should return to the center for her first pregnancy ultrasound one week after the pregnancy test. At this time we will usually see the pregnancy sac or sacs. By two weeks after the pregnancy test we should see some evidence of fetal development and usually fetal heart motion. We will know, with some degree of accuracy, how many pregnancies are present. The main reason for doing these scans is to alert us to the chance of a tubal pregnancy if we do not see a normally placed sac with a fetus in the uterus.

   If the scan indicates a normal single pregnancy or twins we usually refer the patient on to her own obstetrician. The question of whether her own obstetrician is well equipped to take care of an IVF pregnancy is frequently asked by successful IVF patients. In general, we feel that any well-trained and experienced obstetrician is qualified to manage a single or twin IVF pregnancy. In the case of triplets, we would recommend discussing the resources available in her community to handle high-risk pregnancy. In the unlikely event of quadruplets or more, we feel that referral to a high-risk specialist is advisable.

IS THERE A GREATER CHANCE OF MISCARRIAGE?

As we indicated above when we cited the four possible outcomes from a positive pregnancy test, there is a significant risk of early loss of clinical pregnancy through miscarriage. There is some variation among programs in the incidence of early pregnancy loss. Just as with ART procedures, there is also a significant rate of first trimester pregnancy loss of 10 % to 20% in couples who conceive without assistance. In May 2003 the American College of Obstetricians and Gynecologists conducted a survey comparing the miscarriage rate from the 1996 through 1998 ART Registry with the miscarriage rates from the U.S. population-based National Survey of Family Growth and found similar rates in both. Therefore, any increase in early pregnancy loss attributable to these procedures is very small. The largest variation was based on age. The spontaneous abortion risk in ART pregnancies ranged from 10.1% among women 20 to 29 years of age to 39.3% among women older than 43 years. The 2001 results from the SART/CDC report indicate an overall miscarriage of 15.5% in all non-donor fresh ART pregnancies conceived that year.

ARE IVF PREGNANCIES HIGH RISK?

It is apparent that with multiple pregnancies involving three or more fetuses there is substantially more risk to the pregnancy than if there were just one or two fetuses present. Even the occurrence of twins increases the chance of obstetrical problems such as premature labor. But aside from the increased risk from multiple births, are IVF pregnancies in themselves at higher risk than those occurring naturally?

Some studies have found a small but detectable increase in premature labor and poor fetal growth aside from that which occurs with multiple pregnancy. In one study early pregnancy bleeding, hypertension and placenta previa (placenta over the opening of the uterus) were also slightly more common than in pregnancies conceived without assistance. It is not clear whether this is related to the underlying infertility problem or to the ART procedure itself.

A 1996 French study of the outcome of twin pregnancies conceived by IVF, ovarian stimulation and "unassisted" conception found no difference in the outcome in these three groups. Another report from Mount Sinai in New York published in the March 1997 issue of *Obstetrics and Gynecology* compares twin pregnancies conceived through IVF and GIFT with those occurring spontaneously. They concluded that low birth weight and a difference in birth weight between the two babies is more frequent in ART pregnancies, but the well-being of the babies is the same as those conceived naturally. This suggests that the procedures, medications or underlying fertility problem are not responsible for premature labor or poor fetal growth.

MULTIPLE PREGNANCY

In the 2001 SART/CDC data, the incidence of multiple deliveries was 35.8% of the ongoing pregnancies using fresh, non-donor eggs, with 3.8% ending with the delivery of triplets or greater. Almost half the babies born through ART cycles that year were part of a multiple birth. During the same time period, the multiple birth rate of the general population was 3%. A study published by the Centers for Disease Control in February 1997 showed that twin births in the U.S. increased 42% between 1980 and 1994. In the same time period the rate of triplets jumped a spectacular 214%. The reason? You guessed it: ART procedures. Connecticut was the state with the highest rate of multiple births, followed by Massachusetts, New Jersey, Rhode Island and Illinois.

The twin pregnancies can be managed fairly easily within most community resources. In a recent review of twin pregnancies, preterm labor was observed in 58.8% of the cases, with 52% of the mothers delivering before 36 weeks. It is the high-level multiple pregnancy that leads to concern about complications. With triplets or more, the obstetrical outcome is significantly worse than in single or even twin pregnancies. In a review of multiple pregnancies in the U.S. from 1991 to 1995, the mean gestation age of twins was 35.77 weeks, and for triplets 32.48 weeks. It is the more significant prematurity of the triplet babies that results in increased problems in the neonatal period, potential life-long disabilities and markedly increased neonatal costs. For example, the same review showed that the birth of infants born at 25 to 27 weeks gestation cost 28 times more than those born at 39 to 42 weeks gestation ($280,146 versus $9,803 U.S.). The overriding issues with extreme prematurity are the potential for physical or developmental deficits, or both, and the need for life-long therapeutic interventions.

One often overlooked aspect of multiple births is the quality of life for the families of multiples. An article in the August 2003 *Fertility and Sterility* addressed significant quality-of-life issues for mothers of multiples. More than half (58%) of the mothers interviewed had undergone ART procedures, but all had experienced social stigma marked by experiences involving family, friends and strangers asking unsolicited, insensitive questions about their fertility status and making assumptions and expressing moral judgments about the conception of their children. There were a variety of different impacts in patients' marriages. Some disintegrated as husbands and wives lost touch with each other under the incredible stress of caring for multiple infants. Other marriages grew stronger as spouses recognized the necessity of working together as a team to care for their children.

For the couple confronted by a multiple pregnancy with more than four fetuses (high-level multiple pregnancy), the options are few. To continue the pregnancy would lead to a very high chance of prematurity with its associated problems. With triplets or quadruplets, continuing the pregnancy with three or four fetuses may still be a realistic alternative. Although aborting some of the fetuses while leaving others to continue (known as multi-fetal pregnancy reduction or selective reduction) will directly harm some of the fetuses, it may offer the only hope of a successful outcome for any. An example of the danger of high-level multiple pregnancy is the highly publicized 1985 California septuplets case. Four of the babies died within one month of delivery, and it was reported that all three survivors have cerebral palsy. Another possibility would be to avoid these serious potential consequences of prematurity by terminating the entire pregnancy. However, it would be a cruel irony for these patients who had tried for so long to conceive to then have to terminate a pregnancy because of a multiple gestation.

It is because of this dilemma facing couples with high-level multiple pregnancies that selective reduction was developed. At first hearing, this sounds abhorrent. But when you realize that this may be the only way to save any of the fetuses, it may become an option to consider.

People generally take the dangers of multiple pregnancy too lightly. There are risks, even though high-risk care has greatly improved.

Based on various reports, it is now generally suggested that a quadruplet pregnancy should be reduced to twins. With a triplet implantation, the outcome can be improved by reduction, with an increase of the length of gestation and therefore fewer neonatal problems. In some cases even reduction of twins to a singleton may be considered, such as when the uterus is abnormal due to DES exposure or an anomaly, when one fetus is genetically abnormal or because of maternal health problems or advanced maternal age, such as with egg donation. In skilled hands selective reduction can be done with very little discomfort and with a low chance of disturbing the pregnancy. Data show that following reduction of a high-level multiple pregnancy to twins, there is a 75% to 80% chance of producing live-born twins with an adequate amount of time in the uterus. As you would expect, the most common complication is miscarriage of the entire pregnancy. Although this is a relatively new procedure, there are doctors with sufficient experience for the chance of complications to be very low. One expert called selective reduction "a lousy solution but the best hope for this problem." An international registry has been established to learn about the natural history of high-level multiple pregnancies and the operative statistics for selective reduction. In the quality-of-life study discussed above, selective reduction was identified as a particularly troubling experience.

As with most medical conditions, the best treatment is prevention. Although this problem cannot be prevented in all cases, proper monitoring of fertility drugs and limitation of numbers of eggs or embryos to be transferred will go a long way toward preventing high-level multiple pregnancy.

WILL MY BABY BE NORMAL?

One of the most frequent questions we hear regarding ART pregnancies is, "Will my baby be normal?" The answer in initial studies was that the incidence of birth defects was no different than in pregnancies conceived normally. For example, in the 1994 data from the IVF Registry, the rate of defects was 2.7 defects per 100 newborns, roughly the same rate as in the general population. A reassuring study in the February 1997 issue of the journal *Fertility and Sterility* followed a large group of IVF children aged 6 to 13 years. Physical growth in 97.8% was within the normal range. The rate of malfor-

mations was no different from the general population. School performance was good in 92.2%. The most surprising finding was that in the group
of children aged 6 to 10 years, over half the children were not informed that
they had been conceived through IVF. Over one-quarter of the parents also
kept the IVF a secret from their families. Among the children aged 11 to 13
years, one-third of the children were not told about the circumstances of
their conception. A 2001 European study of 400 11- and 12-year-olds showed
them to be just as healthy psychologically and emotionally as their naturally-conceived peers.

However, over the past several years a number of issues have
emerged questioning the belief that children born as the result of ART are
no different from those conceived naturally. Several studies addressed the
issue of increased congenital abnormalities and low birth weight in connection with ART. The CDC found in 2002 that assisted reproduction singleton
infants who were not born prematurely were 2.6 times as likely to have low
birth weights as the general population. In another 2002 study from the
University of Western Australia, funded by the March of Dimes, roughly 9%
of children conceived through either IVF or ICSI had birth defects at one
year of age, compared to 4.2% of children born through natural conception.
In 2003, new research from the United Kingdom revealed a 4 times higher
incidence of a rare genetic disorder, Beckwith-Wiedemann Syndrome, in
babies born from assisted reproduction. The theoretical reason for this possible association is that it results from a genetic imprinting disorder resulting in faulty copies of genes occurring during early cell division while in
culture rather than in the fallopian tube or uterus in nature. On the other
hand, in March 2003, researchers from the United Kingdom and Australia
found that the developmental process and incidence of congenital defects
in children conceived using ICSI, compared to a group of sociodemograph-
ically matched children conceived naturally, did not result in any difference between the two groups. The bottom line is that more research is
needed. In responding to the news of the possible association of ART with
Beckwith-Wiedemann Syndrome (an overgrowth syndrome characterized
by excess growth of the cellular, tissue and organ levels associated with
large organs, including a large tongue, hypoglycemia and an increased risk
of cancer), Dr. Joe Leigh Simpson, chairman of the ob-gyn department at

Baylor College of Medicine and a prominent geneticist, said the number of cases is so small that they will not dissuade infertile couples considering assisted reproduction. "There have been a million IVF babies born now," he told WebMD, "and there has not been a trace of concern that the overall frequency of genetic disorders with standard IVF is any different than the population as a whole."

Another issue of concern to doctors and couples alike is the question of what, if any, effect hormones used to support ART pregnancies may have on the offspring. We know that synthetic hormones used in the past for early pregnancy support have been associated with fetal problems. Androgenic hormones and synthetic progestins taken in the first 12 weeks of gestation may masculinize the external genitalia of a female fetus. A rare form of vaginal cancer and future fertility problems were more frequent in women whose mothers used the synthetic estrogen diethylstilbestrol (DES) in early pregnancy. But today, despite the fact that we use only natural forms of hormones, the FDA persists in requiring frightening warnings to be given with the natural forms of these hormones. To date, there is no scientific evidence that natural hormones are associated with birth defects. Even if there were some effect, it must be small, as most reports show no increase in abnormalities in ART pregnancies and virtually all ART procedures require hormonal support in early pregnancy. Until definitive information is available, the most logical approach is to limit the use of support hormones to the lowest effective dose and shortest time possible without endangering the pregnancy itself.

So, how does one answer the question, "Will my baby be normal?" Why are there such conflicting studies? As you evaluate all this information you must remember that in the U.S. 2% to 3% of births are affected by congenital abnormalities. There are many known factors associated with an increased incidence of congenital abnormalities such as advanced maternal age, maternal medical conditions such as diabetes, certain medications, substance abuse and environmental toxic effects, multiple pregnancies and prematurity. If you compare ART babies to the general population it is vital to find appropriate control populations. Women undergoing ART tend to be older, have more multiple gestations and a higher incidence of prematurity. The control group would have to mirror these demographic features.

The other issue to consider is whether any increased incidence of defects is the result of the technique or of the condition requiring the need for ART, such as genetic defects in the male partner requiring ICSI. It is also necessary to remember that few of the vast majority of the perfectly normal children would have been conceived without the technology.

In view of the possibility of an increase in birth defects, we urge women with ART pregnancies to take advantage of all the diagnostic tests that are appropriate and available for them. Women over 34 and those conceiving as the result of ICSI are encouraged to consider amniocentesis for chromosomal evaluation of the pregnancy. Amniocentesis also gives an opportunity to check for open defects of the tissue covering the brain and spinal cord (neural tube defects) by checking the alphafetoprotein levels in the amniotic fluid. For those not having amniocentesis, blood screening tests are now available to check for neural tube defects and, in addition, chromosomal and other abnormalities. One study showed a higher false positive rate in the screening blood tests for chromosomal abnormalities in IVF patients. Nevertheless, if amniocentesis is not necessary, we recommend the blood tests be done routinely and a 12-week ultrasound for signs of chromosomal defects and a thorough 18-week ultrasound examination may be suggested. (Some argue that this should be done in every pregnancy, anyway.) We generally do not recommend chorionic villus sampling to detect chromosomal defects because it has a slightly higher risk of miscarriage, a situation we especially want to avoid in a woman who has only been able to conceive by means of an ART procedure. In fact, in a recent report there was almost a 4% miscarriage rate associated with CVS compared to less than 1% for amniocentesis in women carrying ICSI pregnancies.

IVF children have now been followed up to age 13 with findings of normal physical growth and school performance.

FINDING AN OBSTETRICIAN

Since you have probably spent years in your quest for this pregnancy, it is very likely that you already know a general obstetrician/gynecologist. Assuming that you like and have confidence in him or her and that you have a single or twin pregnancy, you have no more looking to do. A well-trained obstetrician is experienced in dealing with such cases.

If you do not have your own physician who can take care of your pregnancy, you can use most of the criteria in chapter 9 to make a list of physicians who may become your new Dr. Perfect, the obstetrician. It is most likely that the physicians who participated in your ART procedure do not deliver babies, although there are exceptions. However, your fertility doctor will probably be a good resource to obtain a referral to an obstetrician. He or she naturally wants to be sure you receive good care.

In choosing a doctor to deliver your baby, there are some specific considerations that differ from those in selecting a fertility specialist. Many obstetricians offer a free consultation for you to become acquainted before you sign on the dotted line. This is an opportunity for you to become familiar with the doctor's philosophy and demeanor. There are many choices to be made with regard to your obstetrical care. These choices relate not only to the mechanics of delivery but also in the selection of prenatal testing, location of hospital for delivery, method of analgesia and anesthesia, and availability of consultation in case of complications, to name a few. You will want to make sure that the physician who will guide you through this pregnancy starts with the same basic philosophy you do.

When you do get to meet with the physician, you should plan to get as much information as you can in a period of 5 to 10 minutes. We suggest you focus your limited time on three areas that will give you a pretty good idea of his or her philosophy regarding:

- availability
- coverage by a substitute physician
- flexibility

1. How available are you to answer my questions?

The ideal answer would be total availability—a patient's dream, but in reality an impossibility. Even a doctor has a private life, with its duties and crises and even some time off for good behavior. What you are trying to establish here is to what extent your calls for information will be fielded by the doctor. Or will you be speaking to a nurse or receptionist and not have access to the doctor except in medical emergencies? Some women prefer discussing most things with the nurse; others prefer the physician. It's wise to obtain the office policy on that in advance, as it may avoid potential hassles and feelings of neglect later on.

2. How available are you for deliveries? When you're not available, who covers for you?

Needless to say, this is an extremely important issue. Usually you will be told that the doctor has a regular coverage arrangement with physicians who follow the same general philosophy and that your care will be the same no matter which physician happens to be on call. Unfortunately, some physicians who regularly deliver babies do not have formalized coverage arrangements with other equally qualified physicians. When they do, often it's with a friend or acquaintance who may not share the doctor's or (more importantly) your philosophy. For example, there can be differences in the use of pain medications during labor, the types of anesthetics and different views as to the need for caesarean deliveries.

In answer to this question, you want to hear that there *is* a coverage policy and that you have the option to meet one or all of the doctors who provide this service. You should flinch if the doctor says, "Don't worry…I'll be there." Too many women have been burned by this insincere promise. We know of one woman, a lawyer, who was carrying twins and kept asking her physician who would be there if he were unable to attend the delivery. He kept insisting that he delivered all of his own patients. Well, you guessed it! When she had an emergency necessitating the delivery of the twins, he was nowhere to be found and she had to rely on the luck of the draw. A physician who happened to be in the hospital responded and fortunately all turned out well. Remember that when it comes to delivering babies, the selection of a doctor is often only as good as his or her backup physician.

The techniques to find an obstetrician are the same as we recommend to find a fertility specialist. The questions are a little different, however.

3. What are your routine procedures for patients in labor?

Actually, no procedures are routine in labor. You don't want to hear the doctor rattle off a list of routines pertaining to enema, shave, IV and other predelivery procedures. What you want to hear is that the doctor applies a degree of flexibility in dealing with patients in labor and that the patient's individual needs are an important consideration. You may be told that the hospital calls for specific routines during labor. Don't believe it. Chances are this doctor is hiding behind "hospital rules" in order to apply his or her own preferences. Inflexibility is not what you're looking for in a physician, despite the best credentials.

Those are the three big questions. The doctor's answers and any discussion surrounding them will, in all likelihood, consume the bulk of your allotted time, but should the meeting continue and the doctor has more time to answer questions, here are some more worthwhile ones.

4. How often do you perform a caesarean section?

The question can also be phrased, "What is your c-section rate?" You're looking for a straightforward answer, for example, "My c-section rate is 25%, which is consistent with what we do in the community" or "My rate is a little higher because I see many patients who are at high risk for complications, patients with diabetes, for example." Currently an acceptable rule of thumb is a primary c-section rate (not including repeat caesareans) between 25% and 30%.

5. What are the reasons you induce labor? How often do you induce?

This issue refers to the use of drugs (Pitocin or prostaglandin) to trigger the onset of labor. You'd like to hear the doctor say, "I seldom do elective inductions. But I do induce occasionally for medical reasons such as diabetes, high blood pressure, premature rupture of the membranes or when someone goes too far past her due date." If the doctor says, "I like to induce everybody, it's much more convenient," that's not what you want to hear. It's a very questionable routine practice.

6. What is your fee?

The answer to this question is readily available at the front office. If you're comparison shopping, it might be wise to conduct a small survey in the community. Check with several offices and establish a range of fees. We do not recommend that you select a physician primarily on the basis of the lowest or highest fee. Just make sure that the fees you are being charged are within the range in your community.

The subject of fees raises the issue of medical insurance coverage, an issue that could determine if you have any choice of physician at all. In this era of prepaid health plans and preferred provider arrangements, your choice may be severely limited to those health professionals who are affiliated with the plan. If you belong to a health maintenance organization

(HMO), this will certainly be the case. With a preferred provider organization (PPO) plan, you stand to lose a portion of your insurance reimbursement if you see a physician who is not affiliated with your PPO. Unfortunately, many women discover too late that they're locked into the physician-access system that falls within their husband's health insurance package from work, the 2- or 3-year-old plan he may have forgotten to tell his wife about.

While many physicians in these HMO plans are dedicated to practicing quality medicine, they may differ from each other in regard to the management of obstetric patients. It may be difficult to ensure that all your needs are being met under these conditions and you may have to lobby strongly for what you want. For example, many HMOs have rules that you cannot see an obstetrician until you are a certain number of weeks pregnant. As an IVF- or GIFT-pregnant patient, the early part of pregnancy is crucial and we feel you should be under a doctor's care at this time. You may, in some situations, have to fight for that right.

A WORD OF ADVICE

There is something amazing about pregnancy. You quickly become a believer in the old saying, "One gives nothing so freely as advice," and begin to understand that free advice is worth what you have paid for it. You'll wonder if the news that someone is pregnant has the effect of triggering the advice-giving gene in people. Sometimes it will be difficult to separate wisdom from ignorance, fact from myth. You can count on being told that you must eat for two. Perhaps someone will caution you against raising your arms over your head since it might cause the umbilical cord to wrap itself around the baby's neck. At least one thoughtless individual will probably tell you that you should not be having a baby through IVF or GIFT because it's unnatural or that they are opposed to people having GIFT triplets because humans were not meant to have litters. You will also find that almost everyone who has had a baby wants to regale you with the gory details of her terrible three days in labor.

We recommend that the last piece of advice you take seriously from anyone other than your own health professionals is this: Don't take any medical advice from anyone other than your own health professionals. Either listen politely and forget it or tell the advice-giver that you are really not interested in what happened to his or her Aunt Tillie. If you have questions or concerns, ask your doctor, read or speak to your childbirth instructors, but don't take the advice of well-meaning friends or relatives.

GOOD LUCK!

You are about to embark upon one of the most exciting adventures of your life. We encourage you to learn as much as you can about pregnancy and the birth process through reading and classes, so you can help make many of the choices that will confront you throughout this pregnancy. Good luck!

CHAPTER 12

Third-Party Reproduction

WHEN THE BEST SCIENCE HAS TO OFFER IS NOT ENOUGH

In this book we have described the latest techniques used to treat a variety of conditions that result in infertility. However, even sophisticated, 21st-century medical technology has its limitations. When the best science has to offer is not enough for other medical problems, we may be forced to rely upon the replacement of faulty organs with donor organs, as when kidney failure requires a kidney transplant or end-stage cardiovascular disease requires a heart or lung transplant. Although for some a living sibling or parent can provide an organ, in many cases the donor organ is donated after the death of a stranger.

Donations of semen or eggs for the treatment of infertility are different. They are more akin to blood donations. There is so much reserve built into the human reproduction system that egg donors (and even more so sperm donors) can donate their gametes on many occasions with essentially no significant depletion of their reserves. Sperm donation can be done every few days without any adverse effects on the donor. Egg donation cannot be done so often, but eggs can certainly be donated more than once.

There are four categories of donation in the treatment of infertility:

1. Sperm donation
2. Egg donation

3. Embryo donation
4. Surrogate parenting—where the use of the uterus with or without eggs is donated

Our discussion will revolve mainly around the first two categories, since they are the ones most closely associated with ART procedures. Embryo donation is a relatively new concept and not yet widely practiced, but it can be very effective. Surrogate parenting is another topic in itself with many legal and ethical ramifications which we will touch on. Adoption is a topic beyond the scope of this book. (References regarding adoption are found in Appendix 2.)

SEMEN DONATION

There is no rejection with egg donation because every fetus is always foreign to the woman's body and is always protected from her immune system.

The donation of semen for artificial insemination has been practiced for well over a century. However, concerns during the last two decades about complications related to the transmission of infectious diseases have resulted in changes to the practice of donor artificial insemination. In February 1993 the American Society for Reproductive Medicine issued revised guidelines for the use of donor insemination. Most of the changes in the guidelines relate to measures to try to avoid the transmission of sexually transmitted diseases, most notably HIV.

Reasons for semen donation

The major indications for donor insemination are:

- The husband is irreversibly sterile from any cause.
- The husband has had a vasectomy and does not want to have it reversed.
- The husband has a low or marginal sperm count, antisperm antibodies or some other condition where the male factor is thought to be the predominant cause of the infertility and cannot be overcome by other means, or the couple does not want to use an ART procedure.
- The husband has, or is a carrier of, a known hereditary disease.
- The husband has a problem with ejaculation that cannot be overcome by current technology.

- The wife is Rh-negative and severely sensitized to Rh-positive blood, and the husband is Rh-positive.
- In ART procedures for all the above reasons and in cases of failure of fertilization in couples with a male factor or unexplained infertility.
- Any woman who wishes to have a baby, but does not have a partner with whom she wishes to conceive.

Making the decision

The decision to use donor insemination is at times difficult, but many couples enter this treatment in a very matter-of-fact fashion.

Consider the case of Lorraine, 24, and Steve, 32. Several years ago Steve was treated for testicular cancer with chemotherapy, which left him with low numbers and quality of sperm. Steve's doctors told him, at the time he received his chemotherapy, that he would never be able to have his own children. When they had been married for two years and decided to start a family, they came in requesting donor insemination with no hesitation whatsoever. After being fully informed about the procedure and about the selection of donors through a regional sperm bank, they quickly signed the consents and went off to the cryobank to choose their donor. It was important to them that the donor have as many physical characteristics in common with Steve as possible.

It can be difficult for many couples to make the decision for semen donation.

When they returned for the first insemination based on Lorraine's positive ovulation predictor kit, they proudly announced that they had chosen "number 43." He had the same ethnic origin, hair and eye color, general build and educational background as Steve. Lorraine became pregnant with her first insemination. They had a baby boy and were so delighted with their son that they called the cryobank and placed some of number 43's semen on reserve so that all of their children would resemble one another. One year after the birth of their first son they decided to have another baby. This time it took two tries before Lorraine became pregnant. They had another son. Again they kept some of number 43's semen on reserve. After the birth of their third child, a girl, they notified the sperm bank that they would release the remaining specimens. They are delighted with their three children and are thankful to number 43.

But the decision for other couples to resort to donor insemination is not so easy. Perhaps it was easier for Lorraine and Steve because Steve's doctors had prepared him when he underwent chemotherapy. Sometimes the news that the man is infertile has such intense emotional consequences that he is unable to accept the thought of donor insemination. At other times a couple may be so concerned about the genetic and medical histories of the donors and the potential spread of disease that they are unable to accept donor insemination despite assurances that proper screening and testing have been done. Cultural and religious influences often come into play.

The couple considering the use of a donor must be fully informed about all aspects of the process and their consequences. Then they must sign an informed consent statement that may include, depending on individual state or provincial laws, many or all of the following:

Make sure you are dealing with an ethical sperm bank adhering to the guidelines.

- The husband is treated in law as if he were the natural father of the child and all children born shall be legitimate children and heirs to the couple's estate.
- They will never seek to identify the donor.
- There is no guarantee that insemination will result in a pregnancy.
- A certain percentage of children are born with physical or mental defects, and the occurrence of such defects is beyond the control of physicians.
- There is a very small risk of infection.
- Any pregnancy carries with it the risk of obstetrical complications or miscarriage.
- Semen from the same donor may not be available for all inseminations.
- Frozen sperm will be used.

Guidelines for semen donation

Once the couple has decided to utilize donor insemination, selecting a sperm bank is the next step in the process. Since there are no objective criteria available to the lay public regarding the operation of sperm banks, the couple will have to rely on the advice of their physician in selecting one. However, there are some universally accepted principles and some of the right questions will let you know if the bank is following accepted guidelines.

1. Does the bank either adhere to screening standards established by the American Association of Tissue Banks (AATB) or follow the guidelines for the selection and screening of donors issued by the American Society for Reproductive Medicine (ASRM) or the Canadian Fertility and Andrology Society (CFAS), or both? The answer should be yes. According to the standards of the AATB, the donor should be screened for fertility, health, intelligence and the absence of infectious disease, including HIV screening. The minimal ASRM or CFAS screen includes insuring the absence in the donor and his close relatives of any nontrivial malformation, genetic disorder, familial disease, recessive genes for any disease or chromosomal abnormalities. In addition, he must be free of psychosis, epilepsy, juvenile diabetes and early coronary disease.

2. How do you screen for HIV? The ASRM and CFAS guidelines exclude as donors any men who have engaged in any of the known high-risk behaviors related to the spread of HIV. In addition, HIV antibody tests should be done periodically and the semen should be quarantined until a follow-up HIV antibody test, done six months after the specimen is provided, is found to be negative for the HIV antibody.

3. Do you use fresh specimens? According to the guidelines published in 1988 and revised in October 1998, it is the position of the ASRM that the use of fresh semen for donor insemination is no longer warranted. Although there may be some decrease in pregnancy rates and increase in the length of time to conceive utilizing frozen (cryopreserved) semen, or both, it is the only way to provide maximum safety against the transmission of HIV. In addition, the AATB, U.S. Food and Drug Administration, and the Centers for Disease Control and Prevention all recommend the exclusive use of frozen semen for donation.

4. Isn't frozen semen less effective than fresh? When frozen specimens are utilized for conventional artificial insemination the overall pregnancy rate appears to be less than with fresh semen and the duration of therapy is therefore prolonged. For example, a study from the University of Kansas comparing characteristics of frozen and fresh donor semen found a marked reduction in all aspects of semen quality in the frozen specimens. However, there was no significant difference in cumulative pregnancy rates and they concluded that if minimum criteria for ejaculate quality are met, cryopreserved ejaculates can provide an effective and safe alternative to the use of

With the danger of sexually transmitted diseases, including HIV, quarantined and tested frozen specimens are the only way to go.

fresh semen. With ART procedures, there is no reduction in success with frozen sperm.

But even if there were a lower pregnancy rate, frozen semen provides several distinct advantages that more than make up for the slightly reduced efficacy. The use of frozen semen reduces the risk of acquiring a sexually transmitted disease by allowing more time for screening as well as providing a quarantine period for diseases such as HIV, hepatitis-B and hepatitis-C. It allows greater flexibility in scheduling inseminations and donor selection. The frozen specimen is available at any time while the donor himself may not be. Finally, it allows one specimen to be divided into several doses, which is very economical. Although the processing and storage adds somewhat to the cost, it is more than made for up by the advantages.

5. Besides HIV, what other diseases do you screen for? The ASRM and the CFAS recommend exclusion of a donor if he has had more than one sexual partner or symptoms of a sexually transmitted disease within 6 months, or a past history at any time of warts, herpes, chronic hepatitis or exclusion as a blood donor unless for a noninfectious reason. For donors continuing to participate in the program, the ASRM and CFAS recommend a physical examination and testing every 6 months for:

- gonorrhea
- chlamydia
- cytomegalovirus (CMV)
- hepatitis-B and hepatitis-C
- syphilis
- HIV

There has been a call for legislation in various states and in Congress to require medical and genetic screening of donors and even to set up a national data bank for semen donors to maintain their medical and genetic histories and make them available to the recipient.

How it is done

Multiple studies have shown higher conception rates when frozen sperm are washed and placed into the uterus (intrauterine insemination). One report showed a monthly conception rate of 24% with an ongoing pregnancy rate of 18%, using intrauterine insemination with specimens containing a minimum of 24 million cryopreserved motile sperm. We recommend timing the insemination by means of the LH surge kit. In this way only one insemination is required, which is more convenient and less costly to the patient.

When donor semen is used in ART procedures, it is prepared in a manner similar to fresh specimens to be used to inseminate the eggs in the laboratory in IVF and ZIFT. With GIFT procedures, the prepared semen is mixed with the eggs to be placed in the fallopian tube.

Costs

The use of cryopreserved donor semen does not significantly increase the costs of conventional infertility treatment or ART procedures. Currently, the average cost of a single frozen specimen from among well-known sperm banks is about $200 to $250 U.S., depending on the extent of preparation. When a number of specimens are ordered, the cost per specimen may be lower. The cost of sperm washing and insemination is approximately $250 U.S.

The sub-group of women with premature ovarian failure have the best success rates with egg donation.

EGG DONATION

While the donation of semen has been practiced for more than a century, the history of egg donation spans only two decades. Initially it was applied only to women with ovarian failure who were unable to produce any eggs. Its use has further expanded with the realization that egg quality and number are critical to IVF outcome. Egg donation will yield much higher success in:

- poor responders to stimulation or women who produce poor-quality eggs or embryos, or both.
- those who have a markedly reduced prognosis due to an elevated Day 3 FSH or estradiol.
- women who are of advanced age.

Reasons for egg donation

Prime candidates for donor eggs are female patients in the following circumstances:

- suffering from amenorrhea or anovulation that has not responded to fertility medications.
- has laboratory evidence of premature ovarian failure, usually manifested in elevated gonadotropin levels (FSH and LH).
- has demonstrated poor follicle development with stimulation due to reduced ovarian tissue because of previous surgery, damage to the ovaries by chemotherapy or radiation during successful therapy for a malignancy, or for unknown reasons.
- carries a genetic disease or chromosomal defect likely to be passed on to her offspring, resulting in miscarriage or an abnormal baby.

Or in which the couple:

Egg donors can be either known or anonymous.

- may have had multiple failed ART procedures, particularly with poor egg quality being found.
- may be over 40 and may choose egg donation because of a dramatically higher rate of success.

Making the decision

The decision to utilize donor eggs can be made in two circumstances. It seems to be an easier decision to make if the patient has a sister or friend who wishes to donate eggs for her. When the donor is unknown, the decision is similar to the decision to use donor semen.

Karen, 32, had a long history of endometriosis, including two operations resulting in the removal of one ovary and about half of the other. After many years of attempting to become pregnant without success, she decided to enter the IVF program. She produced six eggs with her first attempt. Four fertilized and were transferred, but she did not get pregnant. In her second attempt, she had only three eggs, all of which fertilized, but without success. With subsequent cycles, she stimulated poorly. It was felt that pelvic adhesions and lack of ovarian substance were impairing her ability to produce an adequate response to the stimulating hormones. The possibility of using an egg donor was discussed with both Karen and her husband, and she suggested that her sister might be willing to donate. Her sister was 34 and already had two children, but Karen thought that her sister might not want to do it and was a little reluctant to ask. As it turned out, her sister immediately agreed and said that she had been thinking of offering to donate before she was asked. In fact, it has been our experience that sisters of infertile women are usually more than happy to provide this service. Karen became pregnant as the result of her sister's donated eggs.

As with the recipients of donor semen, the recipients of donor eggs must be fully informed of every aspect of the procedure, including all potential risks, and must sign an informed consent outlining the following:

- The anonymous donor will not know the identity of the husband and wife and the husband and wife will not know the identity of the donor.
- The anonymous donor's information is supplied by the donor, so there are limitations to the accuracy of this information. Even though laboratory tests are performed on the donor, the transmission of infection is still possible.
- The recipient is responsible for the medical costs of screening and stimulating the donor and harvesting the eggs as well as financial compensation for the efforts, time and inconvenience of an anonymous donor.
- From the moment of conception, the husband and wife will accept the child as their own legitimate child(ren) and heir(s).
- There is no guarantee that a normal pregnancy will occur.
- The husband and wife understand that a certain percentage of babies are born with defects and that this is beyond the control of the doctors.

Guidelines for egg donation

As already indicated, donors fall into one of two categories: the relative or friend who agrees to donate, and the anonymous donor. Incidentally, the friends and relatives are screened with the same intensity as are the anonymous donors because friends and relatives can have significant histories of genetic problems and can also carry sexually transmitted diseases. Guidelines for the selection and screening of egg donors generally follow the basic principles used in the ASRM guidelines for semen donors. We suggest that you check on the guidelines for selection and screening of the program you are considering. If you are planning to use an egg donor, that prospective donor must:

- have no congenital malformations in herself or close relatives
- have no genetic disorder in herself or her family
- have no familial disease with a genetic component such as juvenile diabetes
- not being in or having a sex partner, in an HIV risk group
- not be, or have a sex partner who is, an IV drug user
- not have a past history of genital herpes, genital warts, chronic hepatitis or have been excluded from giving blood other than for a noninfectious reason
- be under age 35.

If the prospective donor passes this historical scrutiny, she will be subjected to a physical examination and testing to rule out the possibility of congenital anomalies, chronic illness or sexually transmitted disease. Blood tests will be obtained for hepatitis-B, hepatitis-C HTLV-1, syphilis and HIV. She must be in a monogamous relationship and her partner must agree to be tested for HIV. The semen donor's partner does not have to be tested for HIV because the semen can be quarantined for six months and the donor retested before the specimens are released.

Because of a scarcity of egg donors compared to semen donors, the characteristics used to match a donor to a recipient are usually limited to ethnicity, hair and eye color, and, in some cases, education. The recipient couple can ask for any set of criteria, but the stricter their criteria, the less chance that they will find a suitable donor.

The major difference between semen and egg donation is that the egg donor does accept some risk to herself in the process. First, she has to undergo significant stimulation of the ovaries to produce the number of eggs necessary to make the donation cost-effective. Secondly, the egg retrieval does carry with it some risk and discomfort.

Most women who donate eggs anonymously decide to donate their eggs for altruistic reasons. It has been the experience of many centers that it is easier than you might expect to find women who are willing to accept the risk because donating eggs to an infertile couple meets some need of theirs. These women probably represent a philosophically select group, emotionally committed to the idea regardless of the inconvenience and possible risk. They are akin to the large number of people we hear about who come forth to donate a kidney to a complete stranger or the thousands who offer to be tested as bone marrow donors for a young cancer victim. There are people who meet some of their own needs by helping others in this way.

In view of the inconvenience and, more crucially, the potential risk, the donors are thoroughly informed about the procedure and must sign a consent form that includes these points:

In our experience egg donors are a very special group of women who want to help someone in this very special way.

- She will have to undergo tests for sexually transmitted diseases, including HIV.
- She must verify that she has not had contact with a person with HIV, used intravenous drugs or had a sexual partner who, to her knowledge, has ever had a sexual contact with a homosexual male, IV drug user or someone with HIV.
- She agrees not to have sexual intercourse from the start of her menstrual period until one week after the egg retrieval.
- She agrees to take fertility drugs to obtain multiple eggs for donation.
- She understands the risks of the fertility drugs and the retrieval procedure.
- She relinquishes any claim to or jurisdiction over offspring that might result from the use of her eggs in the recipient.

Anonymous donors do receive compensation for their time away from work or their families and for their inconvenience. Known donors usually do not receive compensation. In selecting an amount for this honorarium, we want to give the donor something large enough to compensate her adequately for her services, yet we do not want to make it so high that it would encourage women to donate eggs simply to make money. When IVF centers used to recruit donors, they offered an honorarium of $2,000 to

$3,000 U.S. for anonymous donors. Now most donors are recruited by agencies and the compensation has escalated. According to Michelle Weinbaum-Rosen of the Center for Egg Options in Manhattan Beach, California, donor compensation generally varies from $3,500 to $5,000 U.S., but says some donors rarely may be receiving $10,000 U.S. or more. Most agencies charge from $3,500 U.S. to one half the fee the donor receives for the recruitment and initial screening of the donor.

A bond of sorts is established between the anonymous donor and recipient although they never meet. The donors are frequently concerned about the results and call to find out the outcome of the pregnancy test. They tell us to wish the recipient luck and often ask us to "give her a hug for me." On occasion the recipient will give something to the donor. One donor's egg pickup was scheduled for Valentine's Day and the recipient bought her a gold heart-shaped locket with a ruby surrounded by little diamonds. That recipient had twins. The recipients tell us to "tell her thanks" and to indicate how grateful they are. Perhaps IVF using donor eggs would be better called "GIFT."

From the available pool of donors, we recommend that the couple try to make the best match primarily by ethnicity and hair and eye color. When there are other specific requests, we recommend they try to match them, but they must realize that the pool of egg donors is much more limited than semen donors. Once the donor has been selected by the couple, screened, and is ready to start, the process begins.

How it is done

Since the use of an egg donor is very similar to IVF done with an infertile woman's eggs, the same basic steps are required, although with some modifications in who does what:

1. Ripening of the eggs in the donor while the recipient is being primed.
2. Retrieval of the eggs from the donor.
3. Fertilization of the eggs and growth of the resulting embryos in the laboratory.
4. Transfer of the embryos into the uterus of the recipient.

The financial compensation they receive is not high enough to encourage women to donate eggs strictly for the money, given the time commitment, potential risk, and pain involved.

EGG DEVELOPMENT

The process is very similar to that of a non-donor procedure. The donor is seen on the second day of her menstrual cycle. She comes in for an initial vaginal ultrasound scan to evaluate the baseline appearance of her pelvic organs. If the scan is normal, she is started on a three-week course of birth control pills. After two weeks on the pill, another ultrasound is performed and if normal, she is started on Lupron, usually as a single injection of the long-acting Lupron Depot. Ten days after the injection of Lupron Depot she returns for another scan and a blood test to see if her estrogen level is suppressed. A normal scan and a suppressed estrogen level will allow us to start her on gonadotropin injections. The injections are usually given by a standard protocol based on her age, weight and antral follicle count since it is likely that she has had no previous experience with these drugs. Some of these injections are more difficult to give than Lupron because they are a larger volume and are given deep into the muscle (Pergonal, Repronex). The new versions of pure FSH (Bravelle, Follistim and Gonal-F) can be given subcutaneously and can be self-administered. It is rare that a person can self-administer the intramuscular shot, and if it is prescribed in conjunction with one of the newer drugs, the donor's partner or a friend is generally taught how to do this. In place of the intramuscular drugs, it is now possible to add a small amount of a dilute solution of hCG to provide some supplemental LH subcutaneously.

Basically, the donor goes through the stimulation and retrieval. The recipient experiences the transfer.

On the sixth day of gonadotropins, the donor returns for a scan which may result in a modification of her dosage. Repeat scans are done every one to three days. When the follicles reach close to mature size, daily blood tests for estrogen are done. When the size of the follicles and resulting estrogen level indicate that they are mature, hCG is given and preparations are made to retrieve the eggs.

Meanwhile, the recipient is being prepared for the process. If she is still menstruating, she will have been placed on Lupron to totally suppress her own cycle and will be maintained on Lupron until her donor is ready.

When the donor is on her sixth day of Lupron, the recipient will be started on estrogen, which will be increased every few days to simulate a normal cycle. As the eggs reach maturity and the donor receives the hCG, the recipient will be started on progesterone injections to prime her endometrium to receive the embryos.

A typical cycle when the recipient is still ovulating would look like this:

	Recipient	Donor
After two weeks of birth control pills	Lupron	Lupron Depot
Day 6 of Lupron (donor)	Estrogen	Lupron
Day 12 of Lupron (donor)	Estrogen	Lupron/gonadotropins
When eggs are mature	Estrogen	hCG
Day after hCG	Estrogen Progesterone	Pre-retrieval visit
2 days after hCG	Estrogen Progesterone	Retrieval
3 to 5 days after retrieval	Embryo transfer Estrogen Progesterone	—

EGG RETRIEVAL

The egg retrieval procedure in the donor will be identical to the patient undergoing vaginal ultrasound egg retrieval for non-donor IVF. As an extra precaution, we give a week of antibiotics to make the chance of infection as remote as possible.

FERTILIZATION

The eggs are taken to the laboratory and incubated for a period of time before insemination. The partner of the recipient will deposit a semen specimen in a sterile container by masturbation. The insemination technique and observation of the embryos will be no different from the average IVF cycle.

EMBRYO TRANSFER OR REPLACEMENT

The embryos are now prepared to be transferred into the uterus of the recipient. Again, the transfer will be conducted in exactly the same manner as the transfer in any other IVF cycle.

Frozen embryos (Cryopreservation)

Most donors produce enough eggs so that extra embryos are available for freezing. Frozen embryos from egg donation cycles implant more effectively than in regular IVF. Therefore, pregnancies from these embryos make up a very important component of the total success rate with egg donation. By limiting the fresh transfer to two embryos, the risk of multiple pregnancy can be minimized while maintaining a good overall chance of success.

Costs

The medical costs of an IVF cycle employing donor eggs would be slightly more than any other IVF cycle, but would also include the honorarium for the donor (usually $3,500 to $5,000 U.S.), as well as the costs of advertising, recruitment and screening the donors and testing for infections (upwards of $3,500 U.S.) in the overall cost. All the costs relating to stimulation of the ovaries and retrieval of the eggs would be the same as with the regular IVF patient, except that they are performed on the donor, but paid for by the recipient couple. In fact, the cost of stimulation might be somewhat less in the donor than in an infertile IVF patient since fertile women usually require less stimulation.

Egg donation is the most successful fertility treatment averaging a 47% delivery rate per retrieval in the 2001 survey.

There are expenses related to suppressing and replacing the recipient's menstrual cycle and the hormonal replacement and monitoring of the early pregnancy. These might cost an additional $1,000. The cost for embryo freezing is about $500, and in a subsequent frozen cycle, thawing and transfer is about $2,000 U.S.

Success and failure

In the 2001 report by the SART/CDC Registry, 89% of the 384 clinics reporting performed IVF with donated eggs. A total of 7,722 fresh transfers were performed in 2001. Overall, the delivery rate was 47% per transfer. Of the 4,302 pregnancies 35.5% initially had twins, 8.1% had triplets and the number of fetuses in 4.1% was not able to be determined. By the time of the 3,629 deliveries, there were 58.3% single pregnancies, 38.4% twins, and 3.3% triplets or more. This means that a number of the pregnancies initially having triplets or more were reduced to twins or singletons naturally or by multifetal pregnancy reduction.

The level of persistence of patients who succeed through gamete donation is remarkable. Marcy, in her late thirties, had had three ectopic pregnancies, but by the time IVF was attempted she failed to stimulate and was found to be approaching menopause. Her sister offered to donate eggs; on the second attempt with her sister's eggs, she became pregnant and delivered triplets. At the annual Father's Day celebration at our center, Marcy's husband gave thanks for their success and attributed their triplets to the fact that they went through the anguish of losing three babies to ectopic pregnancies.

Sometimes the margin between success and failure is very small. Carolyn, in her early forties, had only a sliver of an ovary left after repeated surgeries. Her cousin offered to donate. However, the cousin's ovaries were unusually difficult to reach and only two eggs were obtained. Of those, only one fertilized. The transfer of that sole embryo resulted in a healthy pregnancy. Talk about "little miracles."

Effects on Recipients and Donors

In this "brave new world" of reproductive technology, incorporating a third person into a process which traditionally was limited to two individuals raises the question of what effect this has on recipients and donors. Many centers are now performing egg donation on women up to age 55. In fact, there have been successful births in women up to age 63. A reassuring study was reported in 2001 reviewing the outcomes of 72 women aged 50 to 63 who underwent IVF with donor eggs. Except for an increased caesarean section rate and an increased incidence of medical complications related to hypertension and diabetes, the group as a whole stood a good chance of having a term delivery with favorable maternal and neonatal outcomes.

The donors apparently do well, also. A 1998 study in the *Journal of Women's Health* showed that women who have elected to donate eggs anonymously are psychologically well adjusted. The donors' motivations were largely altruistic with the item "helping other woman" scoring as the highest motivator. There was a significant negative correlation between pre-donation financial motivation and post-donation satisfaction. Donor satisfaction with the process was supported by a 2003 study which found that over one-third were willing to donate again. However, in this study all of the donors felt that compensation was important and only 11% would donate if they were not compensated. The study reported that a very important motivator for donation in 77% was "helping another woman," while "financial gain" was cited by 30% of donors.

EMBRYO DONATION

The newest form of gamete donation is embryo donation. Assisted reproductive technology has become so efficient that there are now couples who have completed their childbearing, yet still have viable embryos stored in the freezer. Currently, there are limited options for the couples to deal with these embryos. They could discard them, but for a couple who has struggled with having a family, destroying what they might interpret as potential future children is not an option many would consider. A second option might be donating the embryos for stem-cell research to use them to alleviate human suffering and cure disease. However, the Bush administration has forbidden the use of frozen human embryos for this use. So the couples are left with a dilemma. The only remaining option, which is strongly supported by the U.S. Congress and the administration, is to donate them to another couple.

Obtaining Embryos

Most centers now have couples who wish to offer their extra frozen embryos to another infertile couple. Policies vary greatly among centers offering this option to their infertile patients. The medical and psychological screening process is very similar to recipients for egg donation. Embryo donors need to be screened for genetic conditions in their families and have blood tests for infectious diseases at least six months after the embryos were created.

Some groups are calling the procedure "embryo adoption." This designation originated from Snowflakes, a Christian adoption agency that requires the same social and financial screening for embryos as it does to place babies for traditional adoption. Abortion rights advocates worry that this program lays the legal groundwork for considering embryos human beings with full legal rights. Fertility clinics generally look at the transfer of early embryos as more akin to the transfer of sperm and eggs than to live human beings, and thus generally apply protocols similar to sperm or egg donation.

Preparation for transfer

Starting on the first day of her period, the recipient will be started on estrogen, which will be increased every few days to simulate a normal cycle. Once the endometrium reaches the desired thickness and there is no indication of spontaneous follicle development, the recipient will be started on progesterone injections to prime her endometrium to receive the embryos. This preparation is identical to that in any frozen embryo transfer cycle.

Embryo transfer or replacement

The embryos are thawed and prepared to be transferred into the uterus of the recipient. Again, the transfer will be conducted in exactly the same manner as the transfer in any other IVF cycle.

Costs

The medical costs of a frozen cycle employing donor embryos would be approximately the same as any other frozen cycle, but also includes the costs of obtaining the embryos. These would be limited to screening and administrative costs, as there cannot be any cost for the embryos themselves. The cost of thawing and transfer is about $2,000 U.S.

Success and failure

The 2001 report by the SART/CDC Registry does not report on embryo donation cycles. But one would expect these cycles to be very successful since the couples offering embryos generally have been very successful themselves. In a small study reported in 1999, the "ongoing and delivered" success rate from embryos donated by previously infertile couples was 44.4% in fresh cycles and 57.1% in frozen cycles, strange as that may seem. In cycles in which centers created embryos specifically for donation by using both sperm and egg donors (so-called orphan embryos), fresh cycles yielded a 33.3% "on-going and delivered" rate; the rate in frozen cycles was 47.6%.

The most unusual example of embryo donation we have seen is the story of Judy. After fertility treatments were unsuccessful, she came for a consultation at the age of 51, knowing that she wanted to find embryos from another couple to use so she and her husband could become parents.

She had a career as a television editor and did not meet her husband until it was too late to consider having a baby with her own eggs. Since there were no suitable embryos at Reproductive Partners, she turned to the Internet to find her future children. She found a family willing to donate leftover embryos from a respected center in another state. Four donated embryos resulted in healthy twin boys delivered at age 53. Judy's comment in a television interview when the boys were three years old was, "It's just like any other mom, only it's even better because I'm more mature and I've got these two boys that make me very happy."

SURROGATE PARENTING AND ADOPTION

There are two types of surrogacy. The first, traditional surrogacy, which uses both the eggs and uterus of the surrogate, is not widely used today because the baby carries the genetic material of the surrogate, which can lead to legal questions of custody. IVF with a gestational carrier utilizing the eggs of the infertile woman or a donor is now a common procedure performed in 69% of the 383 clinics reporting in 2001. The only aspect of surrogacy we will mention here is surrogate IVF, where the surrogate is only a gestational carrier and has no genetic connection to the offspring. The subject of adoption is beyond the scope of this book and is covered extensively in other literature on the subject. Consult Appendix 2 for resource recommendations on adoption.

Check the Resources section for information on surrogate parenting and adoption.

SURROGATE IVF

If a woman's ovaries are functioning but she has had her uterus removed or it is abnormal, it is possible to retrieve her eggs, fertilize them with her husband's sperm and transfer them to a surrogate who then carries the pregnancy. This procedure allows the infertile couple to have their own genetic offspring. It also has the potential for a higher pregnancy rate because the embryos can be transferred to a normal unstimulated recipient. Since the pregnancy is genetically unrelated to the surrogate, the potential for emotional attachment and consequent legal entanglements is reduced. Also, because the child is solely the genetic offspring of the infertile couple, the chance for any legal ruling assigning a parental right to the surrogate is remote.

In some instances both surrogate and egg donation is required.

Rather than resort to traditional surrogacy, most couples choose to use a separate egg donor and surrogate in order to have more choice regarding donor characteristics, and to avoid custody issues.

Finding the surrogate

The same agencies that recruit egg donors usually perform the service for surrogates as well. Some agencies may provide only one or the other, but today most do both. The process is very similar to recruitment and screening for an egg donor, except the focus is not on genetic history or physical characteristics, but on previous obstetrical history.

Preparing the surrogate

The surrogate is prepared for the transfer in an identical manner to the recipient of a donor egg; the transfer and follow-up protocol is also similar.

Costs

Any form of reproduction involving a surrogate is very involved and expensive. Surrogates must be carefully screened and the legal documents must be thoroughly and skillfully prepared. We have heard of surrogates charging up to $50,000 U.S. for providing this service. The average is about $25,000 U.S., according to Michelle Weinbaum-Rosen of the Center for Egg Options.

Success and failure

In the 2001 SART/CDC IVF Registry 225 programs reported performing surrogate cycles. Every age category and every type of ART cycle that used a gestational carrier had higher success rates than those cycles that did not. That is not surprising since the surrogates provide a uterus with the proven ability to carry a pregnancy to term. The success rate under age 35 was 45.7% live births per transfer for fresh, non-donor cycles using a surrogate compared to 41.0% when the infertile woman's own uterus was used. The difference was greatest in frozen donor cycles and in the 35 to 37 age group.

The use of a surrogate to overcome an otherwise hopeless situation provides some of the most heartwarming stories in assisted reproduction. First, there is the story of "Ripley's Believe It or Not." Becky Ripley struggled for years to conceive, including undergoing three IVF cycles at another clinic. When we first evaluated her situation, we felt that the problem was her endometrial thickness and that a surrogate would be necessary to overcome this problem. Her sister, Beth, already the mother of four-year-old Madison, volunteered. At the same time we were starting Becky's cycle, we had made a minor modification in our IVF protocol: adding one baby aspirin a day because of studies showing a favorable effect on both ovaries and endometrium. When it came time for the transfer Becky decided to have embryos transferred into her as well, but did not expect that they would work. Well, you guessed it. Both sisters got pregnant, delivering the first set of twins delivered from two different women. That story made *People* magazine.

The second is the story of "Pam and Sam." When Pam was 16 her mother took her to an ob/gyn because she had not yet started to menstruate. The ob/gyn delivered devastating news. Pam was born without a uterus and would never be able to have children. But in a television interview, Pam expressed confidence. "When I found out I couldn't have kids, I always knew in my head I would somehow." Her "somehow" surfaced in the form of Sam. After contacting 10 surrogacy agencies, Pam met Sam and the two seemed to be a good match, sharing similar upbringings and family values, and both had gregarious personalities. Their experience sharing roles (Pam's eggs, Sam's uterus) in two successful pregnancies created a special bond between the women and their families which was chronicled in the May 2003 issue of *Ladies' Home Journal*.

BEYOND DONORS

The use of donor eggs, embryos and surrogates are just some of the more exciting aspects of assisted reproduction that is producing pregnancies for women who were otherwise hopelessly infertile. As this technology moves towards its third decade, we will guide you in chapter 13 through the areas where we see the most promise for progress in the next decade.

CHAPTER 13

The Future Looks Bright

I wish they could all get their children; that's not going to happen. We will be able, in the next seven to eight years, to double our success rate. I know that we can.

Gary Hodgen, Ph.D., scientific director, Jones Institute, on "48 Hours" (CBS News), September 1989

THE FUTURE AND ASSISTED REPRODUCTION

The first quarter-century of assisted reproductive technology has seen tremendous progress from a time when teams of researchers worked for years to achieve just one success, to now when many skilled and experienced teams achieve live births in well over 40% of egg retrievals in women under age 35. Problems with stimulation have been reduced, with cancellation of a treatment cycle becoming less common. Egg retrieval has been vastly simplified by the development of ultrasound-guided follicle aspiration under deep sedation. ICSI has even made it possible for men with very poor sperm quality to have the same success rate as other couples having standard IVF. Assisted hatching has increased positive outcomes for older women to a level achieved in the average patient ten years ago. PGD allows couples in which one member carries the gene for a dreaded inherited disease to eliminate the disease from the family tree. Finally, with embryo freezing, an additional pregnancy can be achieved without the risk or cost of another stimulation and egg retrieval. Can we expect as much progress in the next decade? Probably not, but there are going to be continued breakthroughs.

Uniformity of results

First of all, to say that only a number of skilled and experienced teams achieve good success rates is not enough. All patients can't be treated by these few centers. A continuing challenge for the future is to make results more consistent so that all teams are realizing good results. Since there is currently little agreement over which techniques are preferable, this sort of uniformity can only be achieved by the less successful clinics adopting techniques used by highly successful programs. For the last 16 years, Dr. Meldrum has directed a comprehensive postgraduate course in Santa Barbara, together with the UCLA School of Medicine, on all aspects of ART. Most teams have at least one of their members attend every couple of years. The speakers have been chosen for their knowledge and speaking ability, but also for their excellent results and willingness to share the details responsible for their success. There is little doubt that this yearly course has played a major role in the improved success enjoyed by U.S. programs over the last 10 to 15 years, and in the higher rates of U.S. programs compared with other countries. One of the invited speakers from France has repeatedly commented on the lack of any comparable effort in Europe.

We need to bring the success rates of the less successful centers up to those achieving good success rates.

Financial resources

Besides having IVF in a highly successful program, the next most important factor influencing the chance of success is the number of cycles a couple goes through. Here the problem of lack of insurance coverage, which we discussed in chapter 2, is a major impediment to success. Given adequate financial support, the procedure is now simple enough to allow couples to tolerate going through four or more attempts. With success rates in the 40% range, the ability to go through multiple cycles raises the odds to very high levels (four cycles at 40% = 87%). With the addition of frozen embryo pregnancies, the rate would be even higher, especially taking into account improvements in freezing results.

Laboratory techniques

Laboratory techniques will improve, eliminating the difference for most programs in the chance of pregnancy between IVF, which depends heavily on laboratory quality, and GIFT, which substitutes the fallopian tube environment for the laboratory. Already the rates are equal for the average program.

As techniques for producing pregnancy in women with open tubes continue to improve without having to resort to ART techniques, it seems inevitable to us that GIFT may play a smaller role in the future. Also with the ability to choose the best one or two embryos for transfer with IVF, the ability to limit multiple pregnancies will become an overwhelming factor favoring IVF.

Uterine receptivity

The endometrium in a stimulated cycle is less receptive than in a natural cycle, probably due in part to advancement of the endometrium by the ovarian stimulation. This is one reason why egg donation and surrogacy have higher rates of success than routine IVF. Recent studies using a small biopsy of the endometrium have been correlating this advanced development with aspects of the ovarian stimulation. Modifications to the way that stimulation is conducted may then improve the chances of embryo implantation. New research on an anti-progesterone drug could prevent premature progesterone effects and allow a greater level of egg maturity without affecting implantation. Another curious finding has illuminated a simple way to improve implantation. Researchers doing extensive endometrial biopsies in the cycle before IVF observed a surprising increase in the pregnancy rate, which they later confirmed with a prospective, randomized study. Others have reported a similar effect when hysteroscopy is done in the preceding cycle. It has been speculated that the healing process stimulates growth factors that are critical for implantation.

In other research the measurement of integrin (a marker in the endometrium for uterine receptivity) has shown that certain women with a hydrosalpinx or endometriosis have an altered receptivity of the endometrium marked by reduced integrin levels. Removal or interruption of the hydrosalpinx or treatment of endometriosis can restore the endometrial receptivity and the chance of pregnancy to normal levels. Two recent controlled studies have shown a significant increase in pregnancy in women with a history of stage III or IV endometriosis when the IVF cycle is preceded by 3 to 4 months of suppression with a GnRH agonist.

It is also possible that implantation could be improved by delaying transfer until the embyros are at the blastocyst stage, when they normally reach the endometrial cavity. Using new culture media tailored to the specific requirements of embryos at each stage in their early development may allow a similar pregnancy rate with fewer embryos transferred, thus eliminating the risk of higher-order multiple pregnancy. In younger women it may eventually be possible to limit transfer to only one embryo, while still maintaining a high rate of success.

Other factors may explain why the rate of success still is not as high as one would expect if each embryo has the same 20% to 25% chance as in a normally fertile woman trying to conceive. In some women with IVF, the blood flow to the uterus is reduced. In the future, it may be possible to correct this with medication. In fact there is evidence that low-dose aspirin may improve implantation through this mechanism.

The blastocyst transfer where we can limit the transfer to two embryos is our best hope in reducing high-level multiple pregnancies.

Embryo freezing (Cryopreservation)

Embryo freezing is an area that has the greatest potential to result in much better pregnancy rates per stimulation and retrieval in the future. Better freezing techniques can also result in a lower rate of multiple pregnancies since physicians will not feel so pressed to transfer larger numbers of embryos during the IVF cycle itself, rather than freezing more of the apparently good-quality embryos to be used in future cycles. The occurrence of more than one pregnancy from a single retrieval, as seen with the Mohr "triplets" (conceived at the same time but born years apart), is already becoming commonplace.

Sperm preparation

Advances in semen testing and sperm preparation will gradually reduce the incidence of failed or reduced fertilization in non-ICSI cases and increase pregnancy success in both ICSI and non-ICSI cycles. For example, newer tests examining DNA fragmentation, such as the SCSA (Sperm Chromatin Structure Assay), have shown increased fragmentation of the man's DNA with smoking. Other recent studies showing lower pregnancy rates with both IVF and ICSI with male smokers indicate that some embryos are genetically incompatible with implantation due to this habit. (This is another health effect that should encourage smokers to quit.) Clearly men who have a high level of fragmentation have a reduced prognosis, and future research may uncover various reasons and treatments for this previously undetectable problem. For example, various antioxidants that are concentrated in semen have been reported to improve other aspects of sperm function. Since increased free oxygen radicals are a cause of DNA fragmentation, future research may show benefits of antioxidant therapy on DNA integrity. These various antioxidants are now conveniently combined in a single preparation, as we discuss in chapter 14 (e.g. FertilityBlend).

Sperm preparation techniques may differ in their ability to produce a specimen with a low level of DNA fragmentation. We currently use Puresperm, because of its ability to provide a high-quality specimen using standard sperm parameters. This same method has been shown to produce a four- to five-fold improvement in the DNA fragmentation index.

Use of donor gametes

Advances in diagnosis will allow better recognition of cases where the male or female gametes are of such reduced quality that the outcome of the IVF cycle is destined to be poor. Use of frozen donor sperm restores the outcome to normal, whereas egg donation almost doubles the rate over routine IVF. Given an adequate supply of donors, the use of egg donation will greatly expand for older women, for those who stimulate poorly and for couples with multiple failed IVF cycles who want a much greater chance of success.

Cytoplasm and nuclear transfer

Another method of overcoming poor-quality eggs was announced in the July 19, 1997 issue of the journal *The Lancet*. This startling report from the team at Saint Barnabus Medical Center in Livingston, New Jersey, led by Dr. Jacques Cohen, involved transferring cytoplasm (the material in a cell outside the nucleus) from the egg of a donor into the egg of a woman who had failed IVF many times. This allowed the couple in which the woman had poor eggs to give birth to a child who was her own genetic offspring. A series of other women gave birth after the same procedure, but there has been criticism regarding the mixing of genetic material from two individuals (the cytoplasm contains mitichondrial DNA), and two chromosomal abnormalities occurred in this early series of women. The technique is considered highly experimental.

Nuclear transfer is being investigated in animal models to see if a nucleus from a compromised egg, such as from an older woman, can be placed into a donor egg from which the nucleus has been removed. This allows the woman's own genetic material to function more normally in the environment of the younger cytoplasm, which provides energy for cellular functions that have been shown to be deficient in older eggs. This also involves the mixing of genetic material from two individuals. Generally, an immature nucleus is used, requiring in vitro maturation and ICSI for a good rate of embryo development. It has been found that even in vitro culture of embryos in routine IVF is associated with increases of rare imprinting disorders. This is the abnormal function of a gene due to a chemical change rather than, as in most disorders, a change in the structure of the DNA itself, as in a mutation. This means that extensive investigation will be required in animal models before any thought is given to human application of these extensive manipulations of the female gamete.

Genetic screening

One of the most frequent questions we are asked is if we can tell whether the embryo is a boy or a girl or, in fact, is normal. In some centers, genetic testing and diagnosis of embryos with diseases caused by a single gene defect is now possible. At Reproductive Partners we have successfully screened embryos for myotonic dystrophy, allowing the transfer of only disease-free embryos resulting in two successful, healthy pregnancies. This requires the removal of a single cell from the Day 3 embryo for testing so that only normal embryos can be transferred 2 days later at the blastocyst stage. Many chromosomal and metabolic diseases already have been assessed using this technique. In the future it may be possible to eliminate many more genetic defects using this technology, since the entire human genome structure has now been mapped out. Examples of such genes are:

- the gene that accounts for 50% of the genetic susceptibility to insulin-dependent diabetes

- one that may play a role in connective-tissue diseases, such as rheumatoid arthritis
- a gene that may be important in treating depression

According to Dr. Aubry Milunsky, director of the Center for Human Genetics at the Boston University School of Medicine, every gene that causes serious mental retardation and serious and fatal genetic diseases will have been mapped and cloned by 2005.

Genetic screening is only now being done by very few programs.

This technology will not improve success rates, but it will make IVF safer for couples with a family history of some of the more common genetic diseases. It certainly raises many ethical questions, since the degree of impairment varies from neurological disease causing death in early infancy to genetic transmission of breast cancer requiring mastectomy in older adults. There is little doubt that many couples will choose to have genetically normal offspring when they or their children have suffered serious consequences of genetic mutations, and that society will readily accept their decision. But what about avoiding a genetic susceptibility to depression which is often treatable, or color-blindness or other lesser impairments? This area of IVF will be an important advance for society but it will raise many thorny ethical issues.

Another example is sex determination of the embryo. The ethics committee of the ASRM discourages use of this technique to choose the sex of a couple's offspring, yet the use of sperm separation for this reason is gradually being accepted.

Fertilization enhancement

It may be possible in the future to do ICSI in men who do not produce mature sperm, by removing immature sperm from the testes and maturing them in vitro, or even injecting the immature sperm into the egg.

Use of immature eggs

Techniques have already been developed to harvest immature eggs from small follicles in the unstimulated ovary, and to mature them in vitro using follicular fluid from a mature follicle, or a cocktail of hormones normally present in the growing follicle. As yet the success of this procedure has been limited but could dramatically increase with refinements of laboratory techniques. It may even be possible in the future to take a small biopsy of the ovary and mature microscopic eggs to full development. These techniques will be particularly helpful for women who need chemotherapy or radiation that would damage their eggs. Already it has been shown that ovarian tissue from such women can be frozen and then transplanted under the skin of the arm with production of hormones and growth of follicles. It could also be an almost inexhaustible source of eggs for donation. For routine IVF it avoids the use of fertility drugs, eliminating concerns over whether these medications could have long-term effects on health, such as increased risk of ovarian cancer.

Egg Freezing

Until recently, the freezing of unfertilized eggs was only occasionally successful. The oocyte is a very large cell and the mature egg's chromosomes are in a very delicate stage. The large size of the egg made it difficult to freeze without formation of damaging ice crystals, and there has been concern that chromosomal abnormalities could occur if the freezing process were to damage the extremely fine microtubules that keep the chromosomes organized. Refinements of the freezing techniques and the use of ICSI and assisted hatching have now made egg freezing successful enough for clinical application. Although there still have been only a few hundred births, there has not been any apparent increase of abnormalities in the offspring.

Since embryo freezing is highly successful and there have been many thousands of births, egg freezing is limited to women who wish to store their eggs prior to undergoing chemotherapy or radiation for cancer treatment, or for women who are reaching an age when fertility may be reduced but who do not yet have a partner or the appropriate personal situation for having children. For example, a woman could freeze her eggs at age 35 and if she is not ready to have a child until age 45, she could be successful where otherwise her ability to conceive with her own eggs would be very limited. Another future application of egg freezing could be to develop egg banks like present-day sperm banks. Choice of egg donors would be broader and eggs could be more efficiently utilized, since excess embryos from egg donation cycles are now commonly discarded after the recipient couple has had the children they desire.

CONSUMER AND ETHICAL ISSUES

As we indicated at the outset, some serious consumer and ethical issues need attention:

- the general lack of insurance reimbursement for infertility treatment and, specifically, assisted reproductive procedures
- the limited professional or governmental oversight of IVF clinics and laboratories
- the lack of mandatory standards for physicians and technicians performing these procedures
- the failure of some programs to report their statistics in an approved format to SART/CDC to be included in the SART/CDC Registry
- misleading advertising and marketing schemes
- the high cost of these procedures
- the large number of high-level multiple pregnancies resulting from excessive numbers of embryos being transferred

There have been great strides made over the last decade following Representative Ron Wyden's congressional hearing and survey, but the progress should not stop here.

Lack of insurance

Infertility is a medical problem that can devastate a family no less than another serious medical condition. Sure, you don't die from infertility. But insurance companies are now providing coverage for many other non-lethal medical conditions, and we feel infertility coverage should be mandated by law.

IVF and GIFT are now accepted clinical procedures and are no longer experimental. Insurance should provide coverage, for a reasonable number of cycles in couples who have not been able to achieve pregnancy by other conventional means. In fact it may be financially advantageous for insurance companies to offer coverage, as a study in *Fertility and Sterility* in July 2003 showed that mandated insurance coverage affected transfer practices which ultimately should have a beneficial effect on multiple pregnancy rates. Dealing with multiple pregnancies and the neonatal costs of premature births associated with multiples is a major burden for insurance companies.

Lack of regulation

Despite the passage of the Fertility Clinic Success Rate and Certification Act of 1992, which resulted from the Wyden hearings in 1989, the act has only recently been implemented. The law provides that a model program for laboratory accreditation be implemented, which is the CAP/ASRM program. Accreditation will remain voluntary, but a list of programs that are or are not accredited will be made available to the public. The law also provided for the government, through the Centers for Disease Control and Prevention (CDC), to make public results on individual programs, as well as a list of programs electing not to report their results. This information is now available at the CDC website.

In 1987 the Society for Assisted Reproductive Technology (SART) was founded as an affiliate society of the American Society for Reproductive Medicine (ASRM). To promote the highest possible standards for ART, these two organizations have published extensive guidelines for ethical considerations, laboratory procedures, and sperm and egg donation. In conjunction with the College of American Pathologists (CAP) they have developed the voluntary laboratory accreditation program, which is now a requirement for both laboratory accreditation and reporting of results to maintain SART membership.

There is some mandatory oversight in the form of state control of physicians' licenses, but a physician has to go pretty far afield from the standard of practice to interest state medical boards. Endocrine laboratories are regulated by the Clinical Laboratory Improvement Act (CLIA 88). Programs that are connected to hospitals and universities usually have some oversight by their affiliation with these institutions, but as we follow the alleged events at the University of California at Irvine, we can see that the value of this oversight is limited.

Many groups have different approaches to the need for additional legislation. The American Medical Association (AMA) Task Force has recommended no further need for legislation or regulation. The American Bar Association has established a task force to consider model legislation.

The patient advocate group, Resolve, Inc., would like legislation that protects patients' interests, but will not increase costs or limit access to care. The State of California has already passed into law rules specifying the consent for the donation of eggs and embryos and has made it a felony to knowingly donate them without this specific consent.

At the 1996 conference on "The Ethics of Reproductive Medicine: Responsibilities and Challenges," which was held at the University of California, Irvine, there was a general consensus that professional standards and scientific issues should be left to professionals. But some aspects of ART, such as reporting success rates and accreditation, were felt to require regulation. Stay tuned, as this debate is far from over.

Qualifications

It's shocking that in this day and age of sophisticated medicine, any physician can hold him or herself up as an expert in any field without any qualifications.

We are also no closer to defining the qualifications needed to claim expertise in infertility or to perform high-tech reproductive procedures. Actually, this situation is no different than other areas of medicine. When physicians are issued a license, they can claim to be expert in any field and limit their practice to that field. In general, policing of qualifications has been delegated to hospital medical staffs. But if a hospital would allow it, any physician theoretically could do neurosurgery or heart transplants, not to mention ART procedures, without any formal training. (Review chapter 9 for clues to ensure that the doctor treating you has proper qualifications.) One valuable resource for determining qualifications is the ASRM's booklet "IVF and GIFT: A Guide to Assisted Reproductive Technology."

Objective information

The March 9, 1989 hearing by the subcommittee released to the public, for the first time, a survey comparing the centers that voluntarily chose to report their results. That congressional survey has developed into the SART/CDC Registry. Although clinic-specific data has been available since 1990, the data is not widely disseminated among infertile couples, largely because most of them are unaware of its existence or how to obtain the report of a specific center. In addition it is difficult to compare centers, since the results may somewhat reflect the difficulty of cases performed by a particular center. More difficult problems such as male factor not requiring ICSI, older women within each age category, or couples who have previously failed treatment in other centers will adversely affect a program's success rate.

Advertising

The Federal Trade Commission, in an editorial in the journal *Fertility and Sterility,* has published guidelines for advertising. The most important provision is that a clear indication must be given of what the numerator and denominator are for any success rate quoted. It is not acceptable to say, "Our success rate is 30%." A program must state, for example, "Our success rate is 30% *delivery rate per egg retrieval in the year 2001.*" SART also has guidelines for advertising, and it disciplines programs that step outside of these boundaries. Perhaps the most misleading advertising is to report results over a short period following a period of higher success. We all recognize that success varies with the particular couples going through treatment at any given time. Therefore it is only acceptable to report over a calendar year to avoid this problem. Even results from year to year can vary by chance except in very large programs. This is why we report our results to patients over a 4- or 5-year segment of time so that with hundreds of cycles in each age category, the results are an accurate reflection of what a couple can expect.

Costs

ART procedures are very expensive. But when you put them into the perspective of other high-tech procedures such as MRI scans, transplants or even conventional surgery such as a hysterectomy or gall bladder operation, the costs of ART procedures are quite reasonable considering what is involved. A rough breakdown of costs for an "average cycle" today, not including tests done in preparation for the cycle, additional procedures such as ICSI or AH if needed, or embryo storage, would be about:

Medications	$2000+
Monitoring ovulation	$1300
Retrieval procedure	$2500
Laboratory costs for fertilization	$1500

| Transfer | $1100 |
| Embryo freezing | $500 |

Note: All amounts are in U.S. dollars.

It may not surprise you to learn that we don't expect these costs to go down considerably. Nevertheless, they probably won't go up much either, unless new technology makes the procedure more complicated. We feel that the increasing numbers of programs will create a competitive market, which will tend to stabilize prices.

GOING OUT ON A LIMB

What all this boils down to is, "What will the success rate be 10 years from now when the field of ART reaches into its fourth decade?" In 1989 Dr. Gary Hodgen predicted we would double our success rates in the next 7 to 8 years. Average success rates for IVF have climbed 75% in that period of time; not quite doubling, but pretty close.

With all the anticipated developments, it is possible that the average delivery rate per egg retrieval could approach 50% in the next decade. In that case, surgery for infertility may be relegated to the Dark Ages and we'll tell our young colleagues that we actually used to try to fix damaged tubes. With insurance companies offering ART coverage as a marketing feature, insurance coverage may greatly expand. Then "little miracles" will be so commonplace that the procedures won't be thought of as unusual, but rather as simply one of the many highly successful infertility treatments available to couples to fulfill their potential to have a family.

CHAPTER 14

Alternative Treatments in Infertility

"East is East, and West is West, and never the twain shall meet…"

Rudyard Kipling (1892)

THE TWAIN MEET

When Rudyard Kipling wrote that statement in the late 19th century he did not mean it in the context of early 21st-century reproductive medicine but, until recently, it has applied to the chasm between Western scientific method and Eastern traditional practices. There is probably no issue that raises more vociferous differences of opinion between practitioners of both regimens than the role of alternative methods in the standard medical treatment of the infertile couple. The debate often reaches the pitch of religious fervor.

Before we can examine the potential role of alternative methods we need to define what we are talking about. Western medicine is what we practice. It is also referred to as conventional medicine and includes both allopathy (standard medical practice) and osteopathy and is based on the scientific method. Complementary and alternative methods (CAM) incorporate a group of diverse medical and health care systems, practices and products that are not considered part of conventional medicine. While some scientific evidence may exist for the effectiveness of certain CAM therapies, others have not yet been proven safe or effective through well-designed studies.

Strictly speaking, alternative medicine disciplines are used in place of conventional medicine; complementary medicine is used together with conventional treatments. In the U.S. the National Center for Complementary and Alternative Medicine (NCCAM) is the federal government's lead agency for scientific research on CAM. The NCCAM classifies CAM therapies into five categories:

If you are using alternative methods, let your doctor know, as there are some practices which may be harmful.

- Alternative Medical Systems—these are built on complete systems of theory and practice, such as homeopathic and naturopathic medicine in Western cultures, and Traditional Chinese Medicine and Ayurveda developed in non-Western cultures.
- Mind-Body Interventions—these are techniques designed to enhance the mind's capacity to affect bodily functions, including patient support groups and cognitive-behavioral therapy.
- Biologically Based Therapies—these use substances found in nature, such as food, herbs and vitamins.
- Manipulative and Body-Based Methods—these include chiropractic and osteopathic manipulation and massage.
- Energy Therapies—these involve the use of energy fields by applying pressure such as therapeutic touch, qi gong and Reiki or using electromagnetic fields.

A complete review of all these disciplines is beyond the scope of this book. We will instead focus on the types of complementary practices that most infertility patients use.

Until recently, many conventional physicians would not even discuss CAM with their patients. The attitude of many conventional physicians was expressed in a debate in *Human Reproduction in 2002* by Dr. C.N.M. Renckens, Chairman of the Dutch Union against Quackery (note the rhetoric here), entitled "Alternative Treatments in Reproductive Medicine: Much

Ado About Nothing." The reason for his disdain is that the claims made for alternative medicine in the lay press have not been backed up by studies in peer-reviewed medical journals. In the past, practitioners and advocates of alternative medicine have mostly used philosophical arguments to defend their position. More recently, they acknowledge that the effectiveness of their therapies should be proven in randomized trials, as is considered mandatory in mainstream medicine. Dr. Renckens writes, "There are very few well-designed papers on the effectiveness of alternative medicine with the exception of one kind of paper that is hard for editors of medical journals to resist: seemingly impeccable papers proving absurd claims, whose mechanisms of action are, for instance, completely incomprehensible." He argues that this type of paper should be rejected and cites a quote from W.F. Hermans, "The fact that millions of people do not master arithmetic does not prove that two times two is anything else than four."

On the other hand, some randomized studies on alternative methods reported by conventional physicians do meet the rigorous standards of good mainstream medical journals. In between these two extremes is where most of the literature on the subject falls: non-randomized, poorly controlled or anecdotal reports in less than first-line medical journals.

There are some concepts that make sense and do seem to work. The approach that makes the most sense is what NCCAM calls integrative medicine, combining mainstream medical therapies and CAM therapies for which there is high-quality scientific evidence of safety and effectiveness.

A significant number of couples are using alternative methods, many without their doctor's knowledge or approval. In a 2003 survey of 1038 couples undergoing in vitro fertilization, 33% reported having procedures such as acupuncture and relaxation therapy, while 18% used herbal remedies. As you will learn in this chapter, some common herbal remedies can have an adverse effect on the reproductive process.

To help us navigate through this confusing and often contradictory subject we consulted two well-respected experts who practice in our area and who have helped many of our patients succeed with alternative methods. One of the leading practitioners of Traditional Chinese Medicine (TCM) in infertility is Daoshing Ni, L.Ac., D.O.M., Ph.D. of the Tao of Wellness in Santa Monica, California. After Dr. Dao earned his Doctorate in Oriental Medicine, he received advanced training in China. He is a member of the

American Society for Reproductive Medicine. When our nurse-practitioner Cheirel Gustavis-Person, R.N., CNP learned that we were including a chapter on alternative medicine, she said that we must talk to Tara Perry, L.Ac. who, Cheirel claims, has assisted in getting some of our most difficult cases pregnant. Ms. Perry, a California-licensed acupuncturist who has taken special training in reproductive issues and is certified by the National Commission for Certification in Acupuncture and Oriental Medicine (NC-CAOM), also practices in Santa Monica, which leads us to believe that Santa Monica must be the fertility-acupuncture capital of the free world.

LIFESTYLE ISSUES

When planning a pregnancy, it's really important to "clean up your act" to eliminate potentially harmful substances, plus take supplements like folic acid, which have been shown to reduce the risk of spinal and heart problems.

Both camps agree that, aside from specific treatments, there is probably no issue more important in determining a successful result, no matter what the formal method of treatment, than avoiding noxious elements both in the environment and taken purposely. There are many places in this book where you will find admonitions for both members of a couple trying to get pregnant not to smoke, drink alcohol or caffeine, or use recreational drugs. These admonitions can be easily defended by scientific evidence and are also advocated by practitioners of TCM. Most studies have shown fertility impairment is associated with cigarette smoking. Women who smoke have lower levels of all three major estrogens in the luteal phase, an earlier-than-normal onset of menopause and nicotine accumulating in cervical mucus and in follicular fluid, where it's associated with delayed follicular growth and maturation. Nicotine also may increase spontaneous abortion rates.

In a 1998 article in the *British Medical Journal*, researchers in Denmark showed that there was a 40% reduction in the odds of conceiving in women who consumed 1 to 5 alcoholic drinks a week and a 66% reduction for women who consumed more than 10 drinks per week. This can be explained by the observation that high levels of alcohol use can be associated with altered levels of estrogen and progesterone, irregularities in the menstrual cycle including anovulation and early onset of menopause. The Danish investigators found men's alcohol consumption did not affect time to pregnancy. We still recommend that men abstain when trying to conceive, as alcohol is a toxin and may have effects on the process that are yet to be recognized.

While not all reports show caffeine as a risk factor for delayed conception, the bulk of evidence implicates it in reduced fertility. Animal and human data suggest caffeine use is associated with an increase in spontaneous miscarriages. Recent consumption is more important than previous consumption, suggesting the effects of caffeine on fertility are transient and reversible. A 2002 study from the University of California, San Diego published in the journal *Human Reproduction* measured the effect of caffeine consumption on IVF and GIFT cycles. They found that women who consumed up to the equivalent of a half cup of coffee a day during their lifetime were three times less likely to have a live birth than women who had consumed less than a cup of decaf. Men's consumption of more than one cup a day during their lifetime resulted in their partners having a two times greater likelihood of having a multiple birth. On the other hand, a 1998 report in the *American Journal of Public Health* found that women who drink more than one-half cup of caffeinated tea every day may increase their odds of conceiving.

Polyphenolic compounds in tea may actually promote fertility by inhibiting chromosomal abnormalities, thereby decreasing the number of nonviable embryos. But the major factor may be that tea drinking may simply be a marker for a healthier lifestyle that enhances fertility.

There are environmental issues which a couple trying to conceive may be unaware of and certainly have no control over. An example of this is a 2003 study by the Public Health Institute in Berkeley, California which showed that women who were exposed to DDT in their fetal life are more likely to experience delays getting pregnant. DDT is banned in the United States and most of the world, but is still used in parts of Africa, Southeast Asia, and South and Latin America to control malaria-carrying mosquitos.

There are substances we all take unknowingly which may cause us some harm. Pharmacia Corporation settled an environmental lawsuit and agreed to reformulate all of its antidiarrhea products under the Kaopectate brand so they no longer contain potentially harmful levels of lead. Lead is a substance that, in high levels, can impair learning development, cause neurological damage to fetuses and children, and reduce the fertility of men and women.

Because of the dietary additives and environmental toxins to which we are all exposed, some advocate a detox or cleansing diet. The purpose of detoxification is to neutralize and eliminate any compound in the body that can be toxic. The basic detox diet is a 2-week nutritional diet that emphasizes fresh, simply prepared foods that are easy to digest, absorb and eliminate, minimizing allergenic foods. Increasing "elimination" is an important component of this concept and a variety of substances, such as bentonite clay, flaxseeds and lemon juice, are often recommended to assist in this process. To detoxify the liver a number of vitamins, vegetables and other supplements are usually advocated. Some of the dietary and avoidance aspects of this concept are obviously beneficial. Others, such as the elimination regimen, are not supported by scientific evidence. Specific detox programs or diets for infertility are available in books on the subject. Remember that except for common-sense concepts that we already know, scientific proof of these diets' effectiveness in helping couples to conceive is lacking.

ACUPUNCTURE

If you decide to see an acupuncturist, try to find one who has special training and experience in reproductive issues. Many of them specialize, just as physicians do.

Traditional Chinese Medicine (TCM) has been used to treat both male and female infertility for the past 3,000 to 4,000 years and combines both acupuncture and herbs to bring the body into balance. Acupuncture uses fine needles in specific "points" to stimulate invisible lines of energy called Qi (pronounced "chee") running beneath the surface of the skin. This is believed to create a change in the energy balance of the body which works to restore health. According to advocates, acupuncture can be a powerful adjunct to conventional infertility treatments and assisted reproductive procedures. Traditional Chinese Medicine combines acupuncture with herbs to create homeostasis in the body and bring the yin and yang into balance. The acupuncturist uses history and physical signs to determine the nature of the problem.

In the West, acupuncture is a form of alternative treatment which requires an individual or couple undergoing fertility treatments to seek an additional provider. Couples thinking of trying acupuncture need to consider the effectiveness of the treatment and the qualifications of the practitioner.

Studies of acupuncture in traditional Western peer-reviewed journals are few and far between. A 1978 article from the Institute of East-West

Medicine in New York, published in *Fertility and Sterility*, examined the role of acupuncture in female infertility and reviewed a Medline search of relevant articles. These studies suggest that the effect is mediated through the effect of opioids such as beta endorphins on the central nervous system through the hypothalamic-pituitary-ovarian axis, and works peripherally to affect uterine blood flow. When the topic was re-reviewed 24 years later in 2002, studies of adequate design, sample size and using appropriate controls on the use of acupuncture on ovulation induction were still lacking. Only one randomized controlled study examining the efficacy of acupuncture in IVF has been reported. An article in *Human Reproduction* showed a reduction in uterine artery flow impedance with electro-acupuncture, which should result in increased uterine blood flow. A 1992 study from the University of Heidelberg, Germany showed that auricular (ear) acupuncture in women with oligoamenorrhea or luteal insufficiency had similar outcomes to a matched group of women treated with conventional hormone therapy. The women who became pregnant after acupuncture more often suffered menstrual abnormalities, and luteal insufficiency with lower estrogen levels, TSH and DHEAS levels than those who got pregnant after hormone therapy. The one randomized study looking at the influence of acupuncture on the pregnancy rate in patients who undergo ART was published in *Fertility and Sterility* in April 2002. Clinical pregnancies were documented in 34 out of 80 patients (42.5%) in the acupuncture group, and in 21 of 80 patients (26.3%) of the control group. They concluded that acupuncture seems to be a useful tool for improving pregnancy rate after ART.

When selecting an acupuncturist, use the same care and many of the same criteria that you would in selecting a physician or IVF center.

An investigation of combined alternative treatments in men was published in the *Journal of Traditional Chinese Medicine* in 1997. It showed that the combined use of acupuncture, meditation and pilose antler essence injection to acupoints, along with oral administration of herbs, "cured" 47.8% of cases, was "markedly effective" in 27.3% and "effective" in 17.8%. The difficulty with interpreting a publication such as this is that this study did not have a control group, it was not randomized to matched controls and the definition of success was very vague. A study from about the same time from the Institute of Chinese Medicine in Tel Aviv, Israel utilized a control group and found that the treatment group had a significant increase in fertility index with improvement in total functional sperm fraction, percentage of viability and total motile sperm per ejaculate in the treatment group.

By 2000, the Institute studied the effect of acupuncture on patients with very poor sperm density. A definite increase in sperm count was detected in the ejaculates in 67% of 15 azoospermic men. No changes were observed in the control group.

In order to get the greatest possible benefit from acupuncture, you need to be evaluated and treated by an acupuncturist experienced and skilled in the treatment of male or female infertility. As with medical infertility specialists, all acupuncturists are not created equal. Minimal qualifications include either a state or provincial license, or certification by the National Commission for Certification of Acupuncture and Oriental Medicine (NCCAOM). By 2007, certification will require 4,000 hours of training in Traditional Chinese Medicine. Some practitioners who specialize in gynecology have taken formalized specific training or are self-educated in reproductive issues. But there is no board-certification for acupuncturists or a specific society for those interested. Some may be members of the American Society for Reproductive Medicine or other specialty societies. Beyond that, you can ask about experience in treating infertility and look for a track record. Ask about success rates in situations similar to yours, and how many patients he or she has treated. The best recommendation is your doctor's referral, but many infertility specialists may not look upon your use of alternative practices as a positive step, much less refer for this service. Your backup may be a friend who has had success or a nurse from your doctor's office who might be more enthusiastic about your foray into Traditional Chinese Medicine. In our Beverly Hills office, our nurse-practitioner is often the one who picks up the vibe that a patient may benefit from acupuncture.

In order to restore balance, first you need to know what is out of balance.

HERBS, VITAMINS AND DIET

According to Dr. Dao's literature, "Medicinal herbal therapy works in concert with acupuncture by providing the nourishing support for the energetic 'reprogramming' and 'rebalancing' efforts of acupuncture." Herbs can be categorized into three groups. The first is called "food herbs," which are eaten as part of one's diet for general fortification, prevention and maintenance. The other two groups are "medicinal herbs," which are dispensed to each patient in an individual formula based on a person's individual constitution, environment and medical condition. One of the groups of medicinal herbs actually consists of toxic herbs, so as they say on television, "Don't try this yourself at home." You need a qualified professional to select the herbs suitable for your specific situation. According to Tara Perry the purpose of herbal therapy is to restore balance, for example strengthening that which is deficient and toning down that which is in excess.

There are over 10,000 herbal substances documented in the *Materia Medica*, which is published by the Ministry of Health of China. The Chinese government standardizes herbs and grades them from "A" to "D," with "A" being the most pure and potent. Your TCM doctor may dispense them to you or refer you to a good source. Chinese herbs are generally used in combinations of 8 to 20 herbs and are customarily prescribed for an individual patient's specific condition. For treating infertility, mostly raw herbs are prescribed and taken in the form of brewed tea. It is common to have variations in herbal prescriptions from patient to patient, and in the same patient, formula changes can be made from visit to visit, which is partly why we don't have randomized controlled studies documenting the effectiveness of herbal medicine.

Both our experts emphasized the importance of potent and pure herbs, so you must use a professional on whom you can rely. Dr. Dao obtains most of his herbs from China. Some are gathered in the wild; others are cultivated according to ancient methods. Tara Perry recommends that patients make sure that their practitioner is obtaining the herbs from reliable sources to avoid contamination by potentially toxic substances. Remember, this is not like buying standardized prescription medication which is regulated by the Food and Drug Administration at your neighborhood pharmacy. There are so many individual components of an herbal prescription that it is far more complex than a conventional physician selecting a dose of a standard medication manufactured by a pharmaceutical company. You are totally relying on your practitioner for the quality of the products you are using. Both experts feel that the herbs they prescribe are very safe, and side effects and risks are infrequent. Dr. Dao points out in his literature the possibility of slight stomach discomfort when drinking the tea, and suggests that you avoid drinking it on an empty stomach or add slices of fresh ginger root to the herb during cooking.

Over the years sporadic reports linking herbs to female infertility is-

With thousands of herbs available, this can become very confusing. If you are serious about using herbs, get help from a Chinese Medicine specialist. As they say on the TV reality shows, "Don't try this at home."

sues have appeared. In 1991, a study in the *Journal of Traditional Chinese Medicine* of 60 cases of infertility attributed to luteal phase defect were treated with herbs to "tonify the kidney and regulate the menstrual cycle." Improvement in the luteal phase was judged by improvement in the BBT. The pregnancy rate in 32 treated "uncomplicated cases of luteal phase defect" was 56%. Another report citing the benefit of a Chinese herb on the luteal phase was published in the *American Journal of Chinese Medicine* in 2002. In this study the herb tokishakuyakusan was shown to improve luteal insufficiency, but this time it was confirmed by plasma progesterone levels.

More studies are available for the efficacy of treating men with herbs. In 1996, the *American Journal of Chinese Medicine* reported that 37 patients with varicocele were treated with Guizhi-Fuling-Wan for 3 months. They claimed an 80% disappearance rate for the varicocele and improvement in sperm concentration in 71.4% and motility in 62.1% of patients. No control group was used and pregnancy rates were not reported. As reported in the *Journal of Postgraduate Medicine* in 1997, a prospective placebo-controlled double-blind study was done to evaluate the effects of an herbal formulation "Y-virilin," given for 6 months. In oligospermic males a significant increase in sperm count was seen in 2 to 3 months. However, there were no differences in the percentage or grade of motility at the end of treatment in either treated patients or controls. But, during the therapy period, the incidence of conception in the treated group was 20% and only 5% in the controls. Most recently, a pilot study reported in the journal *Homeopathy* in 2002 evaluated the effect of "individualized" homeopathic therapy for male infertility. It showed that sperm density, progressive motility and the number of sperm with propulsive motility improved significantly "comparable" to improvement achieved by conventional therapy. The authors suggested that a randomized, therapy-controlled clinical study with parallel group design would be useful. We agree, but point out that control groups are difficult to design when "individualized" prescriptions are used.

The Traditional Chinese Medicine view on fertility treatment is largely based on individual clinic experience. For example, at his clinic Dr. Dao reports finding:

- increased follicle development with some patients in an ART cycle
- increased production of eggs or increased fertilization rate

Remember, with herbs, you can't assume "one size fits all."

- reduced thinning of endometrium in clomiphene cycles with IUI
- bounce-back of FSH levels in patients with symptoms of premature menopause
- patients able to conceive again after recurrent pregnancy loss without immunosuppressants
- improved semen analysis in male subfertility with the use of TCM for more than three months

As we have advocated throughout this book, informed consumers need to be aware of potential risks of any treatment. A *U.S. News and World Report* devoted an article in February 2001 to the hazards of supplements. It was found that many herbal preparations have contraceptive effects. These include ginger, cayenne, mother wort, black cohosh, extract of juniper berries, saffron, catnip, aloe, cinnamon, camellia, bee balm, penny oil, St. John's Wort, extract of English ivy and Queen Anne's lace. An article in *Fertility and Sterility* in 1997 looked at the effect of certain herbs on fertilization. Eggs exposed to St. John's Wort resulted in no fertilization while high concentrations of echinacea and ginko reduced fertilization. Exposure of sperm to echinacea and St. John's Wort resulted in DNA denaturation and St. John's Wort also induced mutation of certain genes. Remember, herbs can be potent substances and some are even toxic or harmful to the reproductive process.

And you thought these were all safe to take, didn't you?

In 2000 an article in *Alternative Medicine Review* claimed that a number of nutritional therapies have been shown to improve sperm counts and motility, including carnitine, arginine, zinc, selenium and vitamin B-12. Numerous antioxidants such as vitamins C and E, glutathione and coenzyme Q10 have been associated with a beneficial effect in treating male infertility. All these observations have led to the developments of commercially available products for male and female infertility, such as FertilityBlend and Proxeed.

An unusual agenda item for one of our regular Reproductive Partners doctors' meetings was the product "FertilityBlend." The subject was unusual because the doctor who placed it on the agenda, Dr. Meldrum, was the least likely among us to advocate using an alternative method without rock-solid, double-blind randomized controlled studies proving its efficacy and safety. Dr. Meldrum is the most scientifically oriented of all of us. He is on the editorial board of the prestigious *Fertility and Sterility* and the author of more than 100 scholarly studies, articles and book chapters. We could not wait to hear what he had to say about this product.

He reported that he felt that FertilityBlend for Women and Fertility-Blend for Men were developed based on sound published scientific findings on nutritional components which show benefit to fertility and have a safe history of usage. FertilityBlend for Women includes:

- the herb Vitex (chasteberry), which enhances hormone balance and ovulation frequency
- the amino acid L-arginine, which helps improve circulation to the reproductive area
- the antioxidants green tea, vitamin E and selenium, which help repair oxidative damage due to aging and environment
- vitamins, including folic acid which assists in the reduction of specific birth defects (neural tube defects) in children, B6 and B12, and minerals, iron, zinc and magnesium which help address specific deficiencies and promote fertility health

FertilityBlend for Men includes:

- the amino acid L-carnitine, which has been shown to be critical to the formation of healthy sperm
- vitamins C and E, green tea and selenium, all potent antioxidants that help improve sperm counts and quality
- ferulic acid, an antioxidant found in Dong Quai that has also been shown to improve sperm quality
- zinc and B vitamins (B6, B12 and folate), critical nutrients in male reproductive systems for several benefits, including hormone metabolism, sperm formation and motility

A double-blind, placebo-controlled pilot study of the women's blend showed a pregnancy rate of 33% in the treated group; none of the women in the control group became pregnant. The result reached statistical significance.

Proxeed™ is a dietary supplement for men similar to FertilityBlend for Men, but it includes only L-carnitine and Acetyl-L-carnitine, and doesn't include the vitamins, minerals and antioxidants. Clinical trials have shown that the ingredients in Proxeed™ optimize sperm motility, speed, count and concentration, but most of these studies were not done on men with low sperm parameters. Proxeed™ is a citrus-flavored powder that can be dissolved in juice or other cold beverages. The manufacturers recommend it be taken twice a day, once in the morning and once in the evening, for as long as you're attempting to conceive. And because sperm require 74 days to mature, the makers of Proxeed™ say it should be taken for at least 3 months to see initial improvement in sperm quality.

We cannot give specific recommendations on which herbs to use because an herbal prescription needs to be specific for an individual. One size does not fit all. In addition, you must be sure that any herbs used are excellent quality or they may be harmful. For that reason we are not currently recommending their use during active ART treatment. If you decide to use herbs in conjunction with conventional treatments, see an expert in TCM for specific recommendations and guidance in product selection. In choosing an expert, use the same care you did when deciding on an expert in Western medicine.

Recommendations for changes in one's diet are not generally as specific as the prescription for herbs but that does not mean that much dietary advice is not controversial. In searching for dietary changes relating to infertility we found two basic types of advice. The first is usually based on good nutritional priciples but is far too general to attribute success solely to this lifestyle modification. You have heard this advice a million times, probably starting with your mother: eat more fruit and vegetables, drink more water, stay away from sugar and caffeine. We found such advice on websites and books disguised as specific dietary advice that can help you get pregnant. Is it good advice? Sure. But we don't expect to receive letters from women claiming it was all they needed to do to successfully conceive.

The second category of nutritional advice is more specific, but in the minds of conventional physicians, it does not have any scientific basis and the advice is not offered with any scientific facts to back it up. One popular book, *The Infertility Diet: Get Pregnant and Avoid Miscarriage* by Fern Reiss (Peanut Butter and Jelly Press, 1999), offers general advice that we already know in addition to specific suggestions such as the following:

Pumpkin seeds are particularly high in zinc. Zinc deficiency is linked to low sperm motility. Even a marginal zinc deficiency can cause sperm counts to drop precipitously. Zinc also affects female fertility, particularly in concert with vitamin B6 (vitamin B6 protects against estrogen-progesterone imbalance as well as elevated serum prolactic levels). Additionally, zinc is helpful against candida albicans. Zinc deficiency is also implicated in miscarriage, according to a recent Swedish study.

This is an example of advice that is based on a small, obscure fact which, through convoluted reasoning, mushrooms into a whole new theory. In this case, has anyone ever showed in a scientific study that pumpkin seeds have improved sperm motility or counts? We are not aware of any such studies.

Some dietary considerations for specific causes of infertility have been shown to have a positive effect on the reproductive process. Most important is the question of weight, at both extremes. Women who suffer from anorexia or bulimia, or engage in competitive-level exercise so that their body fat is extremely low, often have ovulation problems that can be reversed by better nutrition and less exercise, with the ultimate effect of increasing their body fat. Women who are very overweight have been shown to have poorer success rates in IVF cycles and would do well to lose a significant amount of weight in a sensible weight-loss program emphasizing good nutritional practices and exercise. Obese PCOS patients can have spontaneous ovulation and return to a more normal menstrual pattern based on weight loss of 5% to 10% of their body weight.

We don't think that you need a specific diet. Try to reach a close to ideal weight before trying to conceive, using good nutritional principles and exercise. Eat a good, balanced diet and take a recommended supplement with folic acid to prevent neural tube defects. All this is probably information, with the exception of folic acid, that your mother taught you a long time ago.

THE MIND-BODY CONNECTION

Mind-body medicine uses a variety of techniques to enhance the capacity of one's mind to affect bodily functions. These techniques may include attending support groups, congnitive-behavior therapy in formal Mind-Body Connection programs, meditation, prayer and guided imagery. The debate over the role of the mind in the reproductive process probably originated when the first rudimentary treatments for infertility were developed, and it has not been settled even now in the third decade of assisted reproductive technology. How many times have we heard or even ourselves given well-meaning advice like, "Just relax, take a vacation, take your mind off it" to a couple struggling to get pregnant? Another favorite story people tell is the mythical couple who adopted a baby and then got pregnant on their own. Of course, we often don't know the couple that happened to, but it sounds like a good thing to say. Surprisingly, it may not be such bad advice. The Mind-Body Connection is the area of alternative treatments that has the best randomized, controlled studies from good institutions to back its conclusions.

In 1990, a report from no less than Harvard Medical School, published in the highly respected journal *Fertility and Sterility*, reported increasing evidence that a behavioral treatment approach might be efficacious in the emotional aspects of infertility and lead to increased conception rates. The first 54 women to complete a behavioral treatment program based on the elicitation of the relaxation response showed statistically significant decreases in anxiety, depression and fatigue as well as increases in vigor. The bottom line was that 34% of these women became pregnant within 6 months of completing the program. By 2000 they had conducted a single-blind randomized study of 184 women who had been trying to get pregnant for 1 to 2 years. One-third of the women participated in cognitive-behavioral group therapy, which included nutritional and exercise counseling, relaxation techniques like meditation, progressive muscle relaxation, imagery, yoga and cognitive restructuring or "attitude adjustment." One-third participated in conventional support groups to discuss how they were coping, and another third served as controls. Twenty percent of the controls became pregnant within one year of follow-up, compared to 55% in the cognitive-behavior group and 54% in the support group. The differences were not due to age differences, duration of infertility or medical interventions, as the groups were similar in these parameters.

In October 2001, researchers from the University of California, San Diego investigated the effects of stress on success rates of IVF and GIFT in a multi-center study. Standard tests were used to evaluate the patients' moods and their fluctuations, optimism, perceptions and feelings about

Of all the alternative methods, Mind-Body type programs have the most scientific evidence to support their efficacy.

infertility, social support networks, self-percieved stress and methods of coping, and correlated these with their impact on ART procedures. Higher levels of baseline stress were correlated with fewer eggs retrieved and fertilized and fewer embryos transferred, and subsequently more negative outcomes in IVF or GIFT. Initial optimism about becoming pregnant was associated with an increased number of eggs fertilized and an increase in the number of embryos transferred. Women who said they "would do anything for a child" had a five times higher chance of having a multiple birth. This might be explained, not by a psychological force, but by the fact that these women may represent those who push for more embryos to be transferred.

What about the male partner? Is there a mind-body connection that relates to sperm production? A June 2003 study by researchers in Rome showed a statistically significant correlation between abnormally low sperm counts and the personality traits of alexthymia (difficulty identifying and describing feelings as well as externally oriented thinking) and psychoticism (disconnection from reality, disorganized and disoriented thinking). The psychological testing was done before the first semen analysis was performed. The correlation was so strong that the researchers could predict the semen analysis from the results of the psychological tests. They felt that these results could indicate that the emotional processes may have an effect on hormones and sperm development.

Another modality that can be used to alter the mind-body balance is clinical hypnosis. A review of the applicability of clinical hypnosis in the treatment of functional infertility in the *American Journal of Clinical Hypnosis* found sparse information on the subject and described two anecdotal cases in which hypnosis based on imagery and a relaxation strategy was successful in facilitating pregnancy. The treatment was considered to have resulted in beneficial modification of attitude, optimism and mind-body interaction. The stated beneficial goals were not unlike those in the formal mind-body connection program and support groups which have been shown to be effective statistically. An October 2003 report in *Fertility and Sterility* reported on a series of 12 patients with hypothalemic amenorrhea, in which 9 of the subjects resumed menstruation after receiving a single 45- to 70-minute session of hypnosis. All subjects reported beneficial side effects, such as increased general feeling of well-being and increased self-confidence.

If there is any benefit to reproductive process from a manipulative method such as therapeutic massage, it is probably mediated through the mind-body connection. Massage therapy is the systematized manipulation of soft tissues with the basic goal of helping the body heal itself. Massage therapists claim massage improves circulation, bringing fresh oxygen to the tissues and assisting in the elimination of waste products. According to advocates, it can be used to promote general well-being and enhance self-esteem. A practitioner may recommend relaxing essential oils of lavender, geranium or rosemary to relieve stress and tension. Rose and lemon balm are believed to have a particular affinity with the female sex organs and to be especially useful for stress-related conditions. Some advocates claim that certain massage oils can restore estrogen levels and that others can treat pelvic infections. Still others claim that massage can unblock closed fallopian tubes. In view of the fact that these claims are supported only by anecdotal reports, we would limit the use of massage to its relaxation properties.

An example of the power of the mind-body interaction is represented in a recent patient. Jennifer and Greg were referred to us by Jennifer's mother's neighbor, a local doctor. Although only 27 years old and off birth control pills for a year, Jennifer was very concerned that she would never conceive. She was hypothyroid and had irregular menstruation, which heightened her anxiety that she would never be successful. After a hormonal evaluation, she was placed on clomiphene to regulate her ovulation. In her third cycle she conceived, but the pregnancy ended in an early biochemical loss. Her anxiety worsened. She then started cycles of gonadotropins with insemination, but after three cycles she wanted to proceed with in vitro fertilization, as she was stressed by the process. Her cycle produced 10 eggs, of which 8 fertilized and 3 embryos were transferred. She did not get pregnant. By this time her stress was palpable.

We recommended that she attend the Mind-Body Connection program before undergoing any further attempts at IVF. The psychologist at the program called to report that she was so depressed that she may need a referral to a psychiatrist for anti-depressant medication. While waiting to start another IVF cycle, she conceived spontaneously. Happily, they now have a baby boy. In fact, at the last meeting of her Mind-Body group she was unaware that she was 3 weeks pregnant. What was the problem here: anovulation, embryo quality or stress? We would have to give substantial credit to the Mind-Body Connection program for helping resolve this problem, including her depression.

HAVE THE TWAIN MET?

Not yet, but they're getting closer. According to Kipling's quotation, they will not meet "Till Earth and Sky stand presently at God's great Judgement Seat." We think they're closer than that. In fact, many reproductive specialists are beginning to refer patients, who they feel would benefit, to trained professionals like Dr. Dao and Ms. Perry. But each couple has to decide for themselves whether they feel that an alternative approach would be a good adjunct to their scientifically oriented Western treatment. A lot of Western medicine professionals object to the fact that TCM is based on feelings, philosophy and anecdotal evidence rather than solid scientific evidence, and so the twain may not meet for reproductive medicine for awhile. However, before you make your decision, let us leave you with a story.

Use every positive force available to you to achieve your dream. Maybe for Esther, her mother's prayers helped, too. They certainly didn't hurt.

Esther was a 41-year-old who married at age 38. Almost a year later, she experienced a miscarriage at age 39. About a year after the miscarriage she began acupuncture treatments and herbs. At age 41, with an FSH of 9.1, she had an unsuccessful IVF cycle at a competing facility. She then came to Reproductive Partners with FSH levels of 11.1 and 12.7. Over the next 3 months she started a 10-week Mind-Body Connection course. After the disappointment of having an FSH level of 22.8 in February, she took a vacation in Florida in mid-April during which time she had a menstrual period. She was lucky that her insurance would pay for seven cycles of IVF, and she was preparing herself for egg donation. Two weeks after she had her psychological evaluation for the egg donation, she called us because she had not gotten another period since her vacation. You guessed it. She was pregnant with a chromosomally normal pregnancy which is now ongoing.

Was it the Mind-Body program, acupuncture, herbs, the vacation or just luck? Another possibility is that after she disclosed the pregnancy to her family she found out from her mother that her mother's church group had been praying for her regularly. She wrote to us, "I can't ignore the power and contribution from a higher authority as well. Thank you for promoting and believing in other non-medical alternatives. Your office has helped me find the path to a miracle pregnancy."

We'll leave it for you to decide which factor or factors helped Esther. More importantly, you need to decide which, if any, alternative treatments may help you find the path to a "miracle pregnancy." We are still skeptical about the role of alternative treatments. After all, they are not based on science and statistics, but philosophy and anecdotal evidence. Remember the first ethical rule is, "First, do no harm." Until we have scientific evidence that herbs are not only helpful, but also not harmful, we will likely continue to recommend against their use during ART cycles. Acupuncture holds little chance of harm, while Mind-Body Connection programs have shown favorable results in IVF cycles and are therefore more likely to be recommended, or at least condoned, by reproductive specialists.

APPENDIX 1

The SART/CDC Assisted Reproductive Technology Success Rate Report

SOME WORDS OF CAUTION

Is there some way to objectively compare ART centers? Well, maybe. Some knowledge about what the figures mean can help you make a reasonably well-informed choice. But don't just peruse the latest report, available at the cdc.gov website, select the center with the best numbers and run right out to sign on the dotted line.

The latest SART/CDC report provides data on statistics from cycles started in the year on the title of that report. More up-to-date information may be available, as it takes approximately 3 years from the start of the cycles being reported, to the publication of the report. First, since the report is based on live births, the pregnancies need to be concluded. Then the data needs to be collected, transmitted and published. By the time that happens, a center's success rate might be very different, or perhaps the personnel have changed. So, you might want to ask for and review the most recent, but unpublished, clinic-specific report on any centers you are considering. Clinics will usually have it prepared for submission by the end of December of the year following the year the cycles were initiated.

INTERPRETING THE SURVEY RESULTS

The full report presents treatment results for the following ART procedures for the calendar year:

- all ART cyles broken down as:
- fresh embryos from nondonor eggs broken down into age groups
- frozen embryos from nondonor eggs broken down into age groups
- donor eggs, fresh and frozen cycles

Keep in mind that many other factors which influence delivery rates are not addressed in the report, including:

- variations in patient selection between centers
- numbers of previous cycles a patient may have had
- variations in the reason (diagnosis) for the need for an ART procedure
- where patients fell within the widely defined categories of age
- the severity of male factor when it was present

It is difficult to compare two centers with widely divergent patient populations and protocols on the basis of the numbers alone. For example, compare these two patients at two different centers who would fall into the same report category:

	Center A	*Center B*
Patient Selection	6 years of infertility	1 year of infertility
	Complete testing	Few tests
Previous cycles	3	0
Diagnosis	Endometriosis	Tubal factor
Age	turns 41 next month	just 38
Male factor	Severe	Minimal
Embryos transferred	3	6

Both of these patients could fall into the "38 to 40" category, but they are not at all comparable, and we would anticipate a very different chance of success for each of them. Yet, they would have the same effect on the success rate of the two centers in exactly the same category. That's why you must be careful to look beyond the numbers.

A new program is wise not to take on difficult cases until those running it are sure everything is going well. Then they won't need to wonder if the fertilization rate in a particular case is low because of some problem in the laboratory. The heads of the various IVF programs just starting out around the country comprised one of the first conferences on ART. One director, who initially had good results to report but had not done remotely as well since that time, said, "Of course we chose these patients to be ideal." He then paused and looked around the room and added, "Didn't everyone?" So, if you are considering a new program, you may be taking a risk that their results are not representative of what *you* can expect. A short-term rate of even 30% or 40% could actually be, over the long haul, compatible with a true rate of 5% to 10% based on favorable patient selection in the initial patients.

At the other extreme, programs that are well known for their expertise tend to gather patients who are concerned about associated problems or their lack of success in other programs, seeking out "the best" to maximize their chance of success.

How can you adjust for this variable? You wouldn't be far off if you subtracted 10% for new programs and added 5% for well-recognized programs, as a rule of thumb.

How about age? Some programs accept women at the higher end of the age categories than those admitted by others. This factor may have a relatively small but significant impact.

Another factor to be considered is that many clinics' percentages are based on a small number of cycles. The report deals with this by giving raw numbers in categories with fewer than 20 cases. Giving a rate on fewer than 10 cycles is almost meaningless, but even with 50 cycles there can be enormous variability based on chance alone. For example, with 50 cycles and a true success rate of 15%, the actual rate could vary anywhere from 5% to 25%, simply based on the fertility potential of the 50 couples who happened to go through the procedure at that time. Even with 200 cases, the 95% confidence limits of a 15% success rate is 10% to 20%. This is why programs experience such wide swings of success rate from time to time; it's simply the chance variation of the inherent fertility potential of the couples treated, as expected from simple statistical calculations. So, in choosing a program in which you can have a reasonable estimate of the true success rate, consider only those with a combined total of at least 100 to 200 cases over a number of years or at least 100 cases for a single year. Ideally, the rate for 500 cycles should be examined, which is why we report our 5-year total to couples interested in our program. At the cdc.gov website you can review a number of previous years for any program to compile enough cases and establish trends.

The final major variable in patient selection depends upon whether it is assured that all other reasonable fertility therapy, including adequate time, has been applied. If so, many of the most fertile women have been removed from the ART population. For example, for several years we have recommended gonadotropins combined with intrauterine insemination for women with open and reasonably normal tubes, before going on to an ART procedure. This has resulted in numerous pregnancies, and we have no doubt that these women would have had a very good chance of being counted among the successes if they had proceeded directly to ART.

For a patient choosing a program, this is a difficult variable to assess. You are probably better off in a program that does IVF as part of a general infertility service. Also, becoming a well-informed consumer will help assure you that everything else has been tried before resorting to ART procedures. If an ART procedure is suggested, ask why any other treatment that seems to apply to you has not been done. Ask what your chance of pregnancy will be if you simply take more time. If you think that ART is suggested prematurely, you may want to downwardly adjust that program's success rate by 10%. Remember, the most basic underlying principle is always to first try to achieve pregnancy in the simplest, least expensive way with the least risk. That should be your goal, too, although impatience due to age, duration of infertility or other personal factors is understandable. You may choose to bypass one of the options offered to you, but it is important that it should be a well-informed choice.

You must also be mindful as you review a center's report that the data has been reported voluntarily and has not been subjected to audit for accuracy and completeness.

There are programs that do not report to SART/CDC or report themselves in a form other than in the format created for the report. We can only conclude that this allows them to report their success rates in a more favorable way. You can draw your own conclusions about the reasons that some centers fail to report their statistics at all. Remember, clinics providing ART services in the U.S. are required to submit ART cycle data under the provisions of the Fertility Clinic Success Rate and Certification Act passed by the U.S. Congress. Centers that reported to the 2001 report are listed in Appendix 2. Any centers not listed either failed to submit data or did not provide verification by the clinic medical director.

It is also good to remember that convenience, personal attention and program organization will influence your chance of success. If the process is not easily tolerated and you decide to quit after one cycle instead of three or four, your chance of success will have been greatly affected. At the same time beware of programs that make it too simple; there is no simple way to achieve a high rate of success. The best way to evaluate this factor is to get a recommendation from a satisfied patient or from a physician whose patients were happy with the care they received.

If you are already in a program that satisfies the above criteria, we do not advise switching merely because you have not yet been successful. Even in the best programs, many patients will require more than one attempt. The loss of continuity may deprive you of the "experience factor" whereby physicians and laboratory personnel can make subtle adjustments to improve your chance of success. Also, you will lose the "comfort factor" in being familiar with the team members who have been caring for you already.

This may all sound complicated, but it's worth the effort. You should be able to make a better initial choice based on all this information. This can be found at http://apps.nccd.cdc.gov/ART2001/nation01.asp.

2001 NATIONAL SUMMARY

Type of ART

		Procedural Factors:	
IVF	99%		
GIFT	<1%	With ICSI	50%
ZIFT	<1%	Unstimulated	<1%
Combination	<1%	Used gestational carrier	<1%

Patient Diagnosis

Tubal factor	14%	Other factor	7%
Ovulatory dysfunction	6%	Unknown factor	10%

Diminished ovarian reserve	9%	*Multiple Factors:*		
Endometriosis	6%	Female factors only	13%	
Uterine factor	1%	Female & male factors	17%	
Male factor	17%			

2001 PREGNANCY SUCCESS RATES

Type of Cycle	*Age of Woman*			
Fresh Embryos from				
Nondonor Eggs	<35	35–37	38–40	41–42
Number of cycles	35,984	17,791	16,283	7,044
Percentage of cycles resulting in pregnancies	40.6	34.4	26.2	17.3
Percentage of cycles resulting in live births	35.2	28.4	19.6	10.4
Percentage of retrievals resulting in live births	38.9	33.1	23.8	13.2
Percentage of transfers resulting in live births	41.1	35.1	25.4	14.5
Percentage of transfers resulting in singleton live births	24.8	22.9	18.5	11.9
Percentage of cancellations	9.6	14.1	17.9	21.4
Average number of embryos transferred	2.8	3.1	3.4	3.7
Percentage of pregnancies with twins	33.1	28.6	22.7	14.5
Percentage of pregnancies with triplets or more	8.1	7.8	6.2	2.9
Percentage of live births having multiple infants	39.7	34.7	27.2	17.9
Frozen Embryos from				
Nondonor Eggs				
Number of transfers	7,053	2,971	2,030	646
Percentage of transfers resulting in live births	26.0	23.3	19.4	15.8
Average number of embryos transferred	2.9	2.9	3.1	3.3

All Ages Combined

Donor Eggs	Fresh Embryos	Frozen Embryos
Number of transfers	7,722	3,028
Percentage of transfers resulting in live births	47.0	27.3
Average number of embryos transferred	2.9	3.0

APPENDIX 2

The Canadian Assisted Reproductive Technology Success Rate Report

On November 8, 2003 The Canadian Fertility and Andrology Society (CFAS) released the third annual nationwide results on assisted reproduction live birth rates in Canada. The rates of pregnancy and live birth in the country's fertility clinics were "on par with other national registries, including the United States."

Under the leadership of the Accreditation Committee of the CFAS, 21 of the 22 in vitro fertilization (IVF) centers in Canada voluntarily participated in the collection of nationwide data on the results of assisted reproduction. But the list of which centers participated is not made public. Live birth rates were reported for 5380 IVF treatment cycles (including intracytoplasmic sperm injection (ICSI)) undertaken in 19 IVF centers in 2001.

- the overall live birth rate was 23% per cycle started
  - 67% of live births were singletons
  - 91% of multiple births were twins
- the live birth rates by age of the mother were:
  - for women under 35 years old, the live birth rate was 30%
  - for women aged 35 to 39 years, the live birth rate was 21%
  - for women 40 years old and over, the live birth rate was 7%

Preliminary results were reported for 6,366 IVF treatment cycles (including ICSI) undertaken in 20 IVF centers in 2002.

- the overall pregnancy rate was 30% per cycle started
- only 1 to 2 embryos were replaced in the uterus in half the cycles
- 63% of pregnancies were singletons
- 89% of the multiple pregnancies were twins
- as expected, the woman's age has a strong influence on pregnancy rate:
  - for women under 35 years old, the pregnancy rate was 37%
  - for women aged 35 to 39 years old, the pregnancy rate was 28%
  - for women 40 years old and over, the pregnancy rate was 15%

Live birth rates for cycles started in 2002 will be released when they become available. The CFAS makes these data available for "reference and education." They state that the information should be reviewed together with an appropriate health care professional. Results vary by center, and specific information can be obtained from each center, as they do not publish each center's individual success rates as SART/CDC does.

APPENDIX 3

Resources

SOURCES OF INFORMATION

General information

The American Society for Reproductive Medicine (ASRM), 1209 Montgomery Highway, Birmingham, AL 35216-2809, (205) 978-5000 Web: http://www.asrm.org

American College of Obstetricians and Gynecologists (ACOG), 409 12th Street SW, P.O. Box 96920, Washington, D.C. 20090-6920 Web: http://acog.org

The Canadian Fertility and Andrology Society/La Société Canadienne de Fertilité et d'Andrologie, 2065 Alexandre de Séve, Suite 409, Montreal, Quebec, Canada H2L 2W5, (514) 524-9009 Web: http://www.cfas.ca

SERONO SYMPOSIA, International, One Technology Place, Rockland, MA 02370, (781) 982-9000, (800) 283-8088

Society for Assisted Reproductive Technology (SART), 1029 Montgomery Highway, Birmingham, AL 35216 (205) 978-5000 Web: http://www.sart.org

Adoption

Adoption Council of Canada, Bronson Centre, 211 Bronson Avenue, #210, Ottawa, Ontario, Canada, K1R 6H5, (613) 235-0344 Web: http://www.adoption.ca

Adoptive Families Magazine, 42 West 38th Street, New York, NY 10018, (646) 366-0830 Web: http://www.adoptivefamilies.com

American Academy of Adoption Attorneys, P.O. Box 33053, Washington, D.C. 20033, (202) 832-2222 Web: http://www.adoptionattorneys.org

California Association of Adoption Agencies Web: http://www.california-adoption.org

Families for Private Adoptions, P.O. Box 6375, Washington, D.C. 20015-0375, (202) 722-0338 Web: http://www.ffpa.org

National Adoption Information Clearinghouse, 330 "C" Street SW, Washington, D. C. 20447, (703) 352-3488, (888) 251-0075 Web: http://www.calib.com

National Council for Adoption, 225 N. Washington Street, Alexandria, VA 22314-2561, (703) 299-6633 Web: http://www.ncfa-usa.org

The National Adoption Foundation, 100 Mill Plain Rd., Danbury, CT 06811, (203) 791-3811 Web: http://www.nafadopt.org

SUPPORT GROUPS

American Infertility Association, 666 Fifth Avenue, Suite 278, New York, NY 10103, (888) 917-3777, (718) 621-5083 Web: http://www.americaninfertility.org

Infertility Awareness Association of Canada (IAAC), National Office, 770 Broadview, Suite 305, Ottawa, Ontario, Canada K2A 3Z3, (613) 244-7222, (800) 263-2929 Web: http://www.iaac.ca

Infertility Network, 160 Pickering Street, Toronto, Ontario M4E 3J7, (416) 691-3611 Web: http://www.infertilitynetwork.org

RESOLVE, Inc., National Office, 1310 Broadway, Somerville, MA 02144-1731, (888) 623-0744, (617) 623-1156, Helpline (617) 623-0744, email: info@resolve.org, Web: http://www.resolve.org

Complementary and alternative medicine

Linus Pauling Institute (Oregon State University)
http://www.lpi.oregon-state.edu

National Center for Complementary and Alternative Medicine (National Institutes of Health) http://www.nccam.nih.gov

National Foundation for Alternative Medicine http://www.nfam.org

CENTERS REPORTING TO THE 2001 SART/CDC REPORT

Adapted from the Society for Assisted Reproductive Technology/CDC Assisted Reproductive Technology Success Rates report for the Year 2001

Geographic data

Note: Since this is data reported from 2001, there may be some changes in addresses, telephone numbers and program directors. We have attempted to provide this information as correctly as possible, but some errors or changes may have occurred. If the clinic name has changed since 2001, the current name is listed in italics directly under the 2001 name. Clinic names preceded by the § symbol have reorganized since 2001. Reorganization is defined as a change in ownership or affiliation, or a change in two of the three key staff positions (practice director, medical director or laboratory director). Contact SART for current clinic information.

Explanation of abbreviations for accrediting agencies used throughout this list:

CAP/ASRM-College of American Pathologists/Society for Assisted Reproductive Technology, Reproductive Laboratory Accreditation Program

JCAHO-Joint Commission of Accreditation of Healthcare Organizations

NYSTB-New York State Tissue Bank Program

ALABAMA

ART Program of Alabama, Women's Medical Plaza, 2006 Brookwood Medical Center Dr., Suite 508, Birmingham, AL 35209, Telephone: (205) 870-9784; Fax: (205) 870-0698. Lab Name: IVF/Andrology Laboratory, Accreditation: CAP/ASRM

University of Alabama at Birmingham, IVF Program, 2000 Sixth Ave. South, Birmingham, AL 35233, Telephone: (205) 801-8225; Fax: (205) 975-5732, Lab Name: UAB Gamete Biology Laboratory, Accreditation: CAP/ASRM

Center for Reproductive Medicine, 3 Mobile Infirmary Cir., Suite 213, Mobile, AL 36607, Telephone: (251) 438-4200; Fax: (251) 438-4211, Lab Name: Center for Reproductive Medicine, Accreditation: CAP/ASRM

University of South Alabama IVF and ART Program, Dept. of OB/GYN, Div. of Reproductive Endocrinology, 307 University Blvd. North, CC/CB 326, Mobile, AL 36688, Telephone: (251) 438-4211; Fax: (251) 460-7251, Lab Name: University of South Alabama IVF and Andrology Lab, Accreditation: CAP/ASRM

ARIZONA

Fertility Treatment Center, 3200 N. Dobson Rd., Suite F-7, Chandler, AZ 85224, Telephone: (480) 831-2445; Fax: (480) 897-1283, Lab Name: Fertility Treatment Center, Accreditation: CAP/ASRM

West Valley Fertility Center, 17612 North 59th Ave., Suite 100, Glendale, AZ 85308, Telephone: (602) 993-8636; Fax: (602) 993-2528, Lab Name: West Valley Fertility Center, Accreditation: CAP/ASRM

Arizona Reproductive Medicine Specialists, 1300 N. 12th St., Suite 520, Phoenix, AZ

85006, Telephone: (602) 343-2767; Fax: (602) 343-2766, Lab Name: Arizona Reproductive Medicine Specialists, Accreditation: JCAHO

Southwest Fertility Center, 3125 N. 32nd St., Suite 200, Phoenix, AZ 85018, Telephone: (602) 956-7481; Fax: (602) 956-7591, Lab Name: Southwest Fertility Center, Accreditation: CAP/ASRM

Arizona Center for Fertility Studies, 8997 E. Desert Cove Ave., 2nd Floor, Scottsdale, AZ 85260, Telephone: (480) 860-4792; Fax: (480) 860-6819, Lab Name: Institute for Reproductive Studies, Accreditation: CAP/ASRM

Mayo Clinic Scottsdale, Center for Reproductive Medicine, 13737 N. 92nd St., Scottsdale, AZ 85260, Telephone: (480) 614-6099; Fax: (480) 614-6011, Lab Name: Mayo Clinic Scottsdale, Accreditation: CAP/ASRM

Arizona Center for Reproductive, Endocrinology & Infertility, 5190 E. Farness Dr., Suite 114, Tucson, AZ 85712, Telephone: (520) 326-0001; Fax: (520) 326-7451, Lab Name: Reproductive Endocrinology and Infertility, Accreditation: CAP/ASRM, NYSTB

ART Laboratory, University Physicians, Inc., The University of Arizona, Arizona Health Science Center, 1501 N. Campbell Ave., Room 8329, Tucson, AZ 85724, Telephone: (520) 626-6923; Fax: (520) 626-2768, Lab Name: Assisted Reproductive Technology Laboratory, Accreditation: JCAHO

ARKANSAS

Intra Vaginal Culture Fertilization Program of Arkansas, 500 S. University, Suite 103, Little Rock, AR 72205, Telephone: (501) 663-5858; Fax: (501) 663-9007, Lab Name: Intra Vaginal Culture Fertilization Program of Arkansas, Accreditation: CAP/ASRM

University of Arkansas for Medical Sciences IVF, 5800 W. 10th St., Suite 705, Little Rock, AR 72204, Telephone: (501) 296-1705; Fax: (501) 296-1710, Lab Name: Arkansas Reproductive Technology, Accreditation: CAP/ASRM

CALIFORNIA

Garfield Fertility Center, 320 S. Garfield Ave., Suite 226, Alhambra, CA 91801, Telephone: (626) 943-9536; Fax: (626) 943-9529, Lab Name: ART Reproductive Center, Inc., Accreditation: CAP/ASRM

Alta Bates In Vitro Fertilization Program, 2999 Regent St., Suite 101-A, Berkeley, CA 94705, Telephone: (510) 649-0440; Fax: (510) 649-8700, Lab Name: Alta Bates IVF Laboratory, Accreditation: CAP/ASRM

Center for Reproductive Health & Gynecology, 99 N. La Cienega Blvd., Suite 109,

Beverly Hills, CA 90211, Telephone: (661) 254-0545; Fax: (661) 254-3221, Lab Name: Center for Reproductive Health and Gynecology, Accreditation: CAP/ASRM

Southern California Reproductive Center, 450 N. Roxbury Dr., 5th Floor, Beverly Hills, CA 90210, Telephone: (310) 277-4948; Fax: (310) 274-5112, Lab Name: A.R.T. Reproductive Center, Inc., Accreditation: CAP/ASRM

Southern California Reproductive Center, 450 N. Roxbury Dr., 5th Floor, Beverly Hills, CA 90210, Telephone: (310) 277-2393; Fax: (310) 274-5112, Lab Name: A.R.T. Reproductive Center, Inc., Accreditation: CAP/ASRM

West Coast Infertility Medical Clinic, Inc., 250 N. Robertson Blvd., Suite 403, Beverly Hills, CA 90211, Telephone: (310) 285-0333; Fax: (310) 285-0334, Lab Name: IVF Laboratory, West Coast Infertility Clinic, Inc., Accreditation: JCAHO

Fertility Care of Orange County, 203 N. Brea Blvd., Suite 100, Brea, CA 92821, Telephone: (714) 256-0777; Fax: (714) 256-0105, Lab Name: Southern California Institute for Reproductive Science, Accreditation: CAP/ASRM

Central California IVF, Women's Specialty, and Fertility Center, 722 Medical Center Dr. E., Suite 105, Clovis, CA 93611, Telephone: (559) 299-7700; Fax: (559) 297-9679, Lab Name: Community Medical Center–Fresno, Accreditation: JCAHO

Zouves Fertility Center, Physicians Medical Center, 901 Campus Dr., Suite 214, Daly City, CA 94015, Telephone: (650) 301-4933; Fax: (650) 301-4939, Lab Name: Zouves Fertility Center, Accreditation: CAP/ASRM

Gil N. Mileikowsky, M.D., 5363 Balboa Blvd., Suite 245, Encino, CA 91316, Telephone: (818) 981-1888; Fax: (818) 981-1994, Lab Name: Dr. Gil Mileikowsky, Accreditation: None

West Coast Fertility Centers, 11160 Warner Ave., Suite 411, Fountain Valley, CA 92708, Telephone: (714) 513-1399; Fax: (714) 513-1393, Lab Name: West Coast Fertility Center Gamete Laboratory, Accreditation: CAP/ASRM

Kathleen L. Kornafel, M.D., Ph.D., 1560 E. Chevy Chase Dr., Suite 200, Glendale, CA 91206, Telephone: (818) 242-9933; Fax: (818) 242-9937, Lab Name: ART Roxbury Surgery Center, Accreditation: JCAHO, Lab Name: Century City Hospital, Accreditation: JCAHO

Marin Fertility Medical Group, Advanced Fertility Associates Medical Group, 1100 S. Eliseo Dr., Suite 107, Greenbrae, CA 94904, Telephone: (415) 464-8688; Fax: (415) 449-3422, Lab Name: NorthBay Fertility Center, Inc., Accreditation: CAP/ASRM

Fertility Center of Southern California, 2192 Martin St., Suite 110, Irvine, CA 92612, Telephone: (949) 955-0072; Fax: (949) 955-0077, Lab Name: Southern California Institute for Reproductive Science, Accreditation: CAP/ASRM

La Jolla IVF, Smotrich Center for Reproductive Enhancement, 9850 Genesee Ave.,

Suite 610, La Jolla, CA 92037, Telephone: (858) 558-2221; Fax: (858) 558-2260, Lab Name: La Jolla IVF, Accreditation: None

Reproductive Partners–San Diego, 9850 Genesee Ave., Suite 800, La Jolla, CA 92037, Telephone: (858) 552-9177; Fax: (858) 552-9188, Lab Name: Reproductive Partners–San Diego, Accreditation: CAP/ASRM

Reproductive Sciences Center, 4150 Regents Park Row, Suite 280, La Jolla, CA 92037, Telephone: (858) 625-0125; Fax: (858) 625-0131, Lab Name: Reproductive Sciences Center, Accreditation: CAP/ASRM

Scripps Clinic Fertility Center, 10666 N. Torrey Pines Rd., La Jolla, CA 92037, Telephone: (858) 554-8680; Fax: (858) 554-9092, Lab Name: Scripps Clinic Fertility Center Laboratory, Accreditation: CAP/ASRM

The Zarutskie Fertility and Endocrine Institute, 25500 Rancho Niguel Rd., Suite 280, Laguna Niguel, CA 92677, Telephone: (949) 448-7818; Fax: (949) 448-7819, Lab Name: Southern California Institute for Reproductive Science, Accreditation: CAP/ASRM, Lab Name: La Jolla IVF, Accreditation: None

Loma Linda University Center for Fertility and IVF, 11370 Anderson St., Suite 3950, Loma Linda, CA 92354, Telephone: (909) 558-2851; Fax: (909) 558-2450, Lab Name: Fertility Science Laboratory, Accreditation: CAP/ASRM

Reproductive Partners–Long Beach, 701 E. 28th St., Suite 202, Long Beach, CA 90806, Telephone: (562) 427-2229; Fax: (562) 427-2751, Lab Name: RPMG IVF & Andrology Laboratory–Long Beach, Accreditation: CAP/ASRM, Lab Name: RPMG IVF & Andrology Laboratory–Redondo Beach, Accreditation: CAP/ASRM

University of California–Los Angeles, Fertility Center, Obstetrics and Gynecology, 10833 Le Conte Ave., Room 22-177 CHS, Los Angeles, CA 90024, Telephone: (310) 825-9500; Fax: (310) 206-9731, Lab Name: Center for Reproductive Medicine IVF Lab, Accreditation: CAP/ASRM

University of Southern California, Reproductive Endocrinology and Infertility, 1127 Wilshire Blvd., Suite 1400, Los Angeles, CA 90017, Telephone: (213) 975-9990; Fax: (213) 975-9997, Lab Name: USC School of Medicine IVF Laboratory, Accreditation: CAP/ASRM (Pending)

Reproductive Specialty Medical Center, 1441 Avocado Ave., Suite 203, Newport Beach, CA 92660, Telephone: (949) 640-7200; Fax: (949) 720-0203, Lab Name: Reproductive Specialty Medical Center, Accreditation: JCAHO (Pending)

Southern California Center for Reproductive Medicine, 361 Hospital Rd., Suite 333, Newport Beach, CA 92663, Telephone: (949) 642-8727; Fax: (949) 642-5413, Lab Name: Southern California Institute for Reproductive Sciences, Accreditation: CAP/ASRM

Northridge Center for Reproductive Medicine, 18546 Roscoe Blvd., Suite 240, Northridge, CA 91324, Telephone: (818) 701-8181; Fax: (818) 701-8100, Lab Name: Northridge Center for Reproductive Medicine, Accreditation: None

IVF–Orange Surgery Center, 845 W. La Veta Ave., Suite 104, Orange, CA 92868, Telephone: (714) 744-2040; Fax: (714) 744-2042, Lab Name: IVF–Orange, Accreditation: None

Nova In Vitro Fertilization, 1681 El Camino Real, Palo Alto, CA 94306, Telephone: (650) 322-0500; Fax: (650) 322-5404, Lab Name: Nova IVF Lab, Accreditation: CAP/ASRM

Huntington Reproductive Center, 301 S. Fair Oaks Ave., Suite 402, Pasadena, CA 91105, Telephone: (626) 440-9161; Fax: (626) 440-0138, Lab Name: Huntington Reproductive Gamete Laboratory, Accreditation: CAP/ASRM

Reproductive Partners–Redondo Beach, 510 N. Prospect, Suite 202, Redondo Beach, CA 90277, Telephone: (310) 318-3010; Fax: (310) 798-7304, Lab Name: Reproductive Partners–Redondo Beach, Accreditation: CAP/ASRM, Lab Name: Reproductive Partners–Long Beach, Accreditation: CAP/ASRM

Northern California Fertility Medical Center, 406-1/2 Sunrise Ave., Suite 310, Roseville, CA 95661, Telephone: (916) 773-2229; Fax: (916) 773-8391, Lab Name: Northern California Fertility Medical Center, Accreditation: CAP/ASRM

University of California–Davis, Assisted Reproductive Technology Program, Div. of Reproductive Endocrinology and Infertility, 2521 Stockton Blvd., Suite 4200, Sacramento, CA 95817, Telephone: (916) 734-6944; Fax: (916) 734-6150, Lab Name: IVF Laboratory, Accreditation: CAP/ASRM

The Fertility and Gynecology Center, 212 San Jose St., Suite 201, Salinas, CA 93901, Telephone: (831) 769-0161; Fax: (831) 759-0939, Lab Name: The Fertility and Gynecology Center, Accreditation: CAP/ASRM

Advanced Fertility Institute, 6719 Alvarado Rd., Suite 108, San Diego, CA 92120, Telephone: (619) 265-1800; Fax: (619) 265-4055, Lab Name: Alvarado Hospital Fertility Center, Accreditation: JCAHO

Fertility Specialists Medical Group, 3003 Health Center Dr., 2nd Floor, San Diego, CA 92123, Telephone: (858) 541-4144; Fax: (858) 541-4114, Lab Name: Sharp Fertility Center, Accreditation: CAP/ASRM, JCAHO

Minh N. Ho, M.D., F.A.C.O.G., XPert Fertility Care of California, 5555 Reservoir Dr., Suite 205, San Diego, CA 92120, Telephone: (619) 286-5858; Fax: (619) 286-1474, Lab Name: Reproductive Science Center, Accreditation: CAP/ASRM, Lab Name: Alvarado Hospital Medical Center, Accreditation: JCAHO

IGO Medical Group of San Diego, 9339 Genesee Ave., Suite 220, San Diego, CA 92121,

Telephone: (858) 455-7520; Fax: (858) 554-1312, Lab Name: IGO Medical Group Laboratory, Accreditation: CAP/ASRM

Infertility Clinic, Naval Medical Center, San Diego, 2650 Stockton Rd., Bldg. 624, San Diego, CA 92106, Telephone: (619) 524-6218; Fax: (619) 524-0118, Lab Name: Reproductive Partners–San Diego, Accreditation: CAP/ASRM

San Diego Fertility Center, 11515 El Camino Real, Suite 100, San Diego, CA 92130, Telephone: (858) 794-6363; Fax: (858) 794-6360, Lab Name: SDFC IVF & Andrology Laboratory, Inc., Accreditation: CAP/ASRM

Fertility Associates of the Bay Area, 1700 California St., Suite 570, San Francisco, CA 94109, Telephone: (415) 673-9199; Fax: (415) 673-8796, Lab Name: California Reproductive Laboratories, Accreditation: CAP/ASRM

Simon R. Henderson, M.D., 390 Laurel St., Suite 200, San Francisco, CA 94118, Telephone: (415) 921-6100; Fax: (415) 563-0922, Lab Name: San Francisco Fertility Centers, Accreditation: CAP/ASRM

San Francisco Fertility Centers, Pacific Fertility Center/San Francisco Center for Reproductive Medicine, 55 Francisco St., Suite 500, San Francisco, CA 94133, Telephone: (415) 834-3095; Fax: (415) 834-3080, Lab Name: San Francisco Fertility Centers, Accreditation: CAP/ASRM

§University of California–San Francisco, In Vitro Fertilization Program, 2356 Sutter St. 7, San Francisco, CA 94115, Telephone: (415) 353-3040; Fax: (415) 353-7744, Contact SART for current clinic information.

Fertility Physicians of Northern California, 2516 Samaritan Dr., Suite A, San Jose, CA 95124, Telephone: (408) 358-2500; Fax: (408) 356-8954, Lab Name: Fertility and Reproductive Health Institute of Northern California, Accreditation: CAP/ASRM

Carmelo S. Sgarlata, M.D., 2505 Samaritan Dr., Suite 208, San Jose, CA 95124, Telephone: (408) 358-1776; Fax: (408) 358-9287, Lab Name: Fertility and Reproductive Health Institute, Accreditation: CAP/ASRM

Reproductive Science Center of the San Francisco Bay Area, 3160 Crow Canyon Rd., Suite 150, San Ramon, CA 94583, Telephone: (925) 867-1800; Fax: (925) 275-0933, Lab Name: Reproductive Science Center of the San Francisco Bay Area, Accreditation: CAP/ASRM

§North Bay Fertility Center, Inc., 1111 Sonoma Ave., Suite 212, Santa Rosa, CA 95405, Telephone: (707) 575-1729; Fax: (707) 575-4379, Contact SART for current clinic information.

Center for Assisted Reproductive Medicine/CFP, California Fertility Partners, 1245 16th Street, Suite 220, Santa Monica, CA 90404, Telephone: (310) 828-4008; Fax: (310) 828-3310, Lab Name: Santa Monica/UCLA Medical Center, Accreditation: CAP/ASRM

Parker–Rosenman–Rodi GYN & Infertility Medical Group, 1450 Tenth St., Suite 404, Santa Monica, CA 90401, Telephone: (310) 451-8144; Fax: (310) 451-3414, Lab Name: Century City Hospital, Center for Reproductive Medicine, Accreditation: CAP/ASRM

Valley Center for Reproductive Health, Tina Koopersmith, M.D., 13320 Riverside Dr., Suite 220, Sherman Oaks, CA 91423, Telephone: (818) 986-1648; Fax: (818) 986-1653, Lab Name: Century City Hospital, Center for Reproductive Medicine, Accreditation: CAP/ASRM, Lab Name: Encino–Tarzana Regional Medical Center, Accreditation: CAP/ASRM, Lab Name: ART, Inc., Accreditation: CAP/ASRM (Pending), NYSTB

Stanford University IVF/ART Program, Dept. of Gynecology and Obstetrics, 300 Pasteur Dr., S-387, Stanford, CA 94305, Telephone: (650) 498-7911; Fax: (650) 498-7294, Lab Name: Stanford University IVF/ART Laboratory, Accreditation: CAP/ASRM

The Center for Fertility and Gynecology, Vermesh/Ben-Ozer Center for Fertility, 18370 Burbank Blvd., Suite 301, Tarzana, CA 91356, Telephone: (818) 881-9800; Fax: (818) 881-1857, Lab Name: Center for Reproductive Medicine, Encino–Tarzana Regional Medical Center, Accreditation: JCAHO

The Fertility Institutes, Jeffrey Steinberg, M.D., Inc., 18370 Burbank Blvd., Suite 414, Tarzana, CA 91356, Telephone: (818) 776-8700; Fax: (818) 776-8754, Lab Name: Century City Hospital, Center for Reproductive Medicine, Accreditation: CAP/ASRM

Infertility and Gynecology Institute, 18370 Burbank Blvd., Suite 514, Tarzana, CA 91356, Telephone: (818) 996-5550; Fax: (818) 996-5725, Lab Name: Assisted Reproductive Technology Medical Group, Inc., Accreditation: JCAHO

Pacific Reproductive Center, 3720 Lomita Blvd., Suite 100, Torrance, CA 90505, Telephone: (310) 376-7000; Fax: (310) 373-0319, Lab Name: Pacific Reproductive Center, Accreditation: CAP/ASRM

San Antonio Fertility Center, 510 N. 13th Ave., Suite 201, Upland, CA 91786, Telephone: (909) 920-4858; Fax: (909) 985-7137, Lab Name: San Antonio Fertility Center, Accreditation: CAP/ASRM

Advanced Reproductive Medicine, University of Colorado Health Sciences Center, Anschutz Outpatient Pavilion, 1635 N. Ursula St., Aurora, CO 80010, Telephone: (720) 848-1690; Fax: (720) 848-1662, Lab Name: Advanced Reproductive Medicine Laboratory, Accreditation: CAP/ASRM, JCAHO

Colorado Springs Center for Reproductive Health, Eric H. Silverstein, M.D., Professional LLC dba Colorado Springs Center for Reproductive Health, 1625 Medical Center Point, Suite 290, Colorado Springs, CO 80907, Telephone: (719) 636-0080; Fax: (719) 636-3030, Lab Name: Colorado Springs Center for Reproductive Health, Accreditation: CAP/ASRM

Reproductive Medicine and Fertility Center of Southern Colorado, 3225 International Cir., Suite 100, Colorado Springs, CO 80910, Telephone: (719) 475-2229; Fax: (719) 475-2227, Lab Name: Reproductive Medicine and Fertility Center of Southern Colorado, LLC, Accreditation: CAP/ASRM

Colorado Reproductive Endocrinology, 4600 E. Hale Pkwy., Suite 350, Denver, CO 80220, Telephone: (303) 321-7115; Fax: (303) 321-9519, Lab Name: Colorado Reproductive Endocrinology, Accreditation: CAP/ASRM

Colorado Center for Reproductive Medicine, 799 E. Hampden Ave., Suite 300, Englewood, CO 80110, Telephone: (303) 788-8300; Fax: (303) 788-8310, Lab Name: Colorado Center for Reproductive Medicine, Accreditation: CAP/ASRM

Rocky Mountain Center for Reproductive Medicine, 1080 E. Elizabeth, Fort Collins, CO 80524, Telephone: (970) 493-6353; Fax: (970) 493-6366, Lab Name: Rocky Mountain Center for Reproductive Medicine IVF Lab, Accreditation: CAP/ASRM

Conceptions Reproductive Associates, 7720 S. Broadway, Suite 580, Littleton, CO 80122, Telephone: (303) 794-0045; Fax: (303) 794-2054, Lab Name: Conceptions Reproductive Associates, Accreditation: CAP/ASRM

The Center for Advanced Reproductive Services, at the University of Connecticut Health Center, Dowling South Bldg., 263 Farmington Ave., Suite A330, Farmington, CT 06030, Telephone: (860) 679-4580; Fax: (860) 679-1499, Lab Name: Lab at the Center for Advanced Reproductive Services, Accreditation: CAP/ASRM

New England Fertility Institute, 1275 Summer St., Suite 201, Stamford, CT 06905, Telephone: (203) 325-3200; Fax: (203) 323-3130, Lab Name: New England Fertility Institute IVF Laboratory, Accreditation: CAP/ASRM

Yale University School of Medicine, In Vitro Fertilization Program, Dept. of OB/GYN, 333 Cedar St., New Haven, CT 06520, Telephone: (203) 785-4708; Fax: (203) 785-3560, Lab Name: Yale University In Vitro Fertilization Laboratory, Accreditation: CAP/ASRM (Pending)

The Stamford Hospital, Shelburne & W. Broad Sts. , Stamford, CT 06904, Telephone: (203) 325-7559; Fax: (203) 325-7259, Lab Name: New England Fertility Institute IVF Laboratory, Accreditation: CAP/ASRM

DELAWARE

Delaware Institute for Reproductive Medicine, P.A., 4745 Ogletown-Stanton Rd., Suite III, Newark, DE 19713, Telephone: (302) 738-4600; Fax: (302) 738-3508, Lab Name: Delaware Institute for Reproductive Medicine, P.A., Accreditation: CAP/ASRM

Reproductive Associates of Delaware, Medical Arts Pavilion Two, 4735 Ogletown-Stanton Rd., Suite 3217, Newark, DE 19713, Telephone: (302) 623-4242; Fax: (302) 623-4241, Lab Name: Reproductive Associates of Delaware, Accreditation: None

DISTRICT OF COLUMBIA

§The A.R.T. Institute of Washington, Inc., Walter Reed Army Medical Center, Dept. of OB/GYN, 6900 Georgia Ave., N.W., Bldg. 2, Rm. 2J06, Washington, D.C. 20307, Telephone: (202) 782-6198; Fax: (202) 782-4833, Contact SART for current clinic information.

Columbia Fertility Associates, 2440 M St. N.W., Suite 401, Washington, D.C. 20037, Telephone: (202) 293-6567; Fax: (202) 778-6190, Lab Name: Columbia Hospital for Women ART Laboratory, Accreditation: JCAHO

The George Washington University Medical Faculty Associates, IVF Program, 2150 Pennsylvania Ave., N.W., Washington, D.C. 20037, Telephone: (202) 741-2520; Fax: (202) 741-2519, Lab Name: George Washington University Medical Faculty Associates, Accreditation: CAP/ASRM

James A. Simon, M.D., P.C., 1850 M St. N.W., Suite 450, Washington, D.C. 20036, Telephone: (202) 293-1000; Fax: (202) 463-6150, Lab Name: George Washington University Medical Faculty Associates, Accreditation: CAP/ASRM

FLORIDA

Boca Fertility, 875 Meadows Rd., Suite 334, Boca Raton, FL 33486, Telephone: (561) 368-5500; Fax: (561) 368-4793, Lab Name: Boca Fertility, Accreditation: CAP/ASRM

Palm Beach Fertility Center, 9970 Central Park Blvd., Suite 300, Boca Raton, FL

33428, Telephone: (561) 477-7728; Fax: (561) 477-7035, Lab Name: Palm Beach Fertility Center Lab, Accreditation: JCAHO

Advanced Reproductive Care Center, P.A., 10301 Hagen Ranch Rd., Boynton Beach, FL 33437, Telephone: (561) 736-6006; Fax: (561) 736-5788, Lab Name: Advanced Reproductive Care Center, Accreditation: JCAHO

Reproductive Health Associates, Catherine L. Cowart, M.D., 2695 Ulmerton Rd., Clearwater, FL 33762, Telephone: (727) 572-5300; Fax: (727) 572-5022, Lab Name: Edward Zbella, M.D., P.A., Accreditation: JCAHO

University Fertility Associates, 2454 McMullen Booth Rd., Suite 601, Clearwater, FL 33759, Telephone: (727) 796-7705; Fax: (727) 796-8764, Lab Name: Edward Zbella, M.D., P.A., Accreditation: JCAHO

F.I.R.S.T., Florida Institute for Reproductive Sciences and Technologies, 9900 Stirling Rd., Suite 300, Cooper City, FL 33024, Telephone: (954) 436-2700; Fax: (954) 436-6663, Lab Name: F.I.R.S.T., Accreditation: JCAHO

Southwest Florida Fertility Center, P.A., 13685 Doctor's Way, Suite 330, Fort Myers, FL 33912, Telephone: (239) 561-3430; Fax: (239) 561-6980, Lab Name: Southwest Florida Fertility Center, P.A., Accreditation: None

Specialists in Reproductive Medicine & Surgery, P.A., 12611 World Plaza Ln., Bldg. 53, Fort Myers, FL 33907, Telephone: (239) 275-8118; Fax: (239) 275-5914, Lab Name: Specialists in Reproductive Medicine & Surgery, P.A., Accreditation: CAP/ASRM

University of Florida/Park Avenue Women's Center, University of Florida Women's Health at Magnolia Parke, 3951 N.W. 48th Terrace 101, Gainesville, FL 32606, Telephone: (352) 265-6200; Fax: (352) 265-9103, Lab Name: In Vitro Fertilization and Andrology Laboratory, Accreditation: JCAHO

Fertility Institute of Northwest Florida, 1110 Gulf Breeze Pkwy., Suite 202, Gulf Breeze, FL 32561, Telephone: (850) 934-3900; Fax: (850) 932-3753, Lab Name: Fertility Institute of Northwest Florida, Accreditation: CAP/ASRM

Assisted Fertility Program of North Florida, 3627 University Blvd. South, Suite 450, Jacksonville, FL 32216, Telephone: (904) 398-1407; Fax: (904) 399-3436, Lab Name: Memorial Reference Lab, Accreditation: CAP/ASRM

Florida Institute for Reproductive Medicine, 836 Prudential Dr., Suite 902, Jacksonville, FL 32207, Telephone: (904) 399-5620; Fax: (904) 399-5645, Lab Name: Florida Institute for Reproductive Medicine, Accreditation: CAP/ASRM

North Florida Center for Reproductive Medicine, 3627 University Blvd. South, Suite 200, Jacksonville, FL 32216, Telephone: (904) 396-3806; Fax: (904) 396-4546, Lab

Name: Memorial's Assisted Reproductive Technology Lab, Accreditation: CAP/ASRM

IVF Florida, Memorial Advanced Fertility Treatment Center, 2825 N. State Rd. 7, Suite 302, Margate, FL 33063, Telephone: (954) 247-6200; Fax: (954) 247-6262, Lab Name: IVF Florida, Accreditation: CAP/ASRM, Lab Name: Memorial Advanced Fertility Treatment Center, Accreditation: CAP/ASRM

Fertility and Reproductive Medicine Center for Women, 95 Bulldog Blvd., Suite 204, Melbourne, FL 32901, Telephone: (321) 724-4410; Fax: (321) 956-9957, Lab Name: Fertility & Reproductive Medicine Center for Women, Accreditation: None

Fertility & IVF Center of Miami, Inc., 8950 N. Kendall Dr., Suite 103, Miami, FL 33176, Telephone: (305) 596-4013; Fax: (305) 596-4557, Lab Name: Fertility & IVF Center of Miami, Inc., Accreditation: CAP/ASRM

Palmetto Fertility Center of South Florida, 7100 W. 20th Ave., Suite 205, Miami, FL 33016, Telephone: (305) 558-0808; Fax: (305) 558-0806, Lab Name: Palmetto Fertility Center of South Florida, Accreditation: CAP/ASRM

South Florida Institute for Reproductive Medicine, 7300 S.W. 62nd Pl., 4th Floor, Miami, FL 33143, Telephone: (305) 662-7901; Fax: (305) 662-7910, Lab Name: South Florida Institute for Reproductive Medicine, Accreditation: CAP/ASRM

Center for Infertility & Reproductive Medicine, P.A., 3435 Pinehurst Ave., Orlando, FL 32804, Telephone: (407) 740-0909; Fax: (407) 740-7262, Lab Name: Center for Infertility & Reproductive Medicine, P.A., Accreditation: CAP/ASRM

Reproductive Health Institute, 22 Underwood St., Orlando, FL 32806, Telephone: (407) 649-6995; Fax: (407) 841-3367, Lab Name: Reproductive Health Institute, Accreditation: JCAHO

Reproductive Medicine and Fertility Center, 615 E. Princeton St., Suite 225, Orlando, FL 32803, Telephone: (407) 896-7575; Fax: (407) 894-2692, Lab Name: Reproductive Medicine and Fertility Center, Accreditation: CAP/ASRM

Frank C. Riggall, M.D., P.A., 2501 N. Orange Ave., Suite 209S, Orlando, FL 32804, Telephone: (407) 898-0254; Fax: (407) 898-6224, Lab Name: The Center for Infertility & Reproductive Medicine, Accreditation: CAP/ASRM, Lab Name: Reproductive Health Institute, Accreditation: JCAHO

§University of Florida–Pensacola, 5147 N. Ninth Ave., Suite 315, Pensacola, FL 32504, Telephone: (850) 857-3733; Fax: (850) 857-0670, Contact SART for current clinic information.

Center for Advanced Reproductive Endocrinology, P.A., 6738 W. Sunrise Blvd.,

Suite 106, Plantation, FL 33313, Telephone: (954) 584-2273; Fax: (954) 587-9630, Lab Name: Laboratory for Implantation Fertilization & Embryology, Accreditation: CAP/ASRM

Fertility Center of Sarasota, Julio E. Pabon, M.D., P.A., 5664 Bee Ridge Rd., Suite 202, Sarasota, FL 34233, Telephone: (941) 342-1568; Fax: (941) 342-8296, Lab Name: Fertility Center of Sarasota, Accreditation: JCAHO

Advanced Reproductive Technologies Program, at University Community Hospital, Drs. Verkauf, Bernhisel, Tarantino, Goodman & Yeko, 3450 E. Fletcher Ave., Suite 280, Tampa, FL 33613, Telephone: (813) 615-7956; Fax: (813) 615-7913, Lab Name: Advanced Reproductive Technologies Program Laboratory, Accreditation: CAP/ASRM

Reproductive Medicine & Genetics, 5500 Village Blvd., Suite 103, West Palm Beach, FL 33407, Telephone: (561) 697-4200; Fax: (561) 686-8525, Lab Name: Reproductive Medicine & Genetics, Accreditation: None

Women's Healthcare Specialists, IVF Miami, 17160 Arvida Pkwy., Suite 2, Weston, FL 33326, Telephone: (954) 349-1460; Fax: (954) 349-6646, Lab Name: Fertility and IVF Center of Miami, Accreditation: CAP/ASRM, Lab Name: Palmetto Fertility Center of South Florida, Inc., Accreditation: CAP/ASRM

GEORGIA

Emory Center for Reproductive Medicine and Fertility, 20 Linden Ave., N.E., Suite 4701, Atlanta, GA 30308, Telephone: (404) 686-8095; Fax: (404) 686-4297, Lab Name: Emory Center for Reproductive Medicine and Fertility, Accreditation: JCAHO

Georgia Reproductive Specialists, 5445 Meridian Mark Rd., Suite 270, Atlanta, GA 30342, Telephone: (404) 843-2229; Fax: (404) 843-0812, Lab Name: Georgia Reproductive Specialists, Accreditation: JCAHO

Reproductive Biology Associates, 1150 Lake Hearn Dr., Suite 400, Atlanta, GA 30342, Telephone: (404) 843-3064; Fax: (404) 256-1528, Lab Name: Reproductive Biology Associates, Accreditation: CAP/ASRM

Augusta Area Reproductive Associates, 812 Chafee Ave., Augusta, GA 30904, Telephone: (706) 724-0228; Fax: (706) 722-2387, Lab Name: Reproductive Laboratories of Augusta, Accreditation: CAP/ASRM

Central Georgia Fertility Institute, 4075 Elnora Dr., Macon, GA 31210, Telephone: (478) 757-7888; Fax: (478) 757-7887, Lab Name: Georgia Reproductive Specialists, Accreditation: JCAHO

Atlanta Center for Reproductive Medicine, 100 Stone Forest Dr., Suite 300, Woodstock, GA 30189, Telephone: (770) 928-2276; Fax: (770) 592-2092, Lab Name: Atlanta Center for Reproductive Medicine, Accreditation: JCAHO

HAWAII

Pacific In Vitro Fertilization Institute, 1319 Punahou St., Suite 980, Honolulu, HI 96826, Telephone: (808) 946-2226; Fax: (808) 943-1563, Lab Name: Pacific In Vitro Fertilization Laboratory, Accreditation: CAP/ASRM

Tripler Army Medical Center IVF Institute, Dept. of OB/GYN, 1 Jarrett White Rd., Tripler AMC, HI 96859, Telephone: (808) 433-6845; Fax: (808) 433-1552, Lab Name: Pacific In Vitro Fertilization Laboratory, Accreditation: CAP/ASRM

IDAHO

Fertility Associates of Idaho, 100 W. State St., Boise, ID 83702, Telephone: (208) 368-0223; Fax: (208) 345-1408, Lab Name: Fertility Associates of Idaho, Accreditation: CAP/ASRM

ILLINOIS

Rush–Copley Center for Reproductive Health, 2020 Ogden Ave., Suite 250, Aurora, IL 60504, Telephone: (630) 978-6254; Fax: (630) 499-2487, Lab Name: Rush–Copley IVF Lab, Accreditation: JCAHO

Life–Women's Health Center, 6425 W. Cermak Rd., Suite 202, Berwyn, IL 60402, Telephone: (708) 484-0500; Fax: (708) 484-4259, Lab Name: Advanced Reproductive Health Center, Accreditation: JCAHO (Pending)

IVF Lincoln Park, 2825 N. Halsted St., Chicago, IL 60657, Telephone: (773) 868-0800; Fax: (773) 868-1500, Lab Name: Reproductive Genetics, Accreditation: CAP/ASRM

Northwestern University, 675 N. St. Clair, Suite 14-200, Chicago, IL 60611, Telephone: (312) 695-7269; Fax: (312) 695-4924, Lab Name: Northwestern University, Accreditation: CAP/ASRM

Rush Center for Advanced Reproductive Care, 1653 W. Congress Pkwy., 720 Pavilion, Chicago, IL 60612, Telephone: (312) 997-2229; Fax: (312) 997-2354, Lab Name: Rush Center for Advanced Reproductive Medicine, Accreditation: JCAHO

§University of Chicago Hospitals, Dept. of OB/GYN, 5841 S. Maryland, Suite R308, Chicago, IL 60637, Telephone: (773) 702-6642; Fax: (773) 702-5848, Contact SART for current clinic information.

University of Illinois at Chicago IVF Program, Dept. of OB/GYN, 820 S. Wood St. (M/C 808), Chicago, IL 60612, Telephone: (312) 996-9820; Fax: (312) 355-3161, Lab

Name: University of Illinois at Chicago, IVF Laboratory, Accreditation: CAP/ASRM

WaterTower Women's Center, L.L.C., 845 N. Michigan Ave., Suite 935E, Chicago, IL 60611, Telephone: (312) 642-6777; Fax: (312) 642-8383, Lab Name: WaterTower Women's Center, Accreditation: None

Midwest Fertility Center, 4333 Main St., Downers Grove, IL 60515, Telephone: (630) 810-0212; Fax: (630) 810-1027, Lab Name: Midwest Fertility Center, Accreditation: CAP/ASRM

The Hoxsey-Rinehart Center for Reproductive Medicine, 2500 Ridge Ave., Suite 200, Evanston, IL 60201, Telephone: (847) 869-7777; Fax: (847) 869-7782, Lab Name: The Hoxsey-Rinehart Center for Reproductive Medicine, Accreditation: CAP/ASRM (Pending), Lab Name: The Oak Brook Fertility Center, Accreditation: None

Advanced Fertility Center of Chicago, 30 Tower Ct., Suite F, Gurnee, IL 60031, Telephone: (847) 662-1818; Fax: (847) 662-3001, Lab Name: Advanced Fertility Center of Chicago, Accreditation: CAP/ASRM

Highland Park IVF Center, 750 Homewood Ave., Suite B400, Highland Park, IL 60035, Telephone: (847) 266-3535; Fax: (847) 266-8838, Lab Name: Highland Park IVF Laboratory, Accreditation: JCAHO (Pending)

Hinsdale Center for Reproduction, 121 N. Elm St., Hinsdale, IL 60521, Telephone: (630) 856-3535; Fax: (630) 856-3545, Lab Name: Hinsdale Center for Reproduction, Accreditation: CAP/ASRM

Center for Human Reproduction–Illinois, American Infertility Group, Center for Human Reproduction, 1585 N. Barrington Rd., Suite 406, Hoffman Estates, IL 60194, Telephone: (847) 884-8884; Fax: (847) 884-8093, Lab Name: American Infertility Group Center for Human Reproduction, Accreditation: CAP/ASRM

Reproductive Health Specialists, Ltd., 310 N. Hammes Ave., Suite 101, Joliet, IL 60435, Telephone: (815) 730-1100; Fax: (815) 730-1066, Lab Name: RHS IVF/Andrology Laboratory, Accreditation: CAP/ASRM

IVFI, 636 Raymond Dr., Suite 303, Naperville, IL 60563, Telephone: (630) 357-6540; Fax: (630) 357-6435, Lab Name: Reproductive Genetics Institute, Accreditation: CAP/ASRM

Reena Jabamoni, M.D., S.C., 120 Oak Brook Center, Suite 308, Oak Brook, IL 60523, Telephone: (630) 574-3633; Fax: (630) 574-3660, Lab Name: Reena Jabamoni, M.D., Laboratory, Accreditation: CAP/ASRM

Oak Brook Fertility Center, 2425 W. 22nd St., Suite 102, Oak Brook, IL 60523, Telephone: (630) 954-0054; Fax: (630) 954-0064, Lab Name: Chicago Fertility Laboratories, Accreditation: JCAHO

Lutheran General Hospital IVF Program, 1775 Dempster St., One South, Park Ridge, IL 60068, Telephone: (847) 998-8200; Fax: (847) 998-0419, Lab Name: Lutheran General Hospital IVF Laboratory, Accreditation: CAP/ASRM

Advanced Reproductive Center, Ltd., 435 N. Mulford Rd., Suite 9, Rockford, IL 61107, Telephone: (815) 229-1700; Fax: (815) 229-1831, Lab Name: Advanced Reproductive Center, Ltd., Accreditation: CAP/ASRM

Reproductive Health and Fertility Center, 973 Featherstone Rd., Suite 100, Rockford, IL 61107, Telephone: (815) 986-3737; Fax: (815) 986-3734, Lab Name: Reproductive Health and Fertility Center Laboratory, Accreditation: CAP/ASRM

Reproductive Endocrinology Associates, S.C., 340 W. Miller St., Springfield, IL 62702, Telephone: (217) 523-4700; Fax: (217) 523-9025, Lab Name: Reproductive Endocrinology Associates, S.C., Accreditation: CAP/ASRM

Seth Levrant, M.D., P.C., Partners in Reproductive Health, 16345 S. Harlem Ave., Suite 1W, Tinley Park, IL 60477, Telephone: (708) 524-0730; Fax: (708) 848-7645, Lab Name: Chicago Fertility Laboratory, Accreditation: CAP/ASRM

INDIANA

Associated Fertility & Gynecology, 7910 W. Jefferson Blvd., Suite 301, Fort Wayne, IN 46804, Telephone: (260) 432-6250; Fax: (260) 436-7220, Lab Name: Associated Fertility & Gynecology Laboratory, Accreditation: CAP/ASRM

Advanced Fertility Group, Methodist Medical Plaza Carmel, 201 Pennsylvania Pkwy., Suite 205, Indianapolis, IN 46280, Telephone: (317) 817-1300; Fax: (317) 817-1306, Lab Name: Reproductive Biology Laboratory, Accreditation: JCAHO

Family Beginnings, P.C., 8051 S. Emerson Ave., Suite 460, Indianapolis, IN 46237, Telephone: (317) 865-0411; Fax: (317) 859-3815, Lab Name: Assisted Fertility Services, Accreditation: JCAHO

Indiana University Hospital, Dept. of OB/GYN, 550 N. University Blvd., Rm. 2440, Indianapolis, IN 46202, Telephone: (317) 274-4875; Fax: (317) 278-3787, Lab Name: Reproductive Biology Laboratory, Accreditation: JCAHO

Midwest Reproductive Medicine, 8081 Township Line Rd., Indianapolis, IN 46260, Telephone: (800) 333-1415; Fax: (317) 872-5063, Lab Name: Midwest Reproductive Medicine ART Lab, Accreditation: JCAHO

Reproductive Surgery & Medicine, P.C., Women's Specialty Health Centers, P.C., 8040 Clearvista Pkwy., Suite 280, Indianapolis, IN 46256, Telephone: (317) 621-2255;

Fax: (317) 621-2265, Lab Name: Assisted Fertility Services–Community Hospitals, Accreditation: JCAHO

Reproductive Endocrinology Associates, 2020 W. 86th St., Suite 310, Indianapolis, IN 46260, Telephone: (317) 872-1515; Fax: (317) 879-2784, Lab Name: Assisted Fertility Services, Accreditation: JCAHO

Reproductive Care of Indiana, 1650 W. Oak St., Suite 206, Zionsville, IN 46077, Telephone: (317) 873-8870; Fax: (317) 873-8875, Lab Name: Reproductive Biology Laboratory, Accreditation: JCAHO

IOWA

McFarland Clinic, P.C., Assisted Reproduction, 1215 Duff Ave., Ames, IA 50010, Telephone: (515) 239-4414; Fax: (515) 239-4786, Lab Name: Assisted Reproduction Laboratory, Accreditation: CAP/ASRM

University of Iowa Hospitals and Clinics, Center for Advanced Reproductive Care, Obstetrics and Gynecology, 200 Hawkins Dr., Iowa City, IA 52242, Telephone: (319) 356-8483; Fax: (319) 353-6659, Lab Name: In Vitro Fertilization & Reproductive Testing Lab, Accreditation: CAP/ASRM

Mid-Iowa Fertility, P.C., 3408 Woodland Ave., Suite 302, West Des Moines, IA 50266, Telephone: (515) 222-3060; Fax: (515) 222-9563, Lab Name: Mid-Iowa Fertility, P.C., Accreditation: CAP/ASRM

KANSAS

University of Kansas Medical Center, Women's Reproductive Center, Bell Bldg., 3901 Rainbow Blvd., 5th Floor, Kansas City, KS 66160, Telephone: (913) 588-6272; Fax: (913) 588-3242, Lab Name: University of Kansas Medical Center, Accreditation: CAP/ASRM

Drs. Marshall & Henning, P.A., IVF Reproductive Services, 1133 College Ave., Bldg. E, Suite 210, Manhattan, KS 66502, Telephone: (785) 537-1414; Fax: (785) 537-0623, Lab Name: IVF Reproductive Services, Accreditation: CAP/ASRM

Reproductive Resource Center of Greater Kansas City, 12200 W. 106th St., Suite 120, Overland Park, KS 66215, Telephone: (913) 894-2323; Fax: (913) 894-0841, Lab Name: IVF Lab of Reproductive Resource Center, Accreditation: CAP/ASRM

Reproductive Medicine & Infertility, Shawnee Mission Medical Center, 8800 W. 75th St., Suite 101, Shawnee Mission, KS 66204, Telephone: (913) 432-7161; Fax: (913) 432-6158, Lab Name: Shawnee Mission Medical Center, Accreditation: CAP/ASRM

The Center for Reproductive Medicine, 9220 E. 29th St. North, Suite 102, Wichita,

KS 67226, Telephone: (316) 687-2112; Fax: (316) 687-1260, Lab Name: The Center for Reproductive Medicine ART Lab, Accreditation: CAP/ASRM

KENTUCKY

Fertility and Endocrine Associates, 1780 Nicholasville Rd., Suite 402, Lexington, KY 40503, Telephone: (859) 278-9151; Fax: (859) 278-8946, Lab Name: Central Baptist Hospital, Accreditation: CAP/ASRM, JCAHO

Kentucky Fertility and Gynecology, 141 N. Eagle Creek Dr., Suite 203, Lexington, KY 40509, Telephone: (859) 263-9600; Fax: (859) 264-9977, Lab Name: Central Baptist Hospital Andrology Lab, Accreditation: CAP/ASRM, JCAHO

Kentucky Women's Specialists, Reproductive Endocrinology and Infertility, 1780 Nicholasville Rd., Suite 201, Lexington, KY 40503, Telephone: (859) 260-1515; Fax: (859) 260-1425, Lab Name: Central Baptist Hospital, Accreditation: CAP/ASRM, JCAHO

University OB/GYN Associates Fertility Center, 315 E. Broadway, Louisville, KY 40202, Telephone: (502) 629-8154; Fax: (502) 629-3713, Lab Name: Fertility Center Embryology Laboratory, Accreditation: JCAHO

LOUISIANA

Fertility and Laser Center, 8585 Picardy Ave., Baton Rouge, LA 70809, Telephone: (225) 763-4800; Fax: (225) 763-4883, Lab Name: Reproductive Resources, Accreditation: CAP/ASRM, NYSTB

Woman's Center for Fertility and Advanced Reproductive Medicine, 9000 Airline Hwy., Suite 670, Baton Rouge, LA 70815, Telephone: (225) 926-6886; Fax: (225) 922-3730, Lab Name: Reproductive Endocrine Laboratory, Accreditation: CAP/ASRM, JCAHO

Fertility Clinic, Tulane University Hospital and Clinic, 1415 Tulane Ave., Suite HC-15, New Orleans, LA 70112, Telephone: (504) 588-2341; Fax: (504) 584-1680, Lab Name: Fertility Institute of New Orleans, Accreditation: CAP/ASRM

Fertility Institute of New Orleans, 6020 Bullard Ave., New Orleans, LA 70128, Telephone: (504) 246-8971; Fax: (504) 246-9778, Lab Name: Fertility Institute of New Orleans, Accreditation: CAP/ASRM

Ochsner Foundation Clinic, 1514 Jefferson Hwy., New Orleans, LA 70122, Telephone: (504) 842-6468; Fax: (504) 842-4156, Lab Name: Reproductive Resources, Accreditation: CAP/ASRM, NYSTB

Center for Fertility and Reproductive Health, 2401 Greenwood Rd., Shreveport,

LA 71103, Telephone: (318) 212-8270; Fax: (318) 212-8230, Lab Name: Center for Fertility and Reproductive Health, Accreditation: CAP/ASRM

MARYLAND

Greater Baltimore Medical Center, Fertility Center, Physicians Pavilion West, 6569 N. Charles St., Suite 406, Baltimore, MD 21204, Telephone: (443) 849-2484; Fax: (443) 849-3067, Lab Name: GBMC Fertility Center ART Laboratory, Accreditation: CAP/ASRM

Helix Center for ART, The Center for ART at Union Memorial Hospital, Union Memorial Hospital—OB/GYN, 201 E. University Pkwy., Baltimore, MD 21218, Telephone: (410) 554-2308; Fax: (410) 554-2900, Lab Name: The Center for ART at Union Memorial Hospital, Accreditation: CAP/ASRM

University of Maryland Medical School, Center for Advanced Reproductive Technology, 405 W. Redwood St., 3rd Floor, Baltimore, MD 21201, Telephone: (410) 328-2304; Fax: (410) 328-8389, Lab Name: University of Maryland Medical School, Accreditation: CAP/ASRM

MidAtlantic Fertility Centers, 10215 Fernwood Rd., Suite 301A, Bethesda, MD 20817, Telephone: (301) 897-8850; Fax: (301) 530-8105, Lab Name: MidAtlantic Fertility Centers, Accreditation: CAP/ASRM

Johns Hopkins Fertility Center, 10753 Falls Rd., Suite 335, Lutherville, MD 21093, Telephone: (410) 847-3650; Fax: (410) 583-2792, Lab Name: Johns Hopkins A.R.T. Laboratories, Accreditation: JCAHO

Center for Reproductive Medicine, 9711 Medical Center Dr., Suite 214, Rockville, MD 20850, Telephone: (301) 424-1904; Fax: (301) 424-1902, Lab Name: George Washington University Medical Faculty Associates, Accreditation: CAP/ASRM

Shady Grove Fertility Reproductive Science Center, 15001 Shady Grove Rd., Suite 400, Rockville, MD 20850, Telephone: (301) 340-1188; Fax: (301) 340-1612, Lab Name: Shady Grove Fertility Reproductive Science Center, Accreditation: JCAHO

Fertility Center of Maryland, 110 West Rd., Suite 102, Towson, MD 21204, Telephone: (410) 296-6400; Fax: (410) 296-6405, Lab Name: Fertility Center of Maryland, Accreditation: JCAHO

MASSACHUSETTS

Brigham and Women's Hospital Center for Assisted Reproduction, Brigham and Women's Hospital, 75 Francis St., ASB1-3, Boston, MA 02115, Telephone: (617) 732-4239; Fax: (617) 975-0825, Lab Name: Brigham and Women's Hospital Center for Assisted Reproduction Embryology Lab, Accreditation: CAP/ASRM, JCAHO

Massachusetts General Hospital Vincent IVF Unit, 55 Fruit St., VBK225, Boston, MA 02114, Telephone: (617) 724-3513; Fax: (617) 724-8882, Lab Name: Massachusetts General Hospital, Vincent IVF Lab, Accreditation: CAP/ASRM, JCAHO

New England Fertility and Endocrinology Associates, 500 Brookline Ave., Suite A, Boston, MA 02215, Telephone: (617) 277-1778; Fax: (617) 734-9951, Lab Name: New England Fertility and Endocrinology Associates, Accreditation: CAP/ASRM

Fertility Center of New England, Inc., New England Clinic of Reproductive Medicine, 20 Pond Meadow Dr., Suite 101, Reading, MA 01867, Telephone: (781) 942-7000; Fax: (781) 942-7200, Lab Name: New England Clinic of Reproductive Medicine, Inc., Accreditation: CAP/ASRM

Baystate IVF, Baystate Medical Center, Div. of Reproductive Endocrinology, 759 Chestnut St., Springfield, MA 01199, Telephone: (413) 794-1950; Fax: (413) 794-1857, Lab Name: Reproductive Biology Laboratory, Accreditation: CAP/ASRM

Boston IVF, 40 Second Ave., Suite 300, Waltham, MA 02451, Telephone: (781) 434-6400; Fax: (781) 890-5016, Lab Name: Boston Fertility Laboratories, Accreditation: CAP/ASRM

Reproductive Science Center of Boston, Sterling Medical Center, 9 Hope Ave., Waltham, MA 02454, Telephone: (781) 647-6263; Fax: (781) 647-6323, Lab Name: Reproductive Science Center, Accreditation: CAP/ASRM,

MICHIGAN

University of Michigan, Women's Hospital, Box 0276, 1500 E. Medical Center Dr., L-4100, Ann Arbor, MI 48109, Telephone: (734) 936-7401; Fax: (734) 647-9727, Lab Name: University of Michigan ART Laboratory, Accreditation: CAP/ASRM

Center for Reproductive Medicine and Surgery, P.C., 300 Park St., Suite 460, Birmingham, MI 48009, Telephone: (248) 593-6990; Fax: (248) 593-5925, Lab Name: Oakwood Hospital IVF Center, Accreditation: JCAHO

Center for Reproductive Medicine, Oakwood Hospital and Medical Center, 18181 Oakwood Blvd., Suite 109, Dearborn, MI 48124, Telephone: (313) 593-5880; Fax: (313) 593-8837, Lab Name: Center for Reproductive Medicine, Accreditation: JCAHO

Grand Rapids Fertility & IVF, P.C., 1900 Wealthy St., Suite 315, Grand Rapids, MI 49506, Telephone: (616) 774-2030; Fax: (616) 774-2053, Lab Name: Grand Rapids Fertility & IVF, P.C., Accreditation: CAP/ASRM

Michigan Reproductive & IVF Center, P.C., 630 Kenmoore Ave., S.E., Grand Rapids, MI 49546, Telephone: (616) 988-2229; Fax: (616) 988-2009, Lab Name: Michigan Reproductive & IVF Center, Accreditation: CAP/ASRM

Infertility and Gynecology Center of Lansing, P.C., 1200 E. Michigan Ave., Suite 305, Lansing, MI 48912, Telephone: (517) 484-4900; Fax: (517) 484-4508, Lab Name: Sparrow Fertility Services, Accreditation: CAP/ASRM

Michigan State University, Center for Assisted Reproductive Technology, 1200 E. Michigan Ave., Suite 700, Lansing, MI 48912, Telephone: (517) 364-5888; Fax: (517) 364-5889, Lab Name: Sparrow Fertility Services, Accreditation: CAP/ASRM

The Center for Reproductive Medicine, Hurley Medical Center, IVF Michigan, 3950 S. Rochester Rd., Suite 2300, Rochester Hills, MI 48307, Telephone: (810) 257-9714; Fax: (810) 762-7040, Lab Name: IVF Michigan Laboratories, Accreditation: CAP/ASRM

IVF Michigan, 3950 S. Rochester Rd., Suite 2300, Rochester Hills, MI 48307, Telephone: (248) 844-8840; Fax: (248) 844-8850, Lab Name: IVF Michigan Laboratories, Accreditation: CAP/ASRM

William Beaumont Fertility Center, 3535 W. Thirteen Mile Rd., Suite 344, Royal Oak, MI 48073, Telephone: (248) 551-0515; Fax: (248) 551-3616, Lab Name: William Beaumont Fertility Center IVF Laboratory, Accreditation: CAP/ASRM

University Women's Care/Wayne State University ART Program, 26400 W. Twelve Mile Rd., Suite 140, Southfield, MI 48034, Telephone: (248) 352-8200; Fax: (248) 356-8255, Lab Name: Hutzel Hospital/Wayne State University IVF Laboratory, Accreditation: CAP/ASRM, JCAHO

Henry Ford Reproductive Medicine, Div. of Reproductive Medicine, 1500 W. Big Beaver Rd., Suite 105, Troy, MI 48084, Telephone: (248) 637-4050; Fax: (248) 637-4025, Lab Name: Henry Ford Reproductive Medicine, Accreditation: CAP/ASRM

MINNESOTA

Center for Reproductive Medicine, 2800 Chicago Ave. South, 3rd Floor, Minneapolis, MN 55407, Telephone: (612) 863-5390; Fax: (612) 863-2697, Lab Name: Allina Andrology Lab, Accreditation: CAP/ASRM, JCAHO

The Midwest Center for Reproductive Health, P.A., Oakdale Medical Bldg., 3366 Oakdale Ave. North, Suite 550, Minneapolis, MN 55422, Telephone: (763) 520-2600; Fax: (763) 520-2606, Lab Name: The Midwest Center for Reproductive Health, P.A., Accreditation: CAP/ASRM

Reproductive Medicine Center, 606 24th Ave. South, Suite 500, Minneapolis, MN 55454, Telephone: (612) 627-4564; Fax: (612) 627-4888, Lab Name: Reproductive Medicine Center, Accreditation: CAP/ASRM

Mayo Clinic Assisted Reproductive Technologies, 200 First St. S.W., Charlton 3A,

Rochester, MN 55905, Telephone: (507) 284-4520; Fax: (507) 284-1774, Lab Name: Mayo Clinic Assisted Reproductive Technologies Laboratory, Accreditation: CAP/ASRM

Reproductive Medicine & Infertility Associates, Woodbury Medical Arts Bldg., 2101 Woodwinds Dr., Suite 100, Woodbury, MN 55125, Telephone: (651) 222-6050; Fax: (651) 222-5975, Lab Name: Reproductive Biology Laboratory, Accreditation: CAP/ASRM

MISSISSIPPI

Mississippi Fertility Institute at Women's Specialty Center, Women's Specialty Center, 501 Marshall St., Suite 600, Jackson, MS 39202, Telephone: (601) 948-6540; Fax: (601) 948-6544, Lab Name: Mississippi Fertility Institute, Accreditation: JCAHO

University of Mississippi Medical Center, IVF Program, Dept. of OB/GYN, 2500 N. State St., Jackson, MS 39216, Telephone: (601) 984-5330; Fax: (601) 984-5965, Lab Name: In Vitro Fertilization Laboratory, Accreditation: CAP/ASRM

MISSOURI

Advanced Reproductive Specialists, St. Luke's Hospital, 226 S. Woods Mill Rd., Suite 64 West, Chesterfield, MO 63017, Telephone: (314) 205-6730; Fax: (314) 205-6800, Lab Name: Advanced Reproductive Specialists, Accreditation: CAP/ASRM

Infertility Institute, 226 S. Woods Mill Rd., Suite 39 West, Chesterfield, MO 63017, Telephone: (314) 205-8809; Fax: (314) 205-8776, Lab Name: Infertility Institute, Accreditation: CAP/ASRM

Mid-Missouri Center for Reproductive Health, Boone Hospital Center, 1502 E. Broadway, Suite 106, Columbia, MO 65201, Telephone: (573) 443-4511; Fax: (573) 443-7860, Lab Name: Mid-Missouri Center for Reproductive Health, Accreditation: CAP/ASRM

§University of Missouri Hospital and Clinics, IVF Embryology Laboratory, Dept. of OB/GYN, One Hospital Dr., N624 HSC, Columbia, MO 65212, Telephone: (573) 882-7937; Fax: (573) 882-9010, Contact SART for current clinic information.

Midwest Women's Healthcare, 6400 Prospect Ave., Suite 598, Kansas City, MO 64132, Telephone: (816) 444-6888; Fax: (816) 444-8430, Lab Name: Research Medical Center ART Laboratory, Accreditation: CAP/ASRM (Pending)

§The Infertility and Reproductive Medicine Center at Washington University School of Medicine , and Barnes-Jewish Hospital, 4444 Forest Park Ave., Suite

3100, St. Louis, MO 63108, Telephone: (314) 286-2400; Fax: (314) 286-2455, Contact SART for current clinic information.

Infertility & IVF Center, 3009 N. Ballas Rd., Suite 359C, St. Louis, MO 63131, Telephone: (636) 225-5483; Fax: (314) 872-9040, Lab Name: Infertility & IVF Center, Accreditation: CAP/ASRM

Infertility Center of St. Louis, 224 S. Woods Mill Rd., Suite 730, St. Louis, MO 63017, Telephone: (314) 576-1400; Fax: (314) 576-1442, Lab Name: Assisted Reproductive Technology Laboratory, Accreditation: CAP/ASRM

NEBRASKA

Heartland Center for Reproductive Medicine, P.C., 7308 S. 142nd St., Omaha, NE 68138, Telephone: (402) 717-4200; Fax: (402) 717-4230, Lab Name: Center for Reproductive Medicine Labs, Accreditation: CAP/ASRM

Nebraska Methodist Hospital REI, 8111 Dodge St., Suite 237, Omaha, NE 68114, Telephone: (402) 354-5210; Fax: (402) 354-5221, Lab Name: Andrology and Embryology Laboratories, Accreditation: CAP/ASRM, JCAHO

NEVADA

Fertility Center of Las Vegas, 8851 W. Sahara, Suite 100, Las Vegas, NV 89117, Telephone: (702) 254-1777; Fax: (702) 254-1213, Lab Name: Fertility Center of Las Vegas, Accreditation: CAP/ASRM

The Nevada Center for Reproductive Medicine, 6630 S. McCarran Blvd., Suite 9, Reno, NV 89509, Telephone: (775) 828-1200; Fax: (775) 828-1785, Lab Name: The Nevada Center for Reproductive Medicine, Accreditation: JCAHO

NEW HAMPSHIRE

Dartmouth–Hitchcock Medical Center, One Medical Center Dr., Lebanon, NH 03756, Telephone: (603) 650-8162; Fax: (603) 650-0842, Lab Name: Reproductive Sciences Laboratory, Accreditation: CAP/ASRM

NEW JERSEY

The Center for Reproductive Endocrinology, One Robertson Dr., Bedminster, NJ 07921, Telephone: (908) 781-0666; Fax: (908) 781-6377, Lab Name: The Center for Reproductive Endocrinology, Accreditation: CAP/ASRM (Pending)

Shore IVF and Reproductive Medicine, 1608 Route 88 West, Suite 117, Brick, NJ 08724, Telephone: (732) 840-1447; Fax: (732) 458-8180, Lab Name: Shore Area IVF Laboratory, Accreditation: JCAHO

Reproductive Gynecologists, P.C., Kennedy Health System, 2201 Chapel Ave. West, Suite 206, Cherry Hill, NJ 08002, Telephone: (856) 662-6662; Fax: (856) 661-0661, Lab Name: South Jersey Fertility Center, P.A., Accreditation: JCAHO

IVF of North Jersey, P.A., 1035 Route 46 East, Clifton, NJ 07013, Telephone: (973) 470-0303; Fax: (973) 916-0488, Lab Name: IVF of North Jersey, Accreditation: CAP/ASRM

Center for Advanced Reproductive Medicine and Fertility, Durham Center, One Ethel Rd., Suite 107B, Edison, NJ 08817, Telephone: (732) 339-9300; Fax: (732) 339-9400, Lab Name: CARMF ART Laboratory, Accreditation: JCAHO

Women's Fertility Center, 106 Grand Ave., Englewood, NJ 07631, Telephone: (201) 569-6979; Fax: (201) 569-0269, Lab Name: Westwood Embryology and Andrology, Accreditation: CAP/ASRM, JCAHO

North Hudson I.V.F., Center for Fertility and Gynecology, 385 Sylvan Ave., Englewood Cliffs, NJ 07632, Telephone: (201) 871-1999; Fax: (201) 871-1031, Lab Name: North Hudson I.V.F., Accreditation: CAP/ASRM

Delaware Valley OB/GYN and Infertility Group, 3131 Princeton Pike, Bldg. 3, Lawrenceville, NJ 08648, Telephone: (609) 896-0777; Fax: (609) 896-3266, Lab Name: Diamond Institute for Infertility, Accreditation: CAP/ASRM

Princeton Center for Infertility & Reproductive Medicine, 3131 Princeton Pike, Bldg. 4, Suite 204, Lawrenceville, NJ 08648, Telephone: (609) 895-1114; Fax: (609) 895-1196, Lab Name: Cooper Center for IVF, P.C., Accreditation: CAP/ASRM

East Coast Infertility and IVF, P.C., 200 White Rd., Suite 214, Little Silver, NJ 07739, Telephone: (732) 758-6511; Fax: (732) 758-1048, Lab Name: East Coast Infertility and IVF, P.C., Accreditation: CAP/ASRM

Institute for Reproductive Medicine and Science, St. Barnabas Medical Center, 94 Old Short Hills Rd., Suite 403 East, Livingston, NJ 07039, Telephone: (973) 322-8286; Fax: (973) 322-8890, Lab Name: Institute for Reproductive Medicine and Science, Accreditation: CAP/ASRM

Cooper Center for In Vitro Fertilization, P.C., 8002-E Greentree Commons, Marlton, NJ 08053, Telephone: (856) 751-5575; Fax: (856) 751-7289, Lab Name: Cooper Center for IVF, P.C., Accreditation: CAP/ASRM

Delaware Valley Institute of Fertility and Genetics, 6000 Sagemore Dr., Suite 6102, Marlton, NJ 08053, Telephone: (856) 988-0072; Fax: (856) 988-0056, Lab Name: Reproductive Laboratories, Accreditation: CAP/ASRM

South Jersey Fertility Center, P.A., 512 Lippincott Dr., Marlton, NJ 08053, Telephone: (856) 596-2233; Fax: (856) 596-2411, Lab Name: South Jersey Fertility Center, P.A., Accreditation: JCAHO

Diamond Institute for Infertility, 89 Millburn Ave., Millburn, NJ 07041, Telephone:

(973) 761-5600; Fax: (973) 761-5100, Lab Name: Diamond Institute for Infertility, Accreditation: CAP/ASRM

Reproductive Medicine Associates of New Jersey, 111 Madison Ave., Suite 100, Morristown, NJ 07962, Telephone: (973) 971-4600; Fax: (973) 290-8370, Lab Name: Reproductive Endocrinology & Andrology Laboratory, Accreditation: CAP/ASRM

Robert Wood Johnson Medical School–IVF Program, 303 George St., Suite 250, New Brunswick, NJ 08901, Telephone: (732) 235-7300; Fax: (732) 235-7318, Lab Name: Robert Wood Johnson Medical School IVF Program, Accreditation: CAP/ASRM

IVF New Jersey, 81 Veronica Ave., Somerset, NJ 08873, Telephone: (732) 220-9060; Fax: (732) 545-1164, Lab Name: IVF New Jersey, Accreditation: CAP/ASRM

Dr. Louis R. Manara, 211 White Horse Rd., Voorhees, NJ 08043, Telephone: (856) 783-2802; Fax: (856) 784-1607, Lab Name: Pennsylvania Reproductive Associates, Accreditation: JCAHO

Fertility Institute of New Jersey, 400 Old Hook Rd., Westwood, NJ 07675, Telephone: (201) 666-4200; Fax: (201) 666-2262, Lab Name: Fertility Institute of New Jersey, Accreditation: CAP/ASRM, JCAHO

NEW MEXICO

Center for Reproductive Medicine of New Mexico, Presbyterian Professional Bldg., 201 Cedar St., S.E., Suite LL20, Albuquerque, NM 87106, Telephone: (505) 247-3333; Fax: (505) 224-7476, Lab Name: IVF and Andrology Laboratories, Accreditation: CAP/ASRM

NEW YORK

Albany IVF, Fertility and Gynecology, 349 Northern Blvd., Albany, NY 12204, Telephone: (518) 434-9759; Fax: (518) 436-9822, Lab Name: Embryology Network, Accreditation: NYSTB

Leading Institute for Fertility Enhancement (L.I.F.E.), 130 Everett Rd., Albany, NY 12205, Telephone: (518) 482-1008; Fax: (518) 489-6210, Lab Name: Fertility Studies Laboratory, Accreditation: JCAHO

The Fertility Institute at New York Methodist Hospital, 506 Sixth St., Suite KP4, Brooklyn, NY 11215, Telephone: (718) 643-6307; Fax: (718) 780-5085, Lab Name: The Fertility Institute at New York Methodist Hospital, Accreditation: NYSTB

Genesis Fertility, Genesis Fertility & Reproductive Medicine, 1355 84th St., Brooklyn, NY 11228, Telephone: (718) 283-8600; Fax: (718) 283-6580, Lab Name: Brooklyn IVF, Accreditation: CAP/ASRM, NYSTB

Health Science Center, State University of New York at Stony Brook, Division of Reproductive Endocrinology and Infertility, 6 Technology Dr., East Setauket, NY 11733, Telephone: (631) 444-4686; Fax: (631) 444-5175, Lab Name: Mather Hospital, Accreditation: CAP/ASRM, NYSTB

Garden City Center for Advanced , Reproductive Technologies, Yu-Kang Ying, M.D., P.C., 300 Garden City Plaza, Suite 420, Garden City, NY 11530, Telephone: (516) 248-8307; Fax: (516) 248-5007, Lab Name: John T. Mather Memorial Hospital, Accreditation: CAP/ASRM, NYSTB

Montefiore's Institute for Reproductive Medicine and Health, 141 South Central Ave., Hartsdale, NY 10530, Telephone: (914) 997-1060; Fax: (914) 997-1099, Lab Name: Lab of Montefiore's Institute for Reproductive Medicine and Health, Accreditation: CAP/ASRM, NYSTB

North Shore University Hospital, Center for Human Reproduction, IVF Program, Ambulatory Bldg., 300 Community Dr., Manhasset, NY 11030, Telephone: (516) 562-2229; Fax: (516) 562-1710, Lab Name: North Shore University Hospital, Accreditation: CAP/ASRM, NYSTB

Reproductive Science Associates, 200 Old Country Rd., Suite 330, Mineola, NY 11501, Telephone: (516) 739-2100; Fax: (516) 739-2178, Lab Name: M.P.D. Medical Associates, Accreditation: NYSTB

Advanced Fertility Services, 1625 Third Ave., New York, NY 10128, Telephone: (212) 369-8700; Fax: (212) 722-5587, Lab Name: Advanced Fertility Services IVF Laboratory, Accreditation: NYSTB

Brooklyn Fertility Center, 55 Central Park West, Suite 1C, New York, NY 10023, Telephone: (212) 721-4545; Fax: (212) 721-4598, Lab Name: Brooklyn Fertility Center, Accreditation: NYSTB

Columbia University Center for Women's Reproductive Care, 1790 Broadway, 2nd Floor, New York, NY 10019, Telephone: (646) 756-8282; Fax: (646) 756-8280, Lab Name: Columbia University, Assisted Reproduction, Accreditation: NYSTB

Nabil Husami, M.D., 550 Park Ave., New York, NY 10021, Telephone: (212) 750-3330; Fax: (212) 750-3334, Lab Name: Nabil W. Husami, M.D., Accreditation: None

MacLeod Laboratory, 65 E. 79th St., New York, NY 10021, Telephone: (212) 717-4444; Fax: (212) 717-1868, Lab Name: MacLeod Laboratory, Accreditation: None

Medical Offices for Human Reproduction, Center for Human Reproduction (CHR), 21 E. 69th St., New York, NY 10021, Telephone: (212) 994-4400; Fax: (212) 994-4499, Lab Name: Medical Offices for Human Reproduction, CHR, Accreditation: NYSTB

Dr. Lillian D. Nash, 315 W. 57th St., Lower Level, New York, NY 10019, Telephone: (212) 247-3111; Fax: (212) 247-3255, Lab Name: IVF Center of New York, Accreditation: NYSTB

New York Fertility Institute, 1016 Fifth Ave., New York, NY 10028, Telephone: (212) 734-5555; Fax: (212) 734-6059, Lab Name: New York Fertility Institute, Accreditation: CAP/ASRM, NYSTB

Offices for Fertility and Reproductive Medicine, P.C., 51 E. 67th St., New York, NY 10021, Telephone: (212) 535-5350; Fax: (212) 535-5080, Lab Name: Embryology Laboratories, Accreditation: NYSTB

Program for In Vitro Fertilization, Reproductive Surgery and Infertility, New York University School of Medicine, 660 First Ave. at 38th St., 5th Floor, New York, NY 10016, Telephone: (212) 263-8990; Fax: (212) 263-7853, Lab Name: NYU-SOM–Program for In Vitro Fertilization, Accreditation: NYSTB

Reproductive Endocrinology Associates of St. Luke's , Roosevelt Hospital, 425 W. 59th St., Suite 5A, New York, NY 10019, Telephone: (212) 523-7751; Fax: (212) 523-8348, Lab Name: IVF New York, Accreditation: NYSTB

Weill Medical College of Cornell University, The Center for Reproductive Medicine & Infertility, 505 E. 70th St., HT340, New York, NY 10021, Telephone: (212) 746-1762; Fax: (212) 746-8860, Lab Name: The Embryology Laboratory, Accreditation: NYSTB

The Capital Region Genetics & IVF Center, Bellevue Woman's Hospital, Center for Fertility and Advanced Reproductive Medicine at Bellevue Woman's Hospital, 2210 Troy Rd., Niskayuna, NY 12309, Telephone: (518) 346-9544; Fax: (518) 347-3392, Lab Name: Bellevue Woman's Hospital Laboratory, Accreditation: JCAHO, NYSTB

Long Island IVF Associates, 625 Belle Terre Rd., Suite 200, Port Jefferson, NY 11777, Telephone: (631) 331-7575; Fax: (631) 331-1332, Lab Name: Mather Hospital, Accreditation: CAP/ASRM, NYSTB

Institute for Reproductive Health and Infertility, 1561 Long Pond Rd., Suite 410, Rochester, NY 14626, Telephone: (585) 453-7760; Fax: (585) 453-7771, Lab Name: Strong Fertility and Reproductive Science Center, Accreditation: NYSTB

Strong Fertility and Reproductive Science Center, 601 Elmwood Ave., Box 668, Rochester, NY 14642, Telephone: (585) 275-1930; Fax: (585) 756-4146, Lab Name: Strong Fertility and Reproductive Science Center, Accreditation: NYSTB

CNY Fertility Center, 195 Intrepid Ln., Syracuse, NY 13205, Telephone: (315) 469-8700; Fax: (315) 469-6789, Lab Name: CNY Fertility Center, Accreditation: NYSTB

Infertility and IVF Medical Associates of Western New York, 4510 Main St., Snyder, NY 14226, Telephone: (716) 839-3057; Fax: (716) 839-1477, Lab Name: Infertility and IVF Medical Associates, Accreditation: NYSTB

Westchester Fertility and Reproductive Endocrinology, 136 S. Broadway, Suite 100, White Plains, NY 10605, Telephone: (914) 949-6677; Fax: (914) 949-5758, Lab Name: New England Fertility Institute IVF Laboratory, Accreditation: CAP/ASRM, Lab Name: The Fertility and Hormone Center of Montefiore, Accreditation: CAP/ASRM

Reproductive Medicine/IVF, 1321 Millersport Rd., Suite 102, Williamsville, NY 14221, Telephone: (716) 634-4351, Lab Name: Reproductive Medicine/IVF, Accreditation: NYSTB

NORTH CAROLINA

North Carolina Center for Reproductive Medicine, The Talbert Fertility Institute, 400 Asheville Ave., Suite 200, Cary, NC 27511, Telephone: (919) 233-1680; Fax: (919) 233-1685, Lab Name: NCCRM Main Lab, Accreditation: CAP/ASRM

University of North Carolina A.R.T. Clinic, 4001 Old Clinic Bldg., CB 7570, Chapel Hill, NC 27599, Telephone: (919) 966-1150; Fax: (919) 966-1259, Lab Name: University of North Carolina A.R.T. Laboratory, Accreditation: CAP/ASRM

§Institute for Assisted Reproduction, 1918 Randolph Rd., Suite 500, Charlotte, NC 28233, Telephone: (704) 343-3400; Fax: (704) 343-3428, Contact SART for current clinic information.

Program for Assisted Reproduction, Carolinas Medical Center, 1000 Blythe Blvd., Charlotte, NC 28203, Telephone: (704) 355-3153; Fax: (704) 355-3141, Lab Name: Program for Assisted Reproduction, Carolinas Medical Center, Accreditation: CAP/ASRM

Duke University Medical Center, Division of Reproductive Endocrinology and Infertility, Dept. of OB/GYN, Box 3143, Durham, NC 27710, Telephone: (919) 684-5327; Fax: (919) 681-7904, Lab Name: Duke University Medical Center, Accreditation: CAP/ASRM

East Carolina University, Women's Physicians, 2305 Executive Park West, Greenville, NC 27834, Telephone: (252) 816-3849; Fax: (252) 816-2016, Lab Name: East Carolina University, ECU Women's Physicians, Accreditation: JCAHO

Reproductive Consultants, PA, 2500 Blue Ridge Rd., Suite 300, Raleigh, NC 27607, Telephone: (919) 881-7795; Fax: (919) 881-7796, Lab Name: IVF-labs, LLC, Accreditation: None

MeritCare Medical Group—Fertility Center, 737 Broadway, Fargo, ND 58122, Telephone: (701) 234-2700; Fax: (701) 234-2783, Lab Name: MeritCare Medical Group, Fertility Center Lab, Accreditation: CAP/ASRM

OHIO

Fertility Unlimited, Inc., 468 E. Market St., Akron, OH 44304, Telephone: (330) 376-8353; Fax: (330) 376-4807, Lab Name: Fertility Unlimited, Inc., Accreditation: JCAHO

Reproductive Gynecology, 185 W. Cedar St., Suite 410, Akron, OH 44307, Telephone: (330) 375-3585; Fax: (330) 375-3986, Lab Name: Reproductive Gynecology Laboratories, L.L.C., Accreditation: JCAHO

Cleveland Clinic Fertility Center, Goldfarb/Desai IVF Program, 26900 Cedar Rd., Suite 220-S, Beachwood, OH 44122, Telephone: (216) 839-3150; Fax: (216) 839-3195, Lab Name: IVF/Andrology Laboratory, Accreditation: CAP/ASRM

Bethesda Center for Reproductive Health & Fertility, Bethesda Hospital, 10506 Montgomery Rd., Suite 303, Cincinnati, OH 45242, Telephone: (513) 745-1675; Fax: (513) 745-1676, Lab Name: Reproductive Studies Laboratory, Accreditation: JCAHO

Center for Reproductive Health, 2123 Auburn Ave., Suite 444, Cincinnati, OH 45219, Telephone: (513) 585-2355; Fax: (513) 585-0808, Lab Name: Center for Reproductive Health, Accreditation: CAP/ASRM

Institute for Reproductive Health, 3805 Edwards Rd., Suite 450, Cincinnati, OH 45209, Telephone: (513) 924-5550; Fax: (513) 924-5549, Lab Name: Christ Hospital Center for Reproductive Studies, Accreditation: CAP/ASRM

MacDonald Fertility and IVF Program, MacDonald Women's Hospital, University Hospitals Health System, 11100 Euclid Ave., Suite 1200, Cleveland, OH 44106, Telephone: (216) 844-1514; Fax: (216) 844-7098, Lab Name: MacDonald Fertility IVF Laboratory, Accreditation: CAP/ASRM

MetroHealth Medical Center Fertility Clinic, Dept. of OB/GYN, 2500 MetroHealth Dr., Cleveland, OH 44109, Telephone: (216) 778-5990; Fax: (216) 778-8847, Lab Name: Cleveland Clinic Foundation IVF Center, Accreditation: CAP/ASRM, JCAHO

Ohio Reproductive Medicine, Ohio State University, 4830 E. Knightsbridge Blvd., Columbus, OH 43214, Telephone: (614) 451-2280; Fax: (614) 451-4352, Lab Name: Reproductive Diagnostics, Inc., Accreditation: CAP/ASRM

Miami Valley Hospital Fertility Center, One Wyoming St., Suite 4110, Dayton, OH 45409, Telephone: (937) 208-2120; Fax: (937) 208-5387, Lab Name: Miami Valley Hospital Fertility Center, Accreditation: CAP/ASRM

Kettering Reproductive Medicine, 3533 Southern Blvd., Suite 4100, Kettering, OH 45429, Telephone: (937) 395-8444; Fax: (937) 395-8450, Lab Name: Kettering Reproductive Medicine Laboratory, Accreditation: CAP/ASRM

Fertility Center of Northwestern Ohio, 2142 N. Cove Blvd., Toledo, OH 43606, Telephone: (419) 479-8830; Fax: (419) 479-6005, Lab Name: Fertility Center of NW Ohio, Accreditation: JCAHO

OKLAHOMA

Henry G. Bennett, Jr., Fertility Institute, 3433 N.W. 56th St., Suite 200B, Oklahoma City, OK 73112, Telephone: (405) 949-6060; Fax: (405) 949-6872, Lab Name: Bennett Fertility Institute, Accreditation: CAP/ASRM

Center for Reproductive Health, P.C., 1000 N. Lincoln Blvd., Suite 300, Oklahoma City, OK 73104, Telephone: (405) 271-9200; Fax: (405) 271-9222, Lab Name: OU Medical Center ART Laboratory, Accreditation: CAP/ASRM

Tulsa Center for Fertility & Women's Health, 1145 S. Utica Ave., Suite 1209, Tulsa, OK 74104, Telephone: (918) 584-2870; Fax: (918) 587-3602, Lab Name: Tulsa Center for Fertility & Women's Health, Accreditation: CAP/ASRM

OREGON

Northwest Fertility Center, 1750 S.W. Harbor Way, Suite 200, Portland, OR 97201, Telephone: (503) 227-7799; Fax: (503) 227-5452, Lab Name: Oregon Health & Science University, Accreditation: CAP/ASRM

Portland Center for Reproductive Medicine, 2222 N.W. Lovejoy St., Suite 304, Portland, OR 97210, Telephone: (503) 274-4994; Fax: (503) 274-4946, Lab Name: The Reproductive Medicine Laboratory, Accreditation: JCAHO

University Fertility Consultants, Oregon Health & Science University, 1750 S.W. Harbor Way, Suite 100, Portland, OR 97201, Telephone: (503) 418-3700; Fax: (503) 418-3708, Lab Name: Andrology/Embryology Laboratory, Oregon Health & Science University, Accreditation: CAP/ASRM

PENNSYLVANIA

Toll Center for Reproductive Sciences, Abington Reproductive Medicine, P.C., 1245 Highland Ave., Suite 404, Abington, PA 19001, Telephone: (215) 887-2010; Fax:

(215) 887-3291, Lab Name: Toll Center for Reproductive Sciences, Accreditation: CAP/ASRM, JCAHO

Infertility Solutions, P.C., 2200 Hamilton St., Suite 105, Allentown, PA 18104, Telephone: (610) 776-1217; Fax: (610) 776-4149, Lab Name: Infertility Solutions, P.C., Accreditation: CAP/ASRM

Reproductive Endocrinology & Infertility Specialists, 401 N. 17th St., Suite 303, Allentown, PA 18104, Telephone: (610) 402-9522; Fax: (610) 402-9649, Lab Name: ART Lab at LVH Muhlenberg Campus, Accreditation: CAP/ASRM (Pending)

Reprotech, Inc., IVF Program, 440 S. 15th St., Allentown, PA 18102, Telephone: (610) 437-7000; Fax: (610) 437-6381, Lab Name: Reprotech, Inc., Accreditation: None

Family Fertility Center, 95 Highland Ave., Suite 100, Bethlehem, PA 18017, Telephone: (610) 868-8600; Fax: (610) 868-8700, Lab Name: Family Fertility Center, Accreditation: CAP/ASRM

IVF Marrero, 80 Emerson Ln., Suite 1301-1302, Bridgeville, PA 15017, Telephone: (412) 221-2300; Fax: (412) 221-0322, Lab Name: The Reproductive Center, Accreditation: JCAHO

Main Line Fertility and Reproductive Medicine, Ltd., 130 S. Bryn Mawr Ave., Suite 1000, D Wing, Bryn Mawr, PA 19010, Telephone: (610) 527-0800; Fax: (610) 527-9868, Lab Name: Center for Reproductive Medicine, Accreditation: CAP/ASRM, JCAHO

Geisinger Medical Center Fertility Program, Dept. of OB/GYN, 100 N. Academy Ave., Danville, PA 17822, Telephone: (570) 271-5620; Fax: (570) 271-5629, Lab Name: Geisinger Medical Center ART—Andrology Laboratory, Accreditation: CAP/ASRM

Advanced Center for Infertility and Reproductive, Medicine, R.P.C., 2708 Commerce Dr., Suite 100, Harrisburg, PA 17110, Telephone: (717) 545-9300; Fax: (717) 540-3700, Lab Name: Center for Reproductive Surgery, LLC, Accreditation: None

Milton S. Hershey Medical Center, 500 University Dr., Hershey, PA 17033, Telephone: (717) 531-6731; Fax: (717) 531-6286, Lab Name: ART Laboratory, Accreditation: JCAHO

Jenkintown Reproductive Endocrine & Gynecology Associates, P.C., 500 Old York Rd., Suite 103, Jenkintown, PA 19046, Telephone: (215) 576-7100; Fax: (215) 576-1544, Lab Name: Reproductive Science Institute of Suburban Philadelphia, Accreditation: CAP/ASRM

Northern Fertility and Reproductive Associates, P.C., Holy Redeemer Medical Office Bldg., 1650 Huntingdon Pike, Suite 154, Meadowbrook, PA 19046, Telephone: (215) 938-1515; Fax: (215) 938-8756, Lab Name: Pennsylvania Reproductive

Associates, Accreditation: JCAHO, Lab Name: Toll Center for Reproductive Sciences, Accreditation: CAP/ASRM, JCAHO

§Pennsylvania Reproductive Associates, Women's Institute for Fertility, Endocrinology, and Menopause, 815 Locust St., Philadelphia, PA 19107, Telephone: (215) 922-3173; Fax: (215) 627-7554, Contact SART for current clinic information.

Thomas Jefferson IVF Program, 834 Chestnut St., Room 400, Philadelphia, PA 19107, Telephone: (215) 955-4018; Fax: (215) 923-1089, Lab Name: Center for Reproductive Medicine, Accreditation: CAP/ASRM, JCAHO

University of Pennsylvania, 106 Dulles Bldg., 3400 Spruce St., Philadelphia, PA 19104, Telephone: (215) 662-6560; Fax: (215) 349-5512, Lab Name: University of Pennsylvania, Accreditation: CAP/ASRM

Reproductive Health Specialists, Inc., 665 Rodi Rd., 2nd Floor, Bldg. 2, Pittsburgh, PA 15235, Telephone: (412) 731-8000; Fax: (412) 731-8399, Lab Name: Reproductive Health Specialists, Inc., Accreditation: CAP/ASRM (Pending)

University of Pittsburgh Physicians, Center for Fertility and Reproductive Endocrinology, Magee Women's Hospital, 300 Halket St., 5th Floor, Pittsburgh, PA 15213, Telephone: (412) 641-4726; Fax: (412) 641-1133, Lab Name: University of Pittsburgh Physicians Center for Fertility and Reproductive Endocrinology, Accreditation: CAP/ASRM

Women's Clinic, Ltd., 301 S. Seventh Ave., Suite 245, Reading, PA 19611, Telephone: (610) 374-2214; Fax: (610) 374-8852, Lab Name: Fertility Medical Labs, Inc., Accreditation: CAP/ASRM

Reproductive Endocrinology and Fertility Center, One Medical Center Blvd., Upland, PA 19013, Telephone: (610) 447-2727; Fax: (610) 447-6549, Lab Name: Crozer–Chester Andrology and IVF Laboratory, Accreditation: CAP/ASRM

Reproductive Science Institute of Suburban Philadelphia, 950 W. Valley Rd., Suite 2401, Wayne, PA 19087, Telephone: (610) 964-9663; Fax: (610) 964-0536, Lab Name: Reproductive Science Institute of Suburban Philadelphia, Accreditation: CAP/ASRM

Fertility and Gynecology Associates, Executive Mews, 2300 Computer Ave., Suite H-44, Willow Grove, PA 19090, Telephone: (215) 706-4090; Fax: (215) 706-4072, Lab Name: Toll Center for Reproductive Sciences, Accreditation: CAP/ASRM, JCAHO

PUERTO RICO

Dr. Pedro J. Beauchamp, Dr. Arturo Cadilla, Bldg. 100, Paseo San Pablo, Suite 503, Bayamon, PR 00959, Telephone: (787) 798-0100; Fax: (787) 740-7250, Lab Name: Dr. Beauchamp's IVF Lab, Accreditation: JCAHO

Centro De Fertilidad Del Caribe, Torre San Francisco, Suite 606, Av. de Diego 369, Rio Piedras, PR 00923, Telephone: (787) 763-2773; Fax: (787) 763-2773, Lab Name: Centro De Fertilidad Del Caribe, Accreditation: CAP/ASRM

GREFI—Gynecology, Reproductive Endocrinology & Fertility Institute, First Bank Bldg., 1519 Ponce de Leon Ave., Suite 705, Santurce, PR 00910, Telephone: (787) 721-3544; Fax: (787) 721-5957, Lab Name: GREFI, Accreditation: CAP/ASRM

RHODE ISLAND

Women & Infants' IVF Program, 101 Dudley St., Providence, RI 02905, Telephone: (401) 453-7500; Fax: (401) 453-7598, Lab Name: Women & Infants' IVF Laboratory, Accreditation: CAP/ASRM

SOUTH CAROLINA

Reproductive Endocrinology and Infertility, 890 W. Faris Rd., Suite 470, Greenville, SC 29605, Telephone: (864) 455-1675; Fax: (864) 455-3095, Lab Name: Reproductive Endocrinology and Infertility, Accreditation: CAP/ASRM, JCAHO

Southeastern Fertility Center, P.A., 1375 Hospital Dr., Mount Pleasant, SC 29464, Telephone: (843) 881-3900; Fax: (843) 881-4729, Lab Name: Southeastern Fertility Center Laboratory, Accreditation: CAP/ASRM

SOUTH DAKOTA

University Physicians Fertility Specialists, 1310 W. 22nd St., Sioux Falls, SD 57105, Telephone: (605) 782-2284; Fax: (605) 782-2770, Lab Name: USD Human Reproduction Laboratory, Accreditation: CAP/ASRM

TENNESSEE

Center for Reproductive Medicine and Fertility, Fertility Center of Chattanooga, 1624 Gunbarrel Rd., Chattanooga, TN 37421, Telephone: (423) 899-0500; Fax: (423) 899-2411, Lab Name: Fertility Center of Chattanooga, Accreditation: JCAHO

Appalachian Fertility and Endocrinology Center, 2204 Pavilion Dr., Suite 307, Kingsport, TN 37660, Telephone: (423) 857-6400; Fax: (423) 857-6404, Lab Name: The Fertility Resources Center, Accreditation: JCAHO

East Tennessee IVF, Fertility and Andrology Center, 1924 Alcoa Hwy., Suite 304, Knoxville, TN 37920, Telephone: (865) 544-6756; Fax: (865) 544-6757, Lab Name: East Tennessee IVF, Fertility, and Andrology Center, Accreditation: JCAHO (Pending)

Southeastern Fertility Center, 1928 Alcoa Hwy., Suite 201-B, Knoxville, TN 37920, Telephone: (865) 544-8800; Fax: (865) 544-6581, Lab Name: IVF Labs, Inc., Accreditation: None

University Fertility Associates, 909 Ridgeway Loop Rd., Memphis, TN 38120, Telephone: (901) 767-6868; Fax: (901) 682-2231, Lab Name: University Fertility Associates, Accreditation: CAP/ASRM

The Center for Reproductive Health, 2011 Murphy Ave., Suite 605, Nashville, TN 37203, Telephone: (615) 321-8899; Fax: (615) 321-8877, Lab Name: Fertility Laboratories of Nashville, Inc., Accreditation: CAP/ASRM

Nashville Fertility Center, 2400 Patterson St., Suite 319, Nashville, TN 37203, Telephone: (615) 321-4740; Fax: (615) 320-0240, Lab Name: Nashville Fertility Center, Accreditation: CAP/ASRM

TEXAS

Dr. Harold W. Brumley, 1301 W. 38th St., Suite 109, Austin, TX 78705, Telephone: (512) 451-8211; Fax: (512) 450-1146, Lab Name: St. David's ART/IVF, Accreditation: JCAHO

Texas Fertility Center, Drs. Vaughn, Silverberg and Hansard, 3705 Medical Pkwy., Suite 420, Austin, TX 78705, Telephone: (512) 451-0149; Fax: (512) 451-0977, Lab Name: St. David's ART/IVF, Accreditation: JCAHO

Dr. Jeffrey Youngkin, Austin Fertility Center, 805 E. 32nd St., Austin, TX 78705, Telephone: (512) 478-3188; Fax: (512) 478-5092, Lab Name: St. David's ART/IVF, Accreditation: JCAHO

Center for Assisted Reproduction, 1701 Park Place Ave., Bedford, TX 76022, Telephone: (817) 540-1157; Fax: (817) 267-0522, Lab Name: Center for Assisted Reproduction, Accreditation: CAP/ASRM

Trinity In Vitro Fertilization Program, 4325 N. Josey Ln., Suite 308, Carrollton, TX 75010, Telephone: (972) 394-3699; Fax: (972) 394-6517, Lab Name: Trinity IVF, Accreditation: CAP/ASRM

Baylor Center for Reproductive Health, 3707 Gaston Ave., Suite 310, Dallas, TX 75246, Telephone: (214) 821-2274; Fax: (214) 821-2373, Lab Name: Baylor Center for Reproductive Health, Accreditation: CAP/ASRM

National Fertility Center of Texas, P.A., 7777 Forest Ln., Bldg. C, Suite 638, Dallas, TX 75230, Telephone: (972) 566-6686; Fax: (972) 566-6670, Lab Name: National Fertility Center of Texas, P.A., Accreditation: CAP/ASRM

University of Texas, Southwestern Fertility Associates, Dept. of OB/GYN, Div. of Reproductive Endocrinology & Infertility, 5323 Harry Hines Blvd., Dallas, TX

75390, Telephone: (214) 648-8846; Fax: (214) 648-2813, Lab Name: UT Southwestern Embryology Laboratory, Accreditation: CAP/ASRM

Presbyterian Hospital ARTS Program, Perot Bldg., 6th Floor, 8160 Walnut Hill Ln., Dallas, TX 75231, Telephone: (214) 345-2624; Fax: (214) 345-8317, Lab Name: Presbyterian Hospital ARTS Program, Accreditation: CAP/ASRM

The Women's Place, 3650 W. Wheatland Rd., Suite B, Dallas, TX 75237, Telephone: (972) 709-9777; Fax: (972) 709-8300, Lab Name: Advanced Reproductive Care Center of Irving, Accreditation: CAP/ASRM

Offices of Frank D. De Leon, M.D., 1325 Pennsylvania Ave., Suite 450, Fort Worth, TX 76132, Telephone: (817) 878-5270; Fax: (817) 878-5294, Lab Name: Advanced Reproductive Care Center of Irving, Accreditation: CAP/ASRM

Baylor Assisted Reproductive Technology, 6550 Fannin St., Suite 821, Houston, TX 77030, Telephone: (713) 798-8232; Fax: (713) 798-8231, Lab Name: Baylor Assisted Reproductive Technology, Accreditation: CAP/ASRM

Center for Women's Health, 7400 Fannin St., Suite 1130, Houston, TX 77054, Telephone: (713) 797-9200; Fax: (713) 797-9276, Lab Name: OB GYN Associates IVF Laboratory, Accreditation: CAP/ASRM

Cooper Institute for Advanced Reproductive Medicine, 7500 Beechnut St., Suite 308, Houston, TX 77074, Telephone: (713) 771-9771; Fax: (713) 771-9773, Lab Name: OB GYN Associates IVF Laboratory, Accreditation: CAP/ASRM

North Houston Center for Reproductive Medicine, P.A., 530 Wells Fargo Dr., Suite 116, Houston, TX 77090, Telephone: (281) 444-4784; Fax: (281) 444-0429, Lab Name: North Houston Center for Reproductive Medicine, P.A., Accreditation: CAP/ASRM

Obstetrical & Gynecological Associates, 7550 Fannin St., Houston, TX 77054, Telephone: (713) 512-7914; Fax: (713) 512-7853, Lab Name: OB & GYN Associates IVF Laboratory, Accreditation: CAP/ASRM

Advanced Reproductive Care Center of Irving, 440 W. Highway 635, Suite 455, Irving, TX 75063, Telephone: (972) 506-9986; Fax: (972) 506-0044, Lab Name: Advanced Reproductive Care Center of Irving, Accreditation: CAP/ASRM

Wilford Hall Medical Center, 59th MDW/MMNO, 2200 Bergquist Dr., Suite 1, Lackland AFB, TX 78236, Telephone: (210) 292-6137; Fax: (210) 292-6158, Lab Name: Wilford Hall Medical Center IVF Laboratory, Accreditation: CAP/ASRM

Institute for Women's Health, Advanced Fertility Laboratory, 7940 Floyd Curl Dr., Suite 900, San Antonio, TX 78229, Telephone: (210) 616-0680; Fax: (210) 616-0684,

Lab Name: Institute for Women's Health, Advanced Fertility Laboratory, Accreditation: JCAHO

Texas Fertility, P.A., 751 Hebron Pkwy., Suite 310, Lewisville, TX 75057, Telephone: (972) 315-3245; Fax: (972) 315-9249, Lab Name: Trinity Medical Center, Accreditation: CAP/ASRM (Pending)

The Centre for Reproductive Medicine, 3506 21st St., Suite 605, Lubbock, TX 79410, Telephone: (806) 788-1212; Fax: (806) 788-1253, Lab Name: The Centre for Reproductive Medicine, Accreditation: CAP/ASRM

Fertility Center of San Antonio, 4499 Medical Dr., Suite 200, San Antonio, TX 78229, Telephone: (210) 692-0577; Fax: (210) 692-1210, Lab Name: Fertility Center Laboratory, Accreditation: CAP/ASRM

Fertility Concepts, 4499 Medical Dr., Suite 380, San Antonio, TX 78229, Telephone: (210) 614-3303; Fax: (210) 615-1052, Lab Name: Institute for Women's Health, Advanced Fertility Laboratory, Accreditation: JCAHO

South Texas Fertility Center, University of Texas Health Science Center–San Antonio, 8122 Datapoint Dr., Suite 1300, San Antonio, TX 78229, Telephone: (210) 567-7575; Fax: (210) 567-7538, Lab Name: South Texas Fertility Center/UTHSCSA, Accreditation: CAP/ASRM

Center of Reproductive Medicine, 450 Medical Center Blvd., Suite 202, Webster, TX 77598, Telephone: (281) 332-0073; Fax: (281) 332-1860, Lab Name: Center of Reproductive Medicine, Accreditation: CAP/ASRM

UTAH

Reproductive Care Center, 1220 E. 3900 South, Suite 4-G, Salt Lake City, UT 84124, Telephone: (801) 268-0306; Fax: (801) 268-6234, Lab Name: Reproductive Care Center, Accreditation: CAP/ASRM

Utah Center for Reproductive Medicine, University of Utah, 675 Arapeen Dr., Suite 205, Salt Lake City, UT 84108, Telephone: (801) 581-4838; Fax: (801) 585-2231, Lab Name: University of Utah Andrology Laboratory, Accreditation: CAP/ASRM

VERMONT

Vermont Center for Reproductive Medicine, University of Vermont–IVF Program, Women's Health Care Service–FAHC, One S. Prospect St., Burlington, VT 05401, Telephone: (802) 847-0986; Fax: (802) 847-0111, Lab Name: Vermont Center for Reproductive Medicine, Accreditation: JCAHO

Fertility and Reproductive Health Center, Washington Fertility Center, 4316 Evergreen Ln., Annandale, VA 22003, Telephone: (703) 658-3100; Fax: (703) 658-3103, Lab Name: Northern Virginia Reproductive Laboratory, Accreditation: CAP/ASRM

Dominion Fertility and Endocrinology, 46 S. Glebe Rd., Suite 301, Arlington, VA 22204, Telephone: (703) 920-3890; Fax: (703) 892-6037, Lab Name: Dominion Fertility and Endocrinology, Accreditation: CAP/ASRM

University of Virginia ART Program, University of Virginia Health System, P.O. Box 801304, Charlottesville, VA 22908, Telephone: (434) 243-4590; Fax: (434) 293-6409, Lab Name: Human Gamete & Embryo Laboratory, Accreditation: JCAHO

Genetics & IVF Institute, 3020 Javier Rd., Fairfax, VA 22031, Telephone: (703) 698-7355; Fax: (703) 204-4617, Lab Name: Genetics & IVF Institute, Accreditation: None

Jones Institute, Northern Virginia/D.C. Center, 8501 Arlington Blvd., Suite 500, Fairfax, VA 22031, Telephone: (703) 876-6311; Fax: (703) 876-6317, Lab Name: Jones Institute Embryology Laboratory, Accreditation: CAP/ASRM

Jones Institute for Reproductive Medicine, Dept. of OB/GYN, 601 Colley Ave., Suite 201, Norfolk, VA 23507, Telephone: (757) 446-7116; Fax: (757) 446-8998, Lab Name: Jones Institute Embryology Laboratory, Accreditation: CAP/ASRM

Fertility Institute of Virginia, 10710 Midlothian Turnpike, Suite 331, Richmond, VA 23235, Telephone: (804) 379-9000; Fax: (804) 379-9031, Lab Name: Virginia IVF and Andrology Center, Accreditation: CAP/ASRM

Lifesource Fertility Center, 7603 Forest Ave., Suite 204, Richmond, VA 23229, Telephone: (804) 673-2273; Fax: (804) 285-3109, Lab Name: Virginia IVF and Andrology Center, Accreditation: CAP/ASRM

The Richmond Center for Fertility and Endocrinology, Ltd., Courtyard Office Bldg., 7603 Forest Ave., Suite 301, Richmond, VA 23229, Telephone: (804) 285-9700; Fax: (804) 285-9745, Lab Name: Virginia IVF and Andrology Center, Accreditation: CAP/ASRM

The New Hope Center for Reproductive Medicine, 1181 First Colonial Rd., Suite 100, Virginia Beach, VA 23454, Telephone: (757) 496-5370; Fax: (757) 481-3354, Lab Name: The New Hope Center for Reproductive Medicine, Accreditation: CAP/ASRM (Pending)

Overlake Reproductive Health Inc., P.S., 1135 116th Ave., N.E., Suite 640, Bellevue, WA 98004, Telephone: (425) 646-4700; Fax: (425) 646-1076, Lab Name: Overlake Reproductive Health Laboratory, LLC, Accreditation: CAP/ASRM (Pending)

Washington Center for Reproductive Medicine, 1370 116th Ave., N.E., Suite 202, Bellevue, WA 98004, Telephone: (425) 462-6100; Fax: (425) 635-0742, Lab Name: Washington Center for Reproductive Medicine, Accreditation: CAP/ASRM

Bellingham IVF, 2980 Squalicum Pkwy., Suite 103, Bellingham, WA 98225, Telephone: (360) 715-8124; Fax: (360) 715-8126, Lab Name: Bellingham IVF, Accreditation: None

Olympia Women's Health, Capital Medical Center, 403 E. Black Hills Ln., S.W., Olympia, WA 98502, Telephone: (360) 786-1515; Fax: (360) 754-7476, Lab Name: Olympia Women's Health, Accreditation: CAP/ASRM

Pacific Gynecology Specialists, 1101 Madison St., Suite 1500, Seattle, WA 98104, Telephone: (206) 215-3200; Fax: (206) 215-6590, Lab Name: Reproductive Technology, Accreditation: CAP/ASRM

University of Washington, Fertility & Endocrine Center, 4225 Roosevelt Way, N.E., Suite 305, Seattle, WA 98105, Telephone: (206) 598-4225; Fax: (206) 598-6081, Lab Name: FEC Gamete Laboratory, Accreditation: CAP/ASRM

Virginia Mason Center for Fertility, and Reproductive Endocrinology, 1100 9th Ave., Suite XII-FC, Seattle, WA 98101, Telephone: (206) 223-6190; Fax: (206) 341-0596, Lab Name: Virginia Mason Center for Fertility, Accreditation: CAP/ASRM, JCAHO

The Center for Reproductive Endocrinology and Fertility, N.W. Obstetrics and Gynecology, 508 W. 6th Ave., Suite 500, Spokane, WA 99204, Telephone: (509) 462-7070; Fax: (509) 444-3894, Lab Name: Center for Reproductive Endocrinology and Fertility, Accreditation: JCAHO

GYFT Clinic, P.L.L.C., 502 South M St., Suite 200, Tacoma, WA 98405, Telephone: (206) 475-5433; Fax: (206) 473-6715, Lab Name: Reproductive Assays Laboratory, Accreditation: CAP/ASRM

WEST VIRGINIA

Center for Reproductive Medicine, West Virginia University Health Science Center, 830 Pennsylvania Ave., Suite 304, Charleston, WV 25302, Telephone: (304) 388-1515; Fax: (304) 388-1570, Lab Name: Charleston Area Medical Center–IVF, Accreditation: CAP/ASRM, JCAHO

WISCONSIN

Reproductive Specialty Center, IVF Columbia, Seton Tower, 2315 N. Lake Dr., Suite 501, Milwaukee, WI 53211, Telephone: (414) 289-9668; Fax: (414) 289-0974, Lab Name: IVF Columbia, Accreditation: CAP/ASRM

Gundersen/Lutheran Medical Center, Reproductive Endocrinology & Fertility Center, 1836 South Ave., La Crosse, WI 54601, Telephone: (608) 782-7300; Fax: (608) 791-6611, Lab Name: Gundersen/Lutheran Medical Center IVF Lab, Accreditation: JCAHO

University of Wisconsin–Madison, Infertility and Women's Endocrine Service, Women's Endocrine Clinic, 600 Highland Ave., H4/630 CSC, Madison, WI 53792, Telephone: (608) 263-1217; Fax: (608) 262-9862, Lab Name: University of Wisconsin–Madison, Accreditation: CAP/ASRM

Medical College of Wisconsin, Department of Ob/Gyn, Froedtert Memorial Lutheran Hospital, 9200 W. Wisconsin Ave., Milwaukee, WI 53226, Telephone: (414) 805-6612; Fax: (414) 805-6622, Lab Name: Waukesha Advanced Regional Fertility Services, Accreditation: CAP/ASRM, JCAHO

Women's Health Care, S.C., 721 American Ave., Suite 304, Waukesha, WI 53188, Telephone: (262) 549-2229; Fax: (262) 549-1657, Lab Name: Advanced Institute of Fertility, Accreditation: CAP/ASRM

FERTILITY CLINICS IN CANADA

Inclusion of these centers in this list does not imply endorsement by the authors. This list was provided by the Infertility Awareness Association of Canada.

Fertility clinics and doctors

ALBERTA

Foothills Regional Fertility Programme, Medical Director: Dr. Calvin Greene, Nurse Manager: Tammy Troute-Wood, 1620-29th Street NW, Suite 300 , Calgary, AB T2N 4L7, Dir Tel: (403) 284-9103, Dir Fax: (403)-284-9293

BRITISH COLUMBIA

Genesis Fertility Centre, Medical Directors: Dr. Margo Fluker, Dr. Albert Yuzpe, Nurse Manager: Janice Copeland, 555 W. 12th Ave, Suite 550, Vancouver, BC V5Z 3X7, Dir Tel: (604) 879-3032 or 1-800-753-0111, Dir Fax: (604) 875-1432

University of British Columbia IVF Program, Medical Director: Dr. Anthony Cheung, Nurse Manager: Susan Wilson, 2nd Floor, Willow Pavilion, 805 W 12th Ave. , Vancouver, BC V5Z 1M9, Dir Tel: (604) 875-5440, Dir Fax: (604) 875-5124

Victoria Fertility Centre, Medical Director: Dr. Stephen Hudson, Clinical Coordinator: Stephanie Hunt, 207-4400 Chatterton Way, Victoria, BC V8X 5J2, Dir Tel: (250) 704-0024, Dir Fax: (250) 704-0034

MANITOBA

Heartland Fertility Clinic, Medical Directors: Dr. Jeremy Kredentser, Dr. Francis Lee & Dr. Gord McTavish, 701-1661 Portage, Winnipeg, MB R3J 3T7, Dir Tel: (204) 779-8888, ext. 221, Dir Fax: (204) 779-8877

NEW BRUNSWICK

Clinique CONCEPTIA Clinic, Pavillion Hotel Dieu Pavilion, Medical Director: Dr. Alfred Robichaud, Nurse Manager: Michelle Gauvin-Leblanc, 35 Providence, Moncton, NB E1C 2Z3, Dir Tel: (506) 862-4217/1-866-381-baby (2229), Dir Fax: (506) 862-7571

NOVA SCOTIA

Reproductive Endocrine Centre, Halifax, Medical Director: Dr. Bruce Dunphy, Nurse Manager: Kate Lively, 5980 University Avenue, PO Box 3070, Halifax, NS B3H 4N1, Dir Tel: (902) 470-7180

ONTARIO

McMaster University IVF Clinic, Medical Director: Dr. Robert Hutchison, Nurse Manager: Susan Ward, McMaster University, 690 Main Street West, Hamilton, ON L8S 1A4, Dir Tel: (905) 521-5080, Dir Fax: (905) 521-2627

University of Western Ontario IVF Clinic, Valter Feyles, MD, MSc, PhD, FRCSC, Associate Professor/Medical Director, REI Program, LHSC UC, Room 9-E21, Clinical Leader: Julie Fisher, Tel. 519-663-2966 Room 9-OP1A, Victoria/University Hospital, 339 Windermere Road, London, ON N6A 5A5, Dir Tel: (519) 663-3019, Dir Fax: (519) 663-3162

Markham Fertility Centre, Medical Director: Dr. Michael Virro, 377 Church Street, Suite 308, Markham, ON L6B 1A1, Dir Tel: (905) 472-7128, Dir Fax: (905) 472-4130

ISIS Regional Fertility Centre, Medical Director: Dr. Mathias Gysler, Nurse Manager: Shira Benson, 7145 West Credit Avenue, Bldg. #3, Mississauga, ON L5N 6J7, Dir Tel: (905) 820-8748, ext 239 or (905) 816-9822 (clinic), Dir Fax: (905) 820-6981

NUSTAR Fertility Centre, Medical Directors: Dr. Essam Michael; Dr. Samuel Soliman, Nurse Manager: Isa Hanna, 4303 Village Centre Court, Mississauga, ON L4Z 1S2, Dir Tel: (905) 896-7827, Dir Fax: (905) 896-1248

Goal Programme/Fertility Centre, Medical Director: Dr. Paul Claman, Nurse Manager: Shelley Zurcher, 737 Parkdale Avenue, Suite 510, Ottawa, ON K1Y 1J8, Dir Tel: (613) 761-4865, Fax: (613) 761-4678

IVF Canada, Medical Director: Dr. S. Batarseh, Nurse Manager: Carole Craig, 304, 2347 Kennedy Road , Scarborough, ON M1T 3T8, Dir Tel: (416) 754-8742 (clinic), Dir Fax: (416) 321-1239 (clinic)

Rouge Valley Fertility Center, Medical Director: Dr. Tanya Williams, Nurse Manager: Carol Jarzabek, Centenary Health Centre, 2863 Ellesmere Road, Suite 417, Scarborough, ON M1E 5E9, Dir Tel: (416) 283-5539, Dir Fax: (416) 283-1636

Mt. Sinai Reproductive Biology Unit, Medical Director: Dr. Ellen Greenblatt, Nurse Manager: Nancy Bryceland, Mt. Sinai Hospital, 600 University Avenue, Toronto, ON M5G 1X5, Dir Tel: (416) 586-5217, Dir Fax: (416) 586-4686

LIFE Programme, Medical Director: Dr. S. Batarseh, Nurse Manager: Julie Tolentino, Toronto East General Hospital, 825 Coxwell Avenue, Toronto, ON M4C 3E7, Dir Tel: (416) 469-6590 (clinic)

Sunnybrook Women's College Hospital Fertility Centre & The CreATe IVF Program, Medical Director: Dr. Cliff Librach, Nurse Manager: Ruth Clarke, 1020 - 790 Bay Street, Toronto, ON M5G 1N8, Dir Tel: (416) 323-7727, Dir Fax: (416) 323-7334

Success through Assisted Reproductive Technologies (START), Medical Director: Dr. Ken Cadesky, IVF Co-ordinator Michelle Todgham, 655 Bay Street, 18th Floor, Toronto, ON M5G 2K4, Dir Tel: (416) 506-0805, Dir Fax: (416) 506-0680

Toronto Centre for Advanced Reproductive Technology (TCART), Medical Director: Dr. Robert F. Casper, Nurse Manager: Lynda Gotleib, 150 Bloor Street West Plaza, Renaissance Plaza, 2nd Floor, Toronto, ON M5GS 2X9, Dir Tel: (416) 972-0110, 1-800-520-0110, Dir Fax: (416) 972-0036

QUEBEC

Montreal Fertility Centre, Medical Director: Dr. M.M. Biljan MD, 5252 DeMaisonneuve West, Montreal, PQ H4A 3S5, Tel (514) 369-6116, Fax (514) 369-2662

McGill Reproductive Centre, Medical Director: Dr. S.L. Tan, Nurse Manager: Francine Belisle, Royal Victoria Hospital, 687 Pine Avenue West, Rm F6.58, Montreal, PQ H3A 1A1, Dir Tel: (514) 843-1650, Dir Fax: (514) 843-1496

OVO Fertility Clinic, Medical Director: Dr. Francois Bissionnette, 8000 Decarie Boulevard, Suite 100, Montreal, PQ H4O 2S4, Dir Tel: (514) 798-2000, Dir Fax: (514) 798-2001

PROCREA Montreal, Medical Director: Dr. Pierre St-Michel, Nurse Manager: Anne Desmarais, 1100 Beaumont Avenue, Suite 305, Montreal, PQ H3P 3H5, Tel: (514) 345-8535 or 1-888-776-2732, Fax: (514) 345-8978

PROCREA Quebec, Medical Director: Dr. Marc Villeneuve, Nurse Manager: Marie Bélanger, 5600, Blvd Des Galeries, Suite 401, Québec, PQ G2K 2H6 , Tel: (418) 260-9555 or 1-877-776-2732, Fax: (418) 260-9556

SASKATCHEWAN

ARTUS, Medical Director: Dr. Allison Case, Nurse Manager: Jackie McVee, Royal University Hospital, Dept. Ob/Gyn/Reproductive Sciences, 103 Hospital Drive, Rm 4544, Saskatoon, SK S7N 0W8, Dir Tel: (306) 966-8033, Dir Fax: (306) 966-8040

APPENDIX 4

Twenty Questions for Information at a Glance

Manufacturers of high-tech electronic products such as sophisticated stereo equipment often provide a section in their instructions designed for consumers who want to "plug it in" and enjoy the music before reading in detail about how many decibels are required to blow out their eardrums. The purpose of this appendix is similar. The answers to the following 20 questions will give you a basic working knowledge of assisted reproductive procedures, but without the details. However, if you are considering entering a program or are in the midst of conventional infertility treatment, this chapter is not enough to help you make informed choices and to know if accepted procedures are being followed. You may want to start here, but we urge you to read the entire book to obtain all of the information you will need.

1. What is assisted reproduction? Assisted reproductive technology (ART) consists of procedures beyond conventional infertility treatment. They have as their common characteristic the technical manipulation of the sperm and the egg outside the body for their replacement into the reproductive organs to achieve a pregnancy. They may be replaced as eggs and sperm or early embryos. They can be placed into the woman's uterus or fallopian tube.

2. What procedures are considered to be ART? Currently the clinically available procedures include:

- IVF (In Vitro Fertilization): This is the cornerstone in the ART repertoire, where the egg and sperm are combined in the laboratory, incubated and the resulting embryos are transferred into the woman's uterus. The acronym sometimes used for this procedure is IVF/ET or IVF/ER, indicating embryo transfer or replacement. In 2001, 99% of all ART was IVF.

- GIFT (Gamete IntraFallopian Transfer): In this procedure the physician transfers a mixture of eggs and sperm into the fallopian tube during a laparoscopy, allowing fertilization to take place in the normal location. GIFT represented less than 1% of all ART in 2001.

- ZIFT (Zygote IntraFallopian Transfer): With this method, which is a mixture of IVF and GIFT, fertilization takes place in vitro, but the resulting fertilized eggs (zygotes) are placed into the fallopian tube. In the 2001 SART/CDC report ZIFT accounted for less than 1% of all ART.

- ICSI (IntraCytoplasmic Sperm Injection): This is a variation of IVF in which fertilization is achieved by direct injection of a single sperm into the egg. It is utilized when the male partner has a significant problem with his sperm or when IVF is planned and there is a significant concern regarding fertilization. ICSI was performed in 50% of ART cases in 2001.

- AH (Assisted Hatching): This is an additional variation of IVF in which a small hole is made in the shell surrounding the embryo to facilitate implantation.

- FET (Frozen Embryo Transfer): The cryopreservation (freezing) of extra embryos and later transfer allows the chance of pregnancy when the "fresh" cycle is unsuccessful, or for an additional pregnancy at a later time. Embryos can be frozen at different stages from the "2PN" stage (the egg is fertilized and shows the male and female pronucleus (PN) through the blastocyst stage). The 2PN stage is used primarily when all conceptuses are frozen, for example when the woman has a high risk of ovarian hyperstimulation. The cleavage stage is used when transfer is done on Day 2 or Day 3, and blastocysts are frozen when a Day 5 transfer is done. There is no known limitation on the duration of storage. The longest storage with a successful pregnancy at Reproductive Partners is 8 years, only because couples rarely wait a long time before returning for another pregnancy. The risk of an abnormal offspring has not been reported to be any different from regular IVF. In fact, in one report it was significantly lower.

- PGD (Preimplantation Genetic Diagnosis): This technique is also a variation of IVF involving removal of a polar body (genetic material next to the maturing egg), or a cell from the dividing embryo for genetic analysis to avoid the transfer of genetically abnormal embryos or embryos carrying a genetic abnormality linked to the sex of the offspring (generally the male).

As you can see, many of these procedures are very similar and some procedures, as defined by certain groups, may overlap. Others may be done in conjunction with IVF. In rare cases, both GIFT and IVF are done, with transfer of eggs and sperm into the tube, and embryos into the uterus.

3. Who is a candidate for ART? By the time you are ready to even approach consideration of these techniques, chances are that you will already have been through years of evaluation and treatment. In fact, one of our most important principles is that all the safer, simpler and less expensive treatments should be considered first before thinking of going on to ART procedures.

Couples who have been through all the proper diagnostic tests and adequate trials of conventional treatment may be considered for ART procedures if:

- the woman has tubal disease which has not been or cannot be overcome by surgery
- the man has a problem which has not been or cannot be treated by conventional measures
- the couple has a problem or problems which have not responded to conservative treatment
- the couple has no apparent cause for their inability to achieve a pregnancy and adequate time has been spent in conventional therapies
- the couple is being evaluated and an ART procedure is being done in conjunction with that evaluation

4. How successful are IVF and GIFT? Although the success rates for these procedures are improving, it is very important to have a realistic expectation of the chance of success. In fact, that's exactly what Dr. J. Benjamin Younger, a past president of the former American Fertility Society (AFS, now the American Society for Reproductive Medicine, or ASRM), said in testimony before the House of Representatives Subcommittee on Regulation and Small Business Opportunities (which released the March 1989 survey of IVF/GIFT programs).

The congressional survey, which was developed in conjunction with the American Fertility Society and its affiliate, the Society for Assisted Reproductive Technology (SART), collected the first published statistics on individual fertility clinics. These figures revealed that back in 1987 the average IVF take-home baby rate was 11.6% per egg retrieval procedure and 13.3% per embryo transfer. The corresponding rate for GIFT was 15% per egg retrieval. By 2000, the average chance of delivery from the transfer of fresh embryos doubled to just above 30%.

These statistics may not sound terribly encouraging on the surface. But, as indicated previously, a reproductively normal couple has only about a 20% chance of delivering a baby as a result of a single month's attempt, and IVF patients are not reproductively normal. When you consider that many of these couples were hopelessly infertile before this technology, 40,687 babies in a single year (2001) in the U.S. alone of ART represents enormous progress.

5. Do all IVF programs have similar results? The quoting of average figures obscures the most important finding in the survey—the vast differences in success from one clinic to another as seen in the clinic-specific rates in the 2001 SART/CDC survey available at *www.cdc.gov*.

6. What sort of doctor am I looking for? Your first determination will be to decide what type of doctor or program you need. To a great extent, this will depend on where you are in the process of investigating your fertility problem. If you have never consulted a physician for your problem or have not had many tests, your own gynecologist is usually well equipped to handle the problem at this level and is probably the best place to begin.

If you have already been through the basic testing and have tried various treatments, it may be time to move on. Now you may want to seek a more specialized level of care from a physician who has had special training in reproductive medicine. He or she will either have specialized training, or be certified or a candidate for certification by the American Board of Obstetrics and Gynecology in the specialized area of reproductive endocrinology, or both. These specialists can be found in individual practice, medical groups, fertility centers and as directors of IVF programs.

7. If not all physicians are created equal, how can we select the best one for us?
Here's a breakdown of the major referral sources ranked from best to worst, according to objectivity and to the extent that each is mindful of your needs.

1. physician or health professional–friend
2. your physician
3. support groups
4. friend who has had good results
5. prestigious hospital referral service
6. county medical society
7. classified telephone directory, Internet or any advertising

8. Once I have several names, how do I check to see which center is best for me? You have to do some investigation by calling or visiting the center to find out the answers to key questions. The first question usually relates to success rate. When that is answered to your satisfaction, other areas of concern will include how many cycles they do a year, the number of live births and the cost. Although all of these are good straightforward questions, the answers from some centers may not always be forthright.

9. How can I, as a layperson, evaluate their quoted success rate? We can never guarantee that the answers to your questions will be honest, but we feel that most centers will answer direct questions honestly. You just have to know the right questions to ask.

First you must understand that pregnancy rates among programs are highly variable, with a number of teams having little success. Therefore, obtain a definite figure for success of the program you are investigating. Do not accept "average" success rates for other programs or for IVF as a whole. Average success rates for other programs have no relationship to the success rate of the particular program you are investigating.

It is important for you to understand how success rates are calculated because there can be a wide variation in rates based on a program's experience just by using different figures in the numerator and denominator.

10. Which rate is the best indicator of our chance to have a baby? In order to define the success rate you have to create a fraction. Ideally, the delivery rate of living babies is the most important numerator. This is because the definition of clinical pregnancy may vary among IVF programs, the level of miscarriage may be higher with poorer technique and a live baby is really what you are striving for. Because of the inherent 9-month delay from embryo transfer to delivery, only well-established IVF programs can give a reasonably accurate take-home baby rate.

In the denominator we suggest egg retrievals rather than embryo transfer rate as the best reflection of IVF program quality, because cases not reaching transfer could reflect deficiencies in egg retrieval or laboratory techniques and may give a falsely high success rate. The rate of cycle cancellation should also be examined because the success rate can be substantially influenced by allowing egg retrievals only when the results of stimulation are ideal. The cancellation rate is usually less than 20%. For practical purposes we suggest:

$$\frac{\text{deliveries}}{\text{egg retrievals}} = \text{success rate}$$

Using this formula, you can use the figure of 30% clinical pregnancy rate per egg retrieval in the under-35 age category as the minimum level of performance to warrant confidence in an ART program. Maximum rates have varied in a number of programs as greater than 50% or even more in the under-35 age category. Keep in mind, you are looking for excellence.

11. I have noticed that some of the very small programs have pretty good success rates. Should I consider a small program? We don't feel that you should necessarily shy away from very small programs. On the contrary, many are excellent and afford you the individualization you may desire. But, because of substantial variation based on chance alone, at least 100 cases are required to be able to quote a success rate that is a reasonably accurate reflection of the quality of the program. The variation based on chance alone and the inherent fertility potential of the couples happening to come through during a particular time, is enormous and vastly underestimated.

For example, in our program we have had streaks of up to seven successful IVF cycles in a row interspersed with occasional "dry spells." Because of this, we always recommend that you consider the success rate based on the last 12 months' experience rather than hearing that in the last month they had a streak, for example, of three pregnancies among 12 retrievals for a rate of 25%. They may not have had any pregnancies in the preceding 2 months. In fact Reproductive Partners now posts success rates cumulatively with up to 5 years of experience.

12. How about a new program? Should I wait until they have some experience? Not necessarily. If a program has not been established for at least several years, inquire about how they learned these procedures and where the personnel were trained or practiced previously. In order to learn the fine details that have proven successful through years of experience, these individuals must have prolonged and extensive experience with an established, successful program. If the individuals have a record they can quote with another program, the clinic may be worth considering although it is fairly new.

Keep in mind that just because a program has been established for several years does not mean that the same people who achieved the results reported are still working there. Ask: "How long has the team been together? Are the current members of the team the same people whose success rate they are quoting?" There is some tendency for personnel in this sophisticated field to move from program to program. ART is a complex process requiring a team of individuals with training and experience in pelvic surgery, reproductive endocrinology, andrology and embryology. The absence of one of these key people could have a devastating effect on an otherwise excellent program. There are instances of previously excellent programs that have no experienced people currently working on the team.

13. What if the program we are considering does not participate in the SART/CDC Registry? In the past some fine IVF and GIFT programs chose not to report to the SART Registry or didn't report in the SART format. Therefore, their statistics were not included in the report. Failure to participate did not necessarily mean that their success rates were not good. Today reporting is required. If you come across a program that does not participate, they are not eligible to be SART members and will be listed as non-reporters. Ask some hard-nosed questions about their lack of participation and evaluate the answers with a healthy dose of skepticism. We don't recommend that you put your confidence in a program that is not a SART member and does not report to the SART/CDC report.

14. We noticed a great deal of variation in the cost of IVF and GIFT among the centers we surveyed. How important is cost in making a decision? Only you can answer this question. Relative costs vary quite a bit. At this writing the estimated cost of an IVF or GIFT cycle, exclusive of medication costs, is about $7,000 to $10,000 U.S. The variation depends on many factors, including which additional procedures such as ICSI and AH may be required at extra cost. There is also great geographic variation in the costs, as well as some differences among programs in different parts of the same city. ZIFT will be more expensive because it requires independent expensive procedures for both egg retrieval and transfer. The cost of freezing and maintaining embryos is relatively small as opposed to going through another complete cycle to get more embryos. It is usually about several hundred dollars for the freezing and storage fee, and $2,000 U.S. for the frozen embryo transfer cycle.

We certainly do not suggest that you "shop around" for the lowest price, but that you fit cost into the equation relative to its importance to you. Do not compromise quality for cost, but if you are considering two similar programs, cost may become the deciding factor.

What hurts most is that insurance usually does not pay for ART. Some insurance companies specifically exclude ART procedures or may argue that ART is elective or not medically necessary or does not treat the underlying problem. See chapter 2 for more information on insurance coverage.

15. How do we decide whether to have IVF, GIFT or ZIFT? The choice of GIFT versus IVF may not be easy. It depends on the success rate achieved with GIFT or IVF in a particular program, the potential for diagnostic information and the patient's attitude toward surgery, anesthesia and tubal pregnancy.

What about ZIFT? It is not clear whether ZIFT carries a significantly higher rate of pregnancy than GIFT or IVF. It may be considered an option when a difficult transfer is anticipated in a patient who otherwise would require IVF.

If your tubes are blocked, the choice is easy: IVF is the only appropriate method for you. If your problem is unrelated to a tubal factor, you have a choice. Now, you also have the facts. To summarize:

	IVF	*GIFT*	*ZIFT*
Laparoscopy mandatory	−	+	+
Anesthesia mandatory	−	+	+
Ultrasound retrieval	+	−	+
Fertilization known	+	−	+

Fertilization in normal location	–	+	–
Requires normal fallopian tube	–	+	+
Diagnostic information	–	+	+

16. What if the program I am considering does only one of these procedures? We feel that a quality program should have all the current methods of treatment available. An example might be embryo freezing. Except when a woman is older or embryo quality is reduced, limiting the number of fresh embryos transferred to two can better control the risk of multiple pregnancy. Freezing additional embryos can reduce costs considerably by allowing multiple embryo transfer procedures from one stimulation and retrieval. In some women, the uterus may not be receptive in the stimulated cycle. If embryo freezing is not available in a particular program, you may be limiting your chances for success.

17. What actually is involved in an IVF cycle? Before a patient is placed in the program, we feel that all other conventional treatments should be exhausted. This may include cycles with stimulation of multiple ovulation with gonadotropins coupled with intrauterine insemination for patients with open tubes. Certain tests should be done if they have not been performed recently. We recommend a current semen analysis and semen culture in the husband, chlamydia culture or antibiotic treatment in both partners and a "trial transfer" in the female partner. We believe that the transfer is the most critical part of the process and that a rehearsal of this process with a mapping of the cervical canal is most useful.

The procedure of in vitro fertilization/embryo transfer itself consists of four basic steps, all of which will be accomplished within the time frame of one menstrual cycle and will take approximately 30 days:

1. Ripening of the egg(s)
2. Retrieval of the egg(s)
3. Fertilization of the eggs and growth of the resulting embryo(s)
4. Transfer of the embryo(s) into the uterus

18. Do I need surgery to have the eggs retrieved? At this time the standard method is vaginal ultrasound-guided egg retrieval. However, there are some patients who require laparoscopy for retrieval for technical reasons.

The ultrasound technique, described elsewhere in the book, can utilize sedation rather than anesthesia and requires less recovery time. Patients who have experienced both uniformly prefer the ultrasound technique. The only drawback to ultrasound aspiration is that the diagnostic and therapeutic aspects of laparoscopy are lost. In some individual cases there may be aspects important enough to justify the additional expense and risk of laparoscopy. Of course, with GIFT and ZIFT, laparoscopy is required.

19. Is there an age limit for ART procedures? We generally recommend IVF with a woman's own eggs for couples in which the woman has not reached her 43rd birthday. We do allow treatment until the 46th birthday provided they understand the very low rate of success after age 42. In cases in which donor eggs are being used, we accept women up to age 52. Some centers have higher age limits with egg donation. We feel that physicians have an obligation to consider the welfare of the offspring, who could be orphaned before they are grown.

20. Is IVF a stressful procedure? It is a very intense and stressful procedure for the couple. For this reason, we feel that an experienced program should have readily available psychological support to optimize the couple's ability to cope with the stresses inherent in the process. Psychological issues can have a major impact on the success of an individual couple, since perseverance is critical to the ultimate chance of a pregnancy. Couples may wish to use one or more of the alternative techniques described in chapter 14. Emotional stability and mutual support help a couple persist in their quest. And as we have said repeatedly, persistence is the key to success!

Remember, the answers to these 20 questions will provide you with only a quick introduction to the subject of assisted reproduction. To be good consumers, learn all you can before making a decision. Make sure you read the chapter on the top 10 misconceptions. Choosing a quality program will have a significant influence on your chances for having a baby. Good luck!

Glossary

AATB   American Association of Tissue Banks

adhesions   scar tissue

AFS   American Fertility Society (now ASRM)

agonist   compound that has stimulating properties (a GnRH agonist first stimulates before it suppresses the reproductive system)

AH   assisted hatching

amenorrhea   lack of menstrual period

amniocentesis   withdrawal of a sample of fluid contained in the pregnancy sac

analogue   compound that is chemically similar to another

andrologist   specialist in male reproductive function

anovulation   lack of ovulation

Antagon   brand of ganerelix, a GnRH antagonist

antiphospholipid antibodies   antibodies to cell components which can inhibit placental development or cause clotting in the blood vessels supplying the implanting embryo/fetus

antisperm antibodies   proteins that can specifically attach to sperm, impairing their function

antral follicles   early follicles capable of stimulation

ART   assisted reproductive technology

aspiration (follicle)   withdrawal of fluid surrounding the egg

ASRM   American Society for Reproductive Medicine

assisted hatching   a variation of IVF in which a small hole is made in the shell of the embryo to facilitate implantation

assisted reproductive technology (ART)   technical manipulation of the sperm and egg outside the body for replacement into the reproductive tract to achieve a pregnancy

asthenospermia   poor movement of sperm

Aygestin   brand of norethindrone, a synthetic progestin

Ayurveda   alternative medical system practiced primarily in the Indian subcontinent, including diet and herbal remedies

azoospermia   the complete absence of sperm in the ejaculate

basal body temperature (BBT)   body temperature upon awakening, before any activity

BBT   basal body temperature

Beckwith-Wiedemann Syndrome   a rare genetic disorder associated in one study with babies born from assisted reproduction. Characterized by excess growth at the cellular tissue and organ levels associated with large organs including large tongue, hypoglycemia and an increased risk of cancer

beta hCG   the specific part of the pregnancy hormone that is measured to diagnose pregnancy

biochemical pregnancy   a positive blood test for hCG but without ultrasound evidence of pregnancy

blastocyst   embryo stage following development of a fluid-filled cavity within the embryo; during this stage cells become specialized to form placental cells and the embryo itself (inner cell mass)

Bravelle   brand name of urinary FSH with higher purity enabling subcutaneous injection

bromocriptine (Parlodel)   drug used to reduce elevated levels of prolactin in treating galactorrhea, amenorrhea and prolactin-secreting tumors of the pituitary

cabergoline (Dostinex)   drug used to reduce elevated levels of prolactin in treating galactorrhea, amenorrhea and prolactin-secreting tumors of the pituitary

CAP   College of American Pathologists

capacitation   development of the ability of sperm to fertilize an egg

CDC   Centers for Disease Control and Prevention

cervical mucus   mucus produced by the cervix that thins before ovulation to assist sperm migration

cervix   the opening of the uterus

cetrorelix   a GnRH antagonist (Cetrotide)

Cetrotide   brand of cetrorelix, a GnRH antagonist

CFAS   Canadian Fertility and Andrology Society

chlamydia   an organism, generally sexually transmitted, that can cause tubal damage

chemical pregnancy   see biochemical pregnancy

chromosomes   tiny collections of genetic material within a cell nucleus

clinical pregnancy   evidence of pregnancy by ultrasound, passage of pregnancy tissue in a miscarriage, or delivery of a fetus or baby

Clomid   brand name of clomiphene citrate

clomiphene citrate (Clomid, Serophene)   an oral medication that stimulates ovulation

coasting   stopping the gonadotropins and continuing the Lupron in an ART patient in danger of hyperstimulation, so the estrogen level may be allowed to fall into the acceptable range

conceptus   the developing zygote, pre-embryo or embryo resulting from the joining of the sperm and egg

corpus luteum   hormone-producing tissue in the ovary that develops from the collapsed follicle, produces hormones and supports early pregnancy

Crinone   brand of progesterone vaginal gel

cryobank   organization for storage of frozen sperm

cryopreservation   deep-freezing by techniques that allow survival and growth of cells after thawing

cumulative (conception) pregnancy rate   the chance of a couple conceiving over a period of time

cumulus   the expanded, clear mucuslike tissue surrounding the egg

cytoplasm transfer   experimental procedure where the material in a cell outside the nucleus from the egg of a donor is transferred into the egg of a woman with egg quality problems

danazol (Danocrine)   drug used to treat endometriosis

Danocrine   brand name of danazol

Depo-Provera   medroxyprogesterone acetate, long acting form

DES   diethylstilbestrol

DHEAS   dehydroepiandrosterone sulphate, an adrenal hormone

diethylstilbestrol   a synthetic estrogen, given to women in the 1950s, 1960s and early 1970s to prevent miscarriage, that resulted in abnormalities of the reproductive tract of female offspring

Dostinex   brand of cabergoline

ectopic pregnancy growth of a pregnancy in any location other than the uterine cavity, known commonly as tubal pregnancy

egg retrieval aspiration of eggs from the ovary

ejaculate the sperm and glandular fluid released when a man reaches sexual climax (ejaculation)

embryo the result of the fertilization of the egg by the sperm; the developing individual from conception to the end of the second month

embryologist a person trained to work with gametes and embryos

embryo transfer (or replacement) placement of embryos into the reproductive tract

endometrial biopsy sample of tissue obtained from the endometrium to assess its maturity and ability to promote implantation of the embryo

endometrioma a cyst within the ovary caused by endometriosis and containing a dark-brown chocolate-like fluid

endometriosis a disease in which endometrium grows outside the uterus

endometrium the tissue lining the cavity of the uterus

epididymis part of the tubular system where sperm collect after leaving the testicles

ER (embryo replacement) placement of an embryo into the reproductive tract

estradiol the principal active estrogen in women

ET (embryo transfer) embryo replacement

fallopian tube a thin tubal structure that picks up the egg from the ovary, supports fertilization and early embryo development, and transports the embryo to the uterus

FertilityBlend commercial product claiming to promote fertility in men and women

fertilization union of the sperm and egg resulting in the development of the zygote

FET frozen embryo transfer

fetus developing individual in the postembryonic period, from 7 to 8 weeks after fertilization until birth

fibroid benign muscle tumor of the wall of the uterus

fimbria delicate fingerlike tissue at the end of the fallopian tube that picks up the egg from the ovary

follicle fluid-filled space and surrounding tissue that envelop the developing egg

follicle-stimulating hormone (FSH)   hormone that stimulates growth of the follicle

Follistim   brand name of FSH manufactured by means of recombinant DNA technology

FSH (Bravelle, Gonal-F, Follistim)   follicle-stimulating hormone

galactorrhea   milklike discharge from the breasts

gamete   reproductive cell; sperm in the male, eggs in the female

gamete intrafallopian transfer (GIFT)   placement of sperm and eggs into the fallopian tube

ganerelix   a GnRH antagonist (Antagon)

germ cells   sperm and egg

GIFT   gamete intrafallopian transfer

GnRH   gonadotropin releasing hormone

GnRH agonist   GnRH analogue with stimulating property

GnRH analogue   compound that is almost identical chemically with GnRH

GnRH antagonist   compound that suppresses pituitary gonadotropins

gonadotropin-releasing hormone   a hormone that stimulates the pituitary to release FSH and LH

gonadotropins   the hormones FSH and LH, which act on the ovary to control its function

gonads   reproductive organs that produce gametes and hormones; the testicles and ovaries

Gonal-F   brand of pure FSH

goserelin acetate   GnRH agonist implant (Zoladex)

granulosa cells   the corona and cumulus layers surrounding the egg that proliferate and produce the hormone estrogen

guaifenesin   old treatment used to thin cervical mucus (Robitussin)

hamster test   sperm penetration assay

hCG   human chorionic gonadotropin

health maintenance organization (HMO)   a form of heath insurance where the premium prepays all expenses and providers are strictly limited to those within the plan. Generally no reimbursement is provided for physicians outside the health plan unless prior arrangements are made, with the plan making the referral.

hMG (Pergonal, Repronex)   human menopausal gonadotropin

HMO   health maintenance organization

HSG   hysterosalpingogram

human chorionic gonadotropin (hCG)   hormone produced by the conceptus and later the placenta that can be measured to diagnose pregnancy

human menopausal gonadotropin (hMG; Pergonal, Repronex)   preparation of FSH and LH derived from menopausal urine

hydrosalpinx   dilated, fluid-filled, obstructed fallopian tube

hyperstimulation   a syndrome of enlarged ovaries, fluid retention and imbalance following an abundant ovarian response

hypothalamus   area of the brain just above the pituitary gland that controls many hormone-producing glands through its effects on the pituitary

hysterosalpingogram (HSG)   X-ray of the inside of the uterus and tubes; employs a radio-opaque dye

hysteroscopy   examination of the inside of the uterus using a telescope placed through the cervix

IAAC   Infertility Awareness Association of Canada

ICSI   intracytoplasmic sperm injection

imprinting disorders   the abnormal function of a gene due to chemical change of the chromatin (all of the material in the nucleus of a cell, including DNA), as opposed to most disorders being due to a change in the structure of DNA itself as in a mutation

infertility   generally, the inability of a couple to conceive within 1 year

integrin   a molecule in the endometrium which is a marker for uterine receptivity

intracytoplasmic sperm injection (ICSI)   a variation of IVF in which fertilization is achieved by direct injection of a single sperm into the egg, utilized in couples when the male partner has a significant problem with his sperm

intrauterine device (IUD)   device worn inside the uterine cavity to prevent pregnancy

intrauterine insemination (IUI)   placement of sperm, usually washed, into the uterine cavity

intravenous immunoglobulin   a preparation of immunoglobulin (antibodies) which is given intravenously and acts to suppress a hyperactive immune system

in vitro fertilization (IVF)   most advanced procedure in the ART repertoire: the sperm and egg are combined in the laboratory, incubated and the resulting embryos are transferred into the woman's uterus; literally, fertilization "in glass"

IUD   intrauterine device

IUI   intrauterine insemination

IVF   in vitro fertilization

IVF/ER   in vitro fertilization/embryo replacement

IVF/ET   in vitro fertilization/embryo transfer

IVIG   intravenous immunoglobulin

laparoscopy   examination of the abdomen and pelvic organs by means of a telescope placed through an incision in the navel

Leydig cells   cells in the testicle that produce male hormone (testosterone)

LH   luteinizing hormone

LH surge   marked increase of release of LH into the blood, which causes final maturation of the egg and its release from the follicle

liquefaction   process by which semen changes consistency from jellylike to liquid

LPD   luteal-phase defect

LUF   luteinized unruptured follicle

Lupron (leuprolide acetate)   medication similar to GnRH, used to suppress the pituitary and, in turn, the ovaries

luteal phase   phase of the menstrual cycle from ovulation until menses

luteal-phase defect (LPD)   poor development of the endometrium in preparation for implantation

luteinized unruptured follicle (LUF)   failure of the follicle to rupture and release the egg

luteinizing hormone   a hormone released from the pituitary that causes ovulation and stimulates the corpus luteum to secrete progesterone

male factor   a term for infertility originating in the male partner

medroxyprogesterone acetate   synthetic progestin used to induce menses (Provera) or as long-term treatment for endometriosis (Depo-Provera)

MESA   microsurgical epididymal sperm aspiration

microsurgery   surgery using fine instruments, magnification and gentle handling of the tissues, usually on the fallopian tubes

microsurgical epididymal sperm aspiration (MESA)   an advanced technique for aspirating sperm from the ductal system to use in ICSI

monthly conception rate   the chance of a couple conceiving within the woman's 1-month cycle

morphology   categorization of sperm by their shape

morula   embryo stage wherein numerous cells are packed together inside the zona but before the blastocyst cavity has formed

motility   categorization of sperm by their movement

multi-fetal reduction   selective termination (reduction)

mycoplasma   an organism that can colonize the reproductive tract and may cause miscarriage

myomectomy   surgical procedure to remove fibroids

norethindrone   synthetic progestin (Aygestin)

nuclear transfer   experimental procedure where nucleus from a compromised egg can be placed into a donor egg

oligomenorrhea   infrequent or scanty menstrual periods

oocytes   eggs

OTA   Office of Technology Assessment

ovary   female reproductive organ that produces eggs and hormones

ovulation   release of an egg from the follicle

PCO   polycystic ovarian syndrome

PCOS   polycystic ovarian syndrome

PCT   post coital test

pelvic adhesions   scar tissue capable of covering or holding together organs; most commonly affect fallopian tubes, ovaries, and bowel

pelvic inflammatory disease (PID)   a general term for pelvic infections resulting from sexually transmitted diseases

pelviscopy   synonym for laparoscopy, although often used to indicate operative laparoscopy

percutaneous epididymal sperm aspiration (PESA)   an advanced technique for aspirating sperm from the ductal system to use in ICSI using a needle

Pergonal   brand of human menopausal gonadotropin (HMG)

PESA   percutaneous epididymal sperm aspiration

PGD   preimplantation genetic diagnosis

phagocytosis   the process by which sperm can get eaten by scavenger cells all along the reproductive tract

PID   pelvic inflammatory disease

pituitary   a hormone-producing gland lying under the base of the brain that controls the function of the adrenals, thyroid, ovaries and testicles

polycystic ovarian syndrome (PCO, PCOS)   condition characterized by hormonal imbalance and lack of ovulation

polyspermia   fertilization of the egg by more than one sperm

post coital test (PCT)   a test of the cervical mucus after intercourse

PPO   preferred provider organization

preferred provider organization   a form of health insurance where the insurance company makes contractual arrangements with "preferred providers" for better rates. The patient is not required to go to a specific provider but will generally get better coverage through a preferred provider—for example, 80% reimbursement rather than 50% through a nonpreferred entity.

premature ovarian failure   cessation of normal ovarian function before the usual age of menopause, generally before age 40

progesterone   hormone that causes the endometrium to develop changes to make it receptive to the embryo

progestin   synthetic hormone with action similar to progesterone

prolactin   hormone released from the pituitary that causes the breasts to secrete milk

proliferative endometrium   growth phase of the endometrial lining during the pre-ovulatory portion of the menstrual cycle

pronucleus   the male and female nuclei that are visible 14 to 18 hours after combining sperm with an egg

propofol   medication used to induce deep sedation for retrieval procedures

prostate gland   contributes to fluid to making up the semen

Provera   brand of medroxyprogesterone, a synthetic progestin

Proxeed   commercial product containing l-carnitine claiming to improve sperm parameters

Qi gong   component of traditional Chinese medicine combining movement, meditation and regulation of breathing to enhance the flow of qi (vital energy)

Reiki   a Japanese word representing Universal Life Energy based on the belief that when spiritual energy is channeled through a Reiki practitioner, the patient's spirit is healed, which in turn heals the body

Repronex   brand of human menopausal gonadotropin (hMG)

retrograde ejaculation   passage of semen back into the bladder during ejaculation

retrograde menstrual flow   flow of menses back through the fallopian tubes into the pelvic cavity

Robitussin   brand of guaifenesin, old treatment used to thin cervical mucus

salpingitis   inflammation (infection) of the fallopian tubes

salpingostomy   a procedure designed to open the fimbriated end of the fallopian tube

SART   Society for Assisted Reproductive Technology

scavenger cells   engage in the process by which sperm can get eaten all along the reproductive tract

secretory endometrium   phase of the endometrial lining during the post-ovulatory portion of the menstrual cycle

selective termination (reduction)   a procedure that aborts one or more fetuses of a multiple pregnancy, usually when there are quadruplets or more

semen   the combination of sperm and glandular fluid released from the penis when a man reaches sexual climax

semen analysis   test of the parameters of concentration, motility and morphology of sperm in a semen specimen

seminal vesicles   glands that add fluid to the semen to assist sperm deposition

Serophene   brand name of clomiphene citrate

sexually transmitted disease (STD)   diseases caused by organisms that are transmitted by sexual contact and activity

SPA   sperm penetration assay

sperm   the male germ cell

sperm penetration assay (SPA)   test of fertilizing capacity of the sperm using zona-free hamster eggs, also known as hamster test

STD   sexually transmitted disease

Stein-Leventhal Syndrome   older term for a severe form of polycystic ovarian syndrome (PCO, PCOS)

subfertility   synonym for infertility implying that the ability to conceive is less than normal

superovulation   the process of using fertility drugs to cause multiple eggs to develop in a cycle

TESE (testicular sperm extraction) an advanced technique for obtaining sperm for use in ICSI utilizing testicular biopsy

testicle male sex organ that produces sperm and hormones

testosterone male hormone responsible for a male's secondary sex characteristics

ultrasound high-frequency sound waves used to make an image of body structures

ureaplasma type of mycoplasma implicated in male infertility and miscarriage

urethra the urinating channel leading from the bladder to the outside through the penis

uterus the womb; a muscular organ that carries the developing fetus

vagina a tubular structure leading from the vulva to the cervix

varicocele dilation of the spermatic veins that causes a backflow of blood to the testes and impaired sperm function

varicocelectomy operation for repair of varicocele

vas deferens muscular tube that carries sperm from the epididymis to the urethra

vasovasostomy operation for reversal of male sterilization (vasectomy)

viscosity the thickness of the semen, evaluated after a period of time following ejaculation

volume the quantity of semen ejaculated

ZIFT zygote intrafallopian transfer

Zoladex brand of goserelin acetate, GnRH implant

zona drilling the making of a hole in the shell (zona pellucida) that surrounds the egg

zona pellucida (zona) the shell that surrounds the egg and protects it during early embryo development

zygote fertilized egg prior to the first division

zygote intrafallopian transfer (ZIFT) transfer of fertilized egg(s) (zygotes) to the fallopian tube

Index

Note: Illustrations and figures are indicated by references in *italics.*

Anosmia, and hormone abnormalities, 96

Anovulation. *See* Ovulation; lack of

Antagon, 139, 185, 187, 188, 189

Antioxidant therapy, and DNA integrity, 244

Anti-progesterone drugs, 242

Antisperm antibodies, 102

Arginine, 263

Arizona, 283–284

Arkansas, 284

ART. *See* Assisted reproductive technology (ART)

Arthritis, 246

Asch, Ricardo, 12, 23

Asherman's syndrome, 130

Aspirin during IVF, 136–137, 239, 243

ASRM. *See* American Society for Reproductive Medicine (ASRM)

Assisted hatching (AH)
  complications, 158
  defined, 135, 157, 159, 325
  micromanipulation, 157–159
  in older women, 240
  three-day transfer, 143

Assisted reproductive technology (ART)
  acupuncture use, 258–260
  advertising guidelines, 251
  age limit for, 12, 17–18, 333
  availability of information about, 1, 250–251
  birth defects in, 210–212
  candidates for, 326
  cost-benefit ratio, 132
  cost of, 31–33, 168, 179, 251–252
  criminal acts, 2, 22–24
  decision to use, 26
  defined, 10–11, 324
  ethical issues, 2, 16–18, 163–164, 248
  fetal eggs, 17
  future of, 240–247
  goal of, 15–16
  as growth industry, 2–3
  herbal treatments, 260–265
  hormone effects in, 212
  insurance coverage for, 31–36, 216–217, 248–249
  legislation, 249–250
  low birth weight occurrences, 211
  mind-body connection, 266–270
  regulation of, 249–250
  risks of, 19–22
  statistics on, 2, 12
  stress effects on, 267–268
  success rates, 3, 105, 136, 175–178, 272–280, 328–330
  thirty-day cycle in, 182
  types of procedures in, 324–326
  vitamin treatments, 260–265

Assisted reproductive technology programs
  activity level, 178
  cost, 179
  established *vs* new, 274, 330
  evaluating, 328–330
  laboratory accreditation, 180
  non-participating programs, 275–276
  psychological support, 180
  selection criteria for, 173–181
  size of, 17
  stability of, 178–179
  success rates of, 175–178, 272–280

Asthenospermia, 70

Aygestin, 121

Azoospermia, 69, 96–97, 116–117

Balmaceda, Jose, 23

Basal body temperature (BBT) Chart, 44–45, 86–88

Beckwith-Wiedermann syndrome, 156, 211

Bee balm, 263

Bentonite clay, in detox diet, 258

Biochemical pregnancy, 203–204